THE COMPLETE

NATURE CURE

5th REVISED EDITION

THE COMPLETE HANDBOOK OF

NATURE CURE

The most comprehensive family guide to health, the natural way

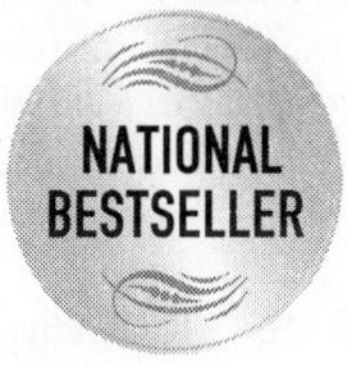

NATIONALLY ACCLAIMED NATUROPATH

DR. H.K. BAKHRU

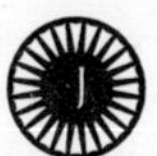

JAICO PUBLISHING HOUSE

Ahmedabad Bangalore Bhopal Bhubaneswar Chennai
Delhi Hyderabad Kolkata Lucknow Mumbai

Published by Jaico Publishing House
A-2 Jash Chambers, 7-A Sir Phirozshah Mehta Road
Fort, Mumbai - 400 001
jaicopub@jaicobooks.com
www.jaicobooks.com

THE COMPLETE HANDBOOK OF NATURE CURE
ISBN 81-7224-229-8

First Jaico Impression: 1991
Twenty-sixth Jaico Impression (Fifth Edition Revised & Enlarged): 2010
Thirty-second Jaico Impression: 2013

Author of:
Yoga for Backache • Yoga and Diabetics • Yoga for High Blood Pressure
Hidden Secrets of Yogic Diet for Weight Loss

Printed by
Anubha Printers
Plot No. 19, Udyog Kendra Extn.1
Ecotech-III,Greater Noida U.P. 201308

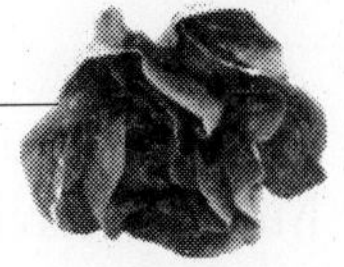

About the Author

Dr. H.K. Bakhru enjoys a countrywide reputation as an expert naturopath and a prolific writer. His well-researched articles on nature cure, health, nutrition and herbs appear regularly in various newspapers and magazines and they bear the stamp of authority.

A diploma holder in naturopathy, all his current 13 books on nature cure, nutrition and herbs titled, *A Complete Handbook of Nature Cure*, *Diet Cure for Common Ailments*, *A Handbook of Natural Beauty*, *Nature Cure for Children*, *Naturopathy for Longevity*, *Healing Through Natural Foods*, *Indian Spices and Condiments as Natural Healers*, *Foods That Heal*, *Herbs That Heal*, *Natural Home Remedies for Common Ailments*, *Vitamins That Heal*, *Conquering Diabetes Naturally* and *Conquering Cancer Naturally* have been highly appreciated by the public and repeatedly reprinted. His first-named book has been awarded first prize in the category *Primer on Naturopathy for Healthy Living* by the jury of judges at the *Book Prize Award* scheme, organized by *National Institute of Naturopathy*, an autonomous body under Govt. of India, Ministry of Health.

Dr. Bakhru began his career with the Indian Railways, holding a first class first postgraduate degree in History from Lucknow University in 1949. He retired in October 1984 as the Chief Public Relations Officer of the Central Railway in Mumbai, having to his credit 35 years of distinguished service in the Public Relations organisations of the Indian Railways and the Railway Board.

An associate member of the All India Alternative Medical Practitioner's Association and a member of the Nature Cure Practitioner's Guild in Mumbai, Dr. Bakhru has extensively studied herbs and natural methods of treating diseases. He has been honoured with 'Lifetime Achievement Award', 'Gem of Alternative Medicines' award and a gold medal in Diet Therapy by the Indian Board of Alternative Medicines, Kolkata, in recognition of his dedication and outstanding contributions in the field of Alternative Medicines. The Board, which is affiliated with the Open International University for Complementary Medicines, established under World Health Organisation and recognised by the United Nations Peace University, has also appointed him as its Honorary Advisor. Dr. Bakhru has also been honoured by Nature Cure Practitioners' Guild, Mumbai with Nature Cure Appreciation Award for his services to Naturopathy.

Dr. Bakhru has founded a registered Public Charitable Trust, known as D.H. Bakhru Foundation, for help to the poor and needy. He has been donating Rs. 25,000 every year to this trust from his income as writer and author.

Contents

Foreword

For people who advocate and recognise the latent healing power of nature like my esteemed friend and fellow practitioner, Shri H.K. Bakhru, naturopathy is a way of life. It is a distinct philosophy and science which strengthens the age-old faith in the correction of bodily disorders and restoration and maintenance of health through elements freely available in nature. It brings home the basic fact that healing is brought about by the inherent curative powers of the body. The simplicity of this method should not deter individuals from its use. The final complete healing will come from within. In short, the naturopath lends intelligent assistance and interprets nature's laws for the patient.

Shri H.K. Bakhru contributed numerous articles to leading newspapers and magazines on various ailments and their cure through dietetics and nature cure treatments.

A news item appeared in newspapers about a famous French folk singer, Rika Zarai, who had never practised naturopathy but her faith, based on her personal experience, turned her into an authority on herbs and nature cure. At the height of her career as a singer, Rika met with an accident, when her car went off the road, due to poor visibility on account of fog and she was taken from the wreckage with four broken vertebrae, one of which was pulverised. The attending doctors indicated that she might not be able to walk again without crutches.

To make matters worse, she had a calcium deficiency. On the brink of suicide, she appealed for help to an eminent homeopath. Clay compresses were smuggled into the hospital and she applied them regularly to her back. Her surgeon was outraged when she attributed her remarkable recovery not to his skill but to the clay. With the zeal of a convert, she applied herself to the wider study of natural medicine.

She has authored two books, titled *Ma Medicine Naturelle*, and *Her Secrets Naturelles*. As many as 2,80,000 copies of the first book were sold. Both the books have challenged the realms of Medical World.

H.K. Bakhru's book titled '*A Complete Handbook of Nature Cure*' is a complete guide to naturopathy. This book offers a way which, if followed, will provide renewed energy, increased vitality and greater satisfaction that comes from living a full and useful life.

The author has advocated that the right food could work wonders and has tremendous curative power. Nutrition is the major problem of human life. This book can also be appropriately titled *Return to Nature*. The aim of naturopathy is to invigorate and stimulate the body's homeostatic mechanism, to restore health structure and function. One can enjoy perfect health by proper regulation of eating, drinking, breathing, bathing, dressing, working, thinking, and other social activities on a normal and natural basis.

I wish the author Shri H.K. Bakhru all success for the publication of this book.

Dr. P.K. Bolar, N.D. (Lon.),
Former Executive Director,
Indian Institute of Drugless Therapy.

Preface to the First Edition

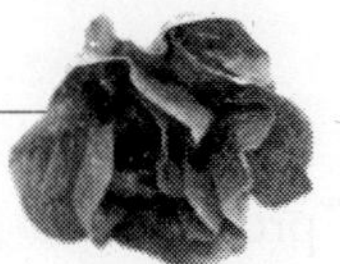

Nature cures, not the physician
—Hippocrates

What, you may ask, is a Public Relations man doing writing a book on nature cure? The answer is simple : good health ought to be everybody's concern, not solely the medical profession's business. More importantly, in my own case, I suffered immensely, for many years, largely due to the shortcomings of the modern medical system. In my despair, I earnestly began my study of natural methods of treatment and cure of disease, as also the ways and means of maintaining good health. Putting the time-tested nature cure methods into practice proved so beneficial in my own case, that I took to studying their application for several other diseases as well. What began as mere jottings was gradually expanded into full-length articles on the subject *Cure without Drugs*, several of which were published in "The Economic Times". The readers' response to the series was overwhelming and several of them suggested that the articles be compiled in book form, to benefit more people. *Health the Natural Way* was the result. This book as well as my second book titled *Diet Cure for Common Ailments* published three years later, was well received by the press and the public. This fact coupled with the immense popularity of my articles on health, nutrition and nature cure being published in several leading newspapers and magazines, have prompted me to write a comprehensive book on nature cure under the present title for the benefit of the general public.

Experience, they say, is the most convincing teacher, and I would like to begin with details of my own case history as a means of indicating the major health problems that nature cure can overcome. While doing my intermediate arts, at the age of 16, I contracted two serious illnesses—pleurisy and typhoid fever—simultaneously. Having run their course for about 45 days, both ailments left me so debilitated that I had to discontinue my studies for one year, on medical advice.

My recovery was gradual but not complete, as I developed heartburn and breathing problems. At 28 came the worst crisis, when I suffered a stroke in the early hours of an extremely hot day in May after acute heartburn throughout the night. The stroke made the left side of my body extremely heavy and weak, and the attending physician referred my case to a well-known neurosurgeon, suspecting a brain tumour. For nearly two months I lay helpless in the special ward of a reputed hospital, undergoing several tests and at the same time observing around me frequent deaths following unsuccessful brain surgery. Finally, having twice failed to inject air through the spinal cord for taking X-rays of the brain, the specialist decided to make holes in my skull for that purpose and even operate if necessary. Fortunately for me, the specialist had to attend a medical conference elsewhere and, therefore, instructed his assistant to try the newly-introduced method of cerebral angiography, which involved injecting dye through an exposed vein in the neck to enable X-raying of veins in the brain. When these X-rays did not reveal anything abnormal, I was allowed to go, but not before the harrowing experience had left me a complete nervous wreck.

However, that was not the end of it, I underwent a barium meal examination which indicated "Chronic duodenitis, may be chronic duodenal ulcer". The numerous drugs prescribed for the treatment of this ailment and the continuing weakness and heaviness of my left side made my condition worse still. I endured this for three years, until the pain and heaviness of the left side was miraculously cured by an astrologer : But nothing could rid me of the heartburn, abdominal pain and occasional severe stomach upsets, which continued to necessitate the use of several drugs. Investigations, from time to time, confirmed the diagnosis of duodenitis or chronic duodenal ulcer. A barium meal examination, done when I was 39, revealed hiatus hernia with peptic oesophegal ulcers.

To add to all of this, at 45, an eminent heart specialist declared me a heart patient following a check-up due to pain on the left side of my chest. The heavy drugging, dieting, etc. that ensued completely ruined my health and resulted in insomnia and a weight loss of 15 kg. Consulting another eminent heart specialist two years later, I was informed that there was no evidence whatsoever of heart trouble, but he confirmed the presence of hiatus hernia and stomach trouble. God alone knows which diagnosis was correct : Then came a host of diseases in rapid succession—spondylosis, myalgia, backache and prostate enlargement, in treating all of which the modern medical system failed to give me any relief, despite taking huge quantities of drugs, especially painkillers, antacid tablets and tranquilisers.

All this time, I was aware of the natural methods of treatment which I had studied from the age of 30 and a few of which I had practised occasionally. I, however, dared not adopt them wholeheartedly because of my heavy dependence on drugs. Rather late in the day, at the age of 55, I made a determined bid to do away with all drugs and take recourse to natural methods. I began collecting and studying a greater deal of data on the subject and also consulted naturopaths. I made drastic changes in my diet and lifestyle and started rigidly observing the laws of nature. I was rewarded sooner than expected so much so, that for one who narrowly escaped death at the age of 28, I can proudly say that today, at 83, I feel healthier, thanks mainly to taking recourse to nature cure methods. Of course, I do not claim that I have cured all my ailments. But I do maintain that I have been able to control them substantially and have obtained a lot of relief without resorting to drugs. This, I feel, is no mean achievement. I am certain that my own success in controlling several dreaded disabilities will serve as inspiration to those readers who are suffering from various ailments and hold out the hope of their deriving real benefits from the natural methods of treatment outlined in this book.

— H.K. BAKHRU

Preface to the Fourth Revised and Enlarged Edition

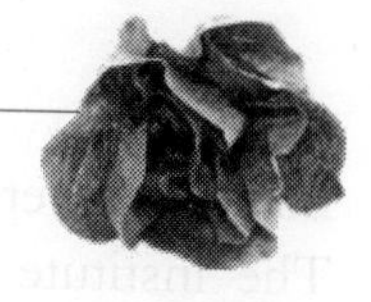

I have great pleasure in presenting the 4th revised and enlarged edition of my book *A Complete Handbook of Nature Cure* which was first published in 1991. It proved to be a great success and received very good response from the readers who benefitted by overcoming their health problems through adoption of various natural methods of treatment prescribed in the book. It also evoked great interest among nature cure practitioners and naturopathic institutions, many of whom prescribed it as a textbook or a reference book for their diploma courses. The book has already gone into twenty-five Jaico Impressions indicating its great popularity.

Naturopathy has taken rapid strides in India in recent years. More and more people are now turning to this system of medicine to treat ailments. They are gradually realising the limitations of the modern medical system and adverse side effects of allopathic drugs. They are becoming increasingly aware that many of our common foods contain valuable natural drugs which can help maintain good health and prevent and treat diseases.

It is gratifying to note that the Government of India has taken cognizance of this growing trend towards Return to Nature. It has established an autonomous body under Ministry of Health called National Institute of Naturopathy which is doing commendable work in the field of Naturopathy. It has initiated several steps to popularise this system of medicine. The institute also organized Book Prize Award scheme to encourage authors and publishers to write books on Naturopathy and Yoga. It is heartening to note that my book *Complete Handbook of Nature Cure* has been awarded first prize under this scheme for the year 1997-98 in the category primer on Naturopathy for Healthy Living by the Jury of Judges.

This decision of the Jury of Judges and encouragement given by the National Institute of Naturopathy, alongwith acclaimation won from the readers, have prompted me to revise this book to help further promote the cause of nature cure. This revised and enlarged edition contains six important additional topics under Nutrition and 50 additional diseases which were not covered in the original book.

— H.K. BAKHRU

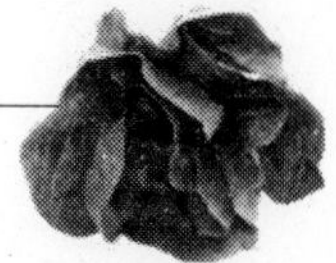

Acknowledgements

My sincere gratitude to Dr. P.K. Bolar, an eminent naturopath and former Executive Director, Indian Institute of Drugless Therapy, for his foreword. I am also grateful to my wife, Draupadi, for her painstaking efforts in going through the typescript of the book and carry out corrections of typographical errors—a task which I possibly could not undertake due to sharp deterioration in my eyesight on account of degeneration of retina of both the eyes.

Part I

Nature Cure and Natural Methods of Treatment

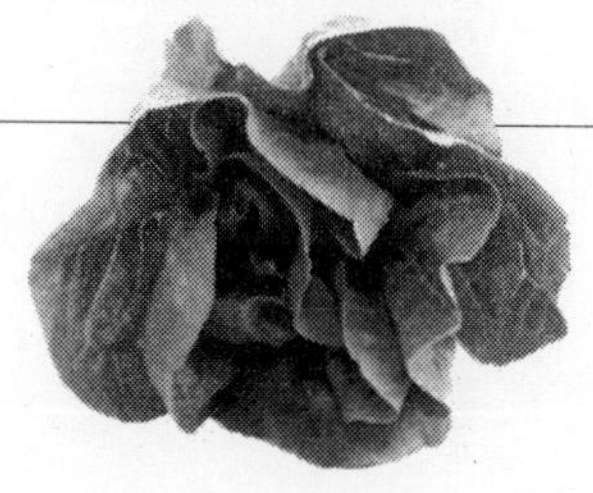

CHAPTER 1

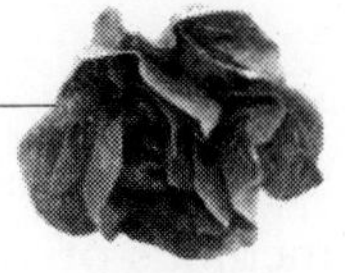

Principles and Practice of Nature Cure

Nature cures, not the physician
—*Hippocrates*

Nature Cure is a constructive method of treatment which aims at removing the basic cause of disease through rational use of elements freely available in nature. It is not only a system of healing, but also a way of life, a complete revolution in the art and science of living.

Although the term 'naturopathy' is of relatively recent origin, the philosophical basis and several of the methods of nature cure treatments are ancient. It was practised in ancient Egypt, Greece and Rome. Hippocrates, the father of medicine (460-357 B.C.) strongly advocated it. India, it appears, was much further advanced in olden days in natural healing system than other countries of the world. There are references in India's ancient sacred books about the extensive use of Nature's excellent healing agents such as air, earth, water and sun. The Great Baths of the Indus Valley civilisation as discovered at Mohenjodaro in old Sind testifies the use of water for curative purposes in ancient India.

The modern methods of nature cure originated in Germany in 1822, when Vincent Priessnitz established the first hydropathic establishment there. With his great success in water cure, the idea of drugless healing spread throughout the civilised world and many medical practitioners from America and other countries became his enthusiastic students and disciples. These students subsequently enlarged and developed the various methods of natural healing in their own way. The whole mass of knowledge was later collected under one name, Naturopathy. The credit for the name Naturopathy goes to Dr. Benedict Lust (1872-1945), and hence he is called the Father of Naturopathy.

Nature cure is based on the realisation that man is born healthy and strong and that he can stay as such by living in accordance with the laws of nature. Even if born with some inherited affliction, the individual can eliminate it by putting to the best use the natural agents of healing. Fresh air, sunshine, a proper diet, exercise, scientific relaxation, constructive thinking and the right mental attitude, along with prayer and meditation all play their part in keeping a sound mind in a sound body.

Nature Cure believes that disease is an abnormal condition of the body resulting from the violation of the natural laws. Every such violation has repercussions on the human system in the shape of lowered vitality, irregularities of the blood and lymph and the accumulation of waste matter and toxins. Thus, through a faulty diet it is not the digestive system alone which is adversely affected. When toxins accumulate, other organs such as the bowels, kidneys, skin and lungs are overworked and cannot get rid of these harmful substances as quickly as they are produced.

Besides this, mental and emotional disturbances cause imbalances of the vital electric field within which cell metabolism takes place, producing toxins. When the soil of this electric field is undisturbed, disease-causing germs can live in it without multiplying or producing toxins. It is only when it is disturbed or when the blood is polluted with toxic waste that the germs multiply and become harmful.

Basic Principles

The whole philosophy and practice of nature cure is built on three basic principles. These principles are based on the conclusions reached from over a century of effective naturopathic treatment of diseases in Germany, America and Great Britain.

The first and most basic principle of nature cure is that all forms of disease are due to the same cause, namely, the accumulation of waste materials and bodily refuse in the system. These waste materials in the healthy individual are removed from the system through the organs of elimination. But in the diseased person, they are steadily piling up in the body through years of faulty habits of living such as wrong feeding, improper care of the body and habits contributing to enervation and nervous exhaustion such as worry, overwork and excesses of all kinds. It follows from this basic principle that the only way to cure disease is to employ methods which will enable the system to throw off these toxic accumulations. All natural treatments are actually directed towards this end.

The second basic principle of nature cure is that all acute diseases such as fevers, colds, inflammations, digestive disturbances and skin eruptions are nothing more than self-initiated efforts on the part of the body to throw off the accumulated waste materials and that all chronic diseases such as heart disease, diabetes, rheumatism, asthma, kidney disorders, are the results of continued suppression of the acute diseases through harmful methods such as drugs, vaccines, narcotics and gland extracts.

The third principle of nature cure is that the body contains an elaborate healing mechanism which has the power to bring about a return to normal condition of health, provided right methods are employed to enable it to do so. In other words, the power to cure disease lies within the body itself and not in the hands of the doctor.

Nature Cure vs Modern System

The modern medical system treats the symptoms and suppresses the disease but does little to ascertain the real cause. Toxic drugs which may suppress or relieve some ailments usually have harmful side-effects. Drugs usually hinder the self-healing efforts of the body and make recovery more difficult. According to the late Sir William Osler, an eminent physician and surgeon, when drugs are used, the patient has to recover twice—once from the illness, and once from the drug. Drugs cannot cure diseases; disease continues. It is only its pattern that changes. Drugs also produce dietary deficiencies by destroying nutrients, using them up, and preventing their absorption. Moreover, the toxicity they produce occurs at a time when the body is least capable of coping with it. The power to restore health thus lies not in drugs, but in nature.

The approach of the modern system is more on combative lines after the disease has set in, whereas nature cure system lays greater emphasis on preventive method and adopts measures to attain and maintain health and prevent disease. The modern medical system treats each disease as a separate entity, requiring specific drug for its cure, whereas the nature cure system treats the organism as a whole and seeks to restore harmony to the whole of the patient's being.

Methods of Nature Cure

The nature cure system aims at the readjustment of the human system from abnormal to normal conditions and functions, and adopts methods of cure which are in conformity with the constructive principles of nature. Such methods remove from the system the accumulation of toxic matter and poisons without injuring the vital organs of the body. They also stimulate the organs of elimination and purification to better functioning.

To cure disease, the first and foremost requirement is to regulate the diet. To get rid of accumulated toxins and restore the equilibrium of the system, it is desirable to completely exclude acid-forming foods, including proteins, starches and fats, for a week or more and to confine the diet to fresh fruits which will disinfect the stomach and alimentary canal. If the body is overloaded with morbid matter, as in acute disease, a complete fast for a few days may be necessary for the elimination of toxins. Fruit juice may, however, be taken during a fast. A simple rule is : do not eat when you are sick, stick to a light diet of fresh fruits. Wait for the return of the usual healthy appetite. Loss of appetite is Nature's warning that no burden should be placed on the digestive organs. Alkaline foods such as raw vegetables and sprouted whole grain cereals may be added after a week of a fruits-only diet.

Another important factor in the cure of diseases by natural methods is to stimulate the vitality of the body. This can be achieved by using water in various ways and at varying temperatures in the form of packs or baths. The application of cold water, especially to the abdomen, the seat of most diseases, and to the sexual organs, through a cold sitting (hip) bath immediately lowers body heat and stimulates the nervous system. In the form of wet packs, hydrotherapy offers a simple natural method of abating fevers and reducing pain and inflammation, without any harmful side-effects. Warm water applications, on the other hand, are relaxing.

Other natural methods useful in the cure of diseases are air and sunbaths, exercise and massage. Air and sunbaths revive dead skin and help maintain it in a normal condition. Exercise, especially yogic asanas, promotes inner health and harmony and helps eliminate all tension : physical, mental and emotional. Massage tones up the nervous system and quickens blood circulation and the metabolic process.

Thus a well-balanced diet, sufficient physical exercise, the observation of the other laws of well-being such as fresh air, plenty of sunlight, pure drinking water, scrupulous cleanliness, adequate rest and right mental attitude can ensure proper health and prevent disease.

CHAPTER 2

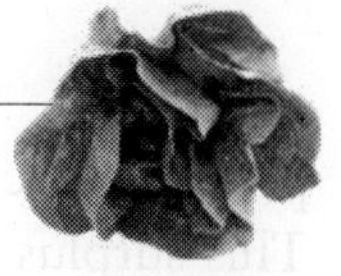

Fasting—The Master Remedy

Fasting refers to complete abstinence from food for a varying length of time. The word is derived from the old English, 'feastan' which means to fast, observe, be strict.

Fasting is nature's oldest, most effective and yet least expensive method of treating disease. It is recognised as the cornerstone of natural healing. Dr. Arnold Eheret, the originator of the mucusless diet healing system, describes it as "nature's only universal and omnipotent remedy of healing" and "nature's only fundamental law of all healing and curing".

The practice of fasting is one of the most ancient customs. It is followed in almost every religion. The Mohammedans, the Buddhists, the Hindus and many others have their periods of strict fasting. The saints of medieval times laid great stress on this method.

Fasting in disease was advocated by the school of natural philosopher, Asclepiades, more than two thousand years ago. Throughout medical history, it has been regarded as one of the most dependable curative methods. Hippocrates, Galen, Paracelsus and many other great authorities on medicine prescribed it. Many noted modern physicians have successfully employed this system of healing in the treatment of numerous diseases.

The common cause of all diseases is the accumulation of waste and poisonous matter in the body which results from overeating. The majority of persons eat too much and follow sedentary occupations which do not permit sufficient and proper exercise for utilisation of this large quantity of food. This surplus overburdens the digestive and assimilative organs and clogs up the system with impurities or poisons. Digestion and elimination become slow and the functional activity of the whole system gets deranged.

The onset of disease is merely the process of ridding the system of these impurities. Every disease can be healed by only one remedy — by doing just the opposite of what causes it, that is, by reducing the food intake or fasting.

By depriving the body of food for a time, the organs of elimination such as the bowels, kidneys, skin and lungs are given opportunity to expel, unhampered, the overload of accumulated waste from the system. Thus, fasting is merely the process of purification and an effective and quick method of cure. It assists nature in her continuous effort to expel foreign matter and disease producing waste from the body, thereby correcting the faults of improper diet and wrong living. It also leads to regeneration of the blood as well as the repair and regeneration of the various tissues of the body.

Duration

The duration of the fast depends upon the age of the patient, the nature of the disease and the amount and type of drugs previously used. The duration is important, because long periods of fasting can be dangerous if undertaken without competent professional guidance. It is, therefore, advisable to undertake a series of short fasts of two to three days and gradually increase the duration of each succeeding fast by a day or so. The period, however, should not exceed a week of total fasting at a time. This will enable the chronically sick body to gradually and slowly eliminate toxic waste matter without seriously affecting the natural functioning of the body. A correct mode of living and a balanced diet after the fast will restore vigour and vitality to the individual.

Fasting is highly beneficial in practically all kinds of stomach and intestinal disorders and in serious conditions of the kidneys and liver. It is a miracle cure for eczema and other skin diseases and offers the only hope of permanent cure in many cases. The various nervous disorders also respond favourably to this mode of treatment.

Fasting should, however, not be resorted to in cases of diabetes, advanced stages of tuberculosis and extreme cases of neurasthenia, long fasts will be harmful. In most cases, however, no harm will accrue to fasting patients, provided they take rest, and are under proper professional care.

Methods

The best, safest and most effective method of fasting is juice fasting. Although the old classic form of fasting was a pure water fast, most of the leading authorities on fasting today agree that juice fasting is far superior to a water fast. According to Dr. Rangar Berg, the world-famous authority on nutrition, "During fasting the body burns up and excretes huge amounts of accumulated wastes. We can help this cleansing process by drinking alkaline juice instead of water while fasting...Elimination of uric acid and other inorganic acids will be accelerated. And sugars in juices will strengthen the heart...Juice fasting is, therefore, the best form of fasting".

Vitamins, minerals, enzymes and trace elements in fresh, raw vegetable and fruit juices are extremely beneficial in normalising all the body processes. They supply essential elements for the body's own healing activity and cell regeneration and thus speeding the recovery. All juices should be prepared from fresh fruit immediately before drinking. Canned or frozen juices should not be used.

A precautionary measure which must be observed in all cases of fasting is the complete emptying of the bowels at the beginning of the fast by enema so that the patient is not bothered by gas or decomposing matter formed from the excrements remaining in the body. Enemas should be administered at least every alternate day during the fasting period. The patient should get as much fresh air as possible and should drink plain lukewarm water when thirsty. Fresh juices may be diluted with pure water. The total liquid intake should be approximately six to eight glasses.

A lot of energy is spent during the fast in the process of eliminating accumulated poisons and toxic waste materials. It is, therefore, of utmost importance that the patient gets as much physical rest and mental relaxation as possible during the fast. In cases of fasts in which fruit juices are taken, especially when fresh grapes, oranges or grapefruit are used exclusively, the toxic wastes enter the blood-stream rapidly, resulting in an overload of toxic matter, which affects normal bodily functions. This often results in dizzy spells, followed by diarrhoea and vomiting. If this physical reaction persists, it is advisable to discontinue the fast and take cooked vegetables containing adequate roughage such as spinach and beets until the body functioning returns to normal.

The overweight person finds it much easier to go without food. Loss of weight causes no fear and the patient's attitude makes fasting almost a pleasure. The first day's hunger pangs are perhaps the most difficult to bear. The craving for food will, however, gradually decrease as the fast progresses. Seriously sick persons have no desire for food and fasting comes naturally to them. The simplest rule is to stop eating until the appetite returns or until one feels completely well.

Only very simple exercises like short walks may be undertaken during the fast. A warm water or neutral bath may be taken during the period. Cold baths are not advisable. Sun and air baths should be taken daily. Fasting sometimes produces a state of sleepelessness which can be overcome by a warm tub bath, hot water bottles at the feet and by drinking one or two glasses of hot water.

Benefits

There are several benefits of fasting. During a long fast, the body feeds upon its reserves. Being deprived of needed nutrients, particularly of protein and fats, it will burn and digest its own tissues by the process of autolysis (breaking down of fat stores in the body in order to produce energy). But it will not do so indiscriminately. The body will first decompose and burn those cells and tissues which are diseased, damaged, aged or dead. The essential tissues and vital organs, the glands, the nervous system and the brain are not damaged or digested in fasting. Here lies the secret of the effectiveness of fasting as a curative and rejuvenative method. During fasting, the building of new and healthy cells are speeded up by the amino acids released from the diseased cells. The capacity of the eliminative organs, that is, lungs, liver, kidneys and the skin is greatly increased as they are relieved of the usual burden of digesting food and eliminating the resultant wastes. They are, therefore, able to quickly expel old accumulated wastes and toxins.

Fasting affords a physiological rest to the digestive, assimilative and protective organs. As a result, the digestion of food and the utilisation of nutrients is greatly improved after fasting. The fast also exerts a normalising, stabilising and rejuvenating effect on all the vital physiological, nervous and mental functions.

Breaking of Fast

The success of the fast depends largely on how it is broken. This is the most significant phase. The main rules for breaking the fast are : do not overeat, eat slowly and chew your food thoroughly; and take several days for the gradual change to the normal diet. If the transition to eating solid foods is carefully planned, there will be no discomfort or damage. The patient should also continue to take rest during the transition period. The right food after a fast is as important and decisive for proper results as the fast itself.

CHAPTER 3

Therapeutic Baths

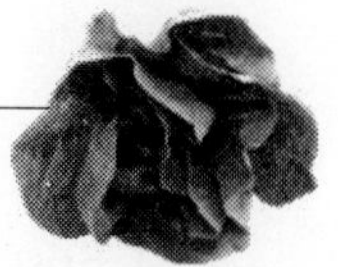

Water has been used as a valuable therapeutic agent since time immemorial. In all major ancient civilizations, bathing was considered an important measure for the maintenance of health and prevention of disease. It was also valued for its remedial properties. The ancient Vedic literature in India contains numerous references to the efficacy of water in the treatment of disease.

In modern times, the therapeutic value of water was popularised by Vincent Priessnitz, Father Sebastian Kneipp, Louis Kuhne and other European water-cure pioneers. They raised water cure to an institutional level and employed it successfully for the treatment of almost every known disease. There are numerous spas and "Bads" in most European countries where therapeutic baths are used as a major healing agent.

Water exerts beneficial effects on the human system. It equalises circulation, boosts muscular tone and aids digestion and nutrition. It also tones up the activity of perspiratory gland and in the process eliminates the damaged cells and toxic matter from the system.

The common water temperature chart is: cold 10°C to 18°C, neutral 32°C to 36°C and hot 40°C to 45°C . Above 45°C, water loses its therapeutic value and is destructive.

The main methods of water treatment which can be employed in the healing of various diseases in a do-it-yourself manner are described below.

Enema

Also known as rectal irrigation, an enema involves the injection of fluid into the rectum. In nature cure treatment, only lukewarm water is used for cleaning the bowels. The patient is made to lie on his left side extending his left leg and bending the right leg slightly. The enema nozzle, lubricated with oil or vaseline, is inserted in the rectum. The enema can containing the lukewarm water is then slowly raised and water is allowed to enter into the rectum. Generally, one to two litres of water is injected. The patient may either lie down on his back or walk a little while retaining the water. After five to 10 minutes, the water can be ejected along with the accumulated morbid matter.

A warm water enema helps to clean the rectum of accumulated faecal matter. This is not only the safest system for cleaning the bowels, but also improves the peristalic movement of the bowels and thereby relieves constipation. A cold water enema is helpful in inflammatory conditions of the colon, especially in cases of dysentery, diarrhoea, ulcerative colitis, haemorrhoids and fever. A hot water enema is beneficial in relieving irritation due to inflammation of the rectum and painful haemorrhoids. It also benefits women in leucorrhoea.

Cold Compress

This is a local application using a cloth which has been wrung out in cold water. The cloth should be folded into a broad strip and dipped in cold water or ice water. The compress is generally applied to the head, neck, chest, abdomen and back. The cold compress is an effective means of controlling inflammatory conditions of the liver, spleen, stomach, kidneys, intestines, lungs, brain, pelvic organs and so on. It is also advantageous in cases of fever and heart disease.

The cold compress soothes dermetitis and inflammations of external portions of the eye. When the eyeball is affected, the cold compress should follow a short fomentation.

Heating Compress

This is a cold compress covered in such a manner as to bring warmth. A heating compress consists of three or four folds of linen cloth wrung out in cold water which is then covered completely with dry flannel or blanket to prevent the circulation of air and help accumulation of body heat. It is sometimes applied for several hours. The duration of the application is determined by the extent and location of the surface involved, the nature and thickness of the coverings and the water temperature. After removing the compress, the area should be rubbed with a wet cloth and then dried with a towel. A heating compress can be applied to the throat, chest, abdomen and joints. A throat compress relieves sore throat, hoarseness, tonsillitis, pharyngitis and laryngitis. An abdominal compress helps those suffering from gastritis, hyperacidity, indigestion, jaundice, constipation, diarrhoea, dysentery and other ailments relating to the abdominal organs. The chest compress, also known as chest pack, relieves cold, bronchitis, pleurisy, pneumonia, fever, cough and so on, while the joints compress is helpful for inflamed joints, rheumatism, rheumatic fever and sprains.

Hip Baths

The hip bath is one of the most useful forms of hydrotherapy. As the name suggests, this mode of treatment involves only the hips and the abdominal region below the navel. A special type of tub is used for the purpose. The tub is filled with water in such a way that it covers the hips and reaches upto the navel when the patient sits in it. Generally, four to six gallons of water are required. If the special tub is not available, a common tub may be used. A support may be placed under one edge to elevate it by two or three inches. Hip bath is given in cold, hot, neutral or alternate temperatures.

Cold Hip Bath

The water temperature should be 10°C to 18°C. The duration of the bath is usually 10 minutes, but in specific conditions it may vary from one minute to 30 minutes. If the patient feels cold or is very weak, a hot foot immersion should be given with the cold hip bath.

The patient should rub the abdomen briskly from the navel downwards and across the body with a moderately coarse wet cloth. The legs, feet and upper part of the body should remain completely dry during and after the bath. The patient should undertake moderate exercise like yogasanas, after the cold hip bath, to warm the body.

A cold hip bath is a routine treatment in most diseases. It relieves constipation, indigestion, obesity and helps the eliminative organs to function properly. It is also helpful in uterine problems like irregular menstruation, chronic uterine infections, pelvic inflammation, piles, hepatic congestion, chronic congestion of the prostate gland, seminal weakness, impotency, sterility, uterine and ovarian displacements, dilation of the stomach and colon, diarrhoea, dysentery, hemorrhage of the bladder and so on. The cold hip bath should not be employed in acute inflammations of the pelvic and abdominal organs, ovaries and in painful contractions of the bladder, rectum or vagina.

Hot Hip Bath

This bath is generally taken for eight to 10 minutes at a

water temperature of 40°C to 45°C. The bath should start at 40°C. The temperature should be gradually increased to 45°C. No friction should be applied to the abdomen. Before entering the tub, the patient should drink one glass of cold water. A cold compress should be placed on the head. A hot hip bath helps to relieve painful menstruation, pain in the pelvic organs, painful urination, inflamed rectum or bladder and painful piles. It also benefits enlarged prostatic gland, painful contractions or spasm of the bladder, sciatica, neuralgia of the ovaries and bladder. A cold shower bath should be taken immediately after the hot hip bath.

Care should be taken to prevent the patient from catching a chill after the bath. The bath should be terminated if the patient feels giddy or complains of excessive pain.

Neutral Hip Bath

The temperature of the water should be 32°C to 36°C. Here too, friction to the abdomen should be avoided. This bath is generally taken for 20 minutes to an hour. The neutral hip bath helps to relieve all acute and sub-acute inflammatory conditions such as acute catarrh of the bladder and urethra and sub-acute inflammations in the uterus, ovaries and tubes. It also relieves neuralgia of the fallopian tubes or testicles, painful spasms of the vagina and pruritus of the anus and vulva. Besides, it is a sedative treatment for erotomanis in both sexes.

Alternate Hip Bath

This is also known as revulsive hip bath. The temperature in the hot tub should be 40°C to 45°C and in the cold tub 10°C to 18°C. The patient should alternately sit in the hot tub for five minutes and then in the cold tub for three minutes. The duration of the bath is generally 10 to 20 minutes. The head and neck should be kept cold with a cold compress. The treatment should end with a dash of cold water to the hips.

This bath relieves chronic inflammatory conditions of the pelvic viscera such as salpingitis, ovaritis, cellulitis and various neuralgias of the genito-urinary organs, sciatica and lumbago.

Spinal Bath

The spinal bath is another important form of hydrotherapic treatment. This bath provides a soothing effect to the spinal column and thereby influences the central nervous system. It is given in a specially designed tub with its back raised so as to provide proper support to the head. The bath can be administered at cold, neutral and hot temperatures. The water level in the tub should be an inch and a half to two inches and the patient should lie in it for three to 10 minutes.

The cold spinal bath relieves irritation, fatigue, hypertension and excitement. It is beneficial in almost all nervous disorders such as hysteria, fits, mental disorders, loss of memory and tension. The neutral spinal bath is a soothing and sedative treatment, especially for the highly strung and irritable patient. It is the ideal treatment for insomnia and also relieves tension of the vertebral column. The duration of this bath is 20 to 30 minutes. The hot spinal bath, on the other hand, helps to stimulate the nerves, especially when they are in a depressed state. It also relieves vertebral pain in spondylitis and muscular backache. It relieves sciatic pain and gastrointestinal disturbances of gastric origin.

Full Wet Sheet Pack

This is a procedure in which the whole body is wrapped in a wet sheet, which in turn is wrapped in a dry blanket for regulating evaporation. The blanket should be spread on the bed with its edges hanging over the edge of the bed. The upper end should be about eight inches from the head of the bed. Then spread a linen sheet wrung out in cold water over the blanket so that its end is slightly below the upper end of the blanket. The patient should lie on the bedsheet with his shoulders about three inches below the upper edge. The wet sheet should be quickly wrapped round the body of the patient, drawn in, tightly tucked between the legs and also between the body and the arms. The sheet should be folded over the shoulders and across the neck. Now the blanket should be drawn tightly around the body and tucked in along the side in a similar manner, pulling it tightly. The ends should be doubled up at the feet. A turkish towel should be placed below the chin to protect the face and neck from coming into contact with the blanket and to exclude outside air more effectively. The head should be covered with a wet cloth so that the scalp remains cold. The feet should be kept warm during the entire treatment. If the patient's feet are cold, place hot water bottles near them to hasten reaction. The pack is administered for half an hour to one hour till the patient begins to perspire profusely. He may be given cold or hot water to drink.

This pack is useful in cases of fever especially in typhoid and continued fevers, and benefits those suffering from insomnia, epilepsy and infantile convulsions. It is useful in relieving chronic cold and bronchitis and helps in the treatment of rheumatism and obesity.

Hot Foot Baths

In this method, the patient should keep his or her legs in a tub or bucket filled with hot water at a temperature of 40°C to 45°C. Before taking this bath, a glass of water should be taken and the body should be covered with a blanket so that no heat or vapour escapes from the foot bath. The head should be protected with a cold compress. The duration of the bath is generally from five to 20 minutes. The patient should take a cold shower immediately after the bath.

The hot foot bath stimulates the involuntary muscles of the uterus, intestines, bladder and other pelvic and abdominal organs. It also relieves sprains and ankle joint pains, headaches caused by cerebral congestion and colds. In women, it helps restore menstruation, if suspended, by increasing supply of blood especially to the uterus and ovaries.

Cold Foot Bath

Three to four inches of cold water at a temperature of 7.2°C to 12.7°C should be placed in a small tub or a bucket. The feet should be completely immersed in the water for one to five minutes. Friction should be continuously applied to the feet during the bath, either by an attendant or by the patient by rubbing one foot against the other.

A cold foot bath, taken for one or two minutes, relieves cerebral congestion and uterine hemorrhage. It also helps in the treatment of sprains, strains and inflamed bunions when taken for longer periods. It should not be taken in cases of inflammatory conditions of the genito-urinary organs, liver and kidneys.

Steam Bath

Steam bath is one of the most important time-tested water treatments which induces perspiration in a most natural way. The patient, clad in minimum loin cloth or underwear, is made to sit on a stool inside a specially designed cabinet. Before entering the cabinet, the patient should drink one or two glasses of cold water and protect the head with a cold towel. The duration of the steam bath is generally 10 to 20 minutes or until profuse perspiration takes place. A cold shower should be taken immediately after the bath.

Very weak patients, pregnant women, cardiac patients and those suffering from high blood pressure should avoid this bath. If the patient feels giddy or uneasy during the steam bath, he or she should immediately be taken out and given a glass of cold water and the face washed with cold water.

The steam bath helps to eliminate morbid matter from the surface of the skin. It also improves circulation of blood and tissue activity. It relieves rheumatism, gout, uric acid problems, and obesity. The steam bath is helpful in all forms of chronic toxemias. It also relieves neuralgias, chronic nephritis, infections, tetanus and migraine.

Immersion Baths

This is also known as full bath. It is administered in a bath tub which should be properly fitted with hot and cold water connections. The bath can be taken at cold, neutral, hot, graduated and alternate temperatures.

Cold Immersion Bath

This may be taken for four seconds to 20 minutes at a temperature ranging from 10°C to 23.8°C. Before entering the bath, cold water should be poured on the patient's head, chest and neck and the head should be protected with a cold moist towel. During the bath, the patient should vigorously rub his or her body. After the bath the body should be quickly dried and wrapped up in a blanket. If the climate is favourable, moderate exercise should be undertaken.

This bath helps to bring down fever. It also improves the skin when taken for five to 15 seconds after a prolonged hot bath, by exhilarating circulation and stimulating the nervous system.

This bath should not be given to young children or very elderly persons, nor be taken in cases of acute inflammation of some internal organs such as acute peritonitis, gastritis, enteritis and inflammatory conditions of uterus and ovaries.

Graduated Bath

The patient should enter the bath at a temperature of 31°C. The water temperature should be lowered gradually at the rate of 1°C per minute until it reaches 25°C. The bath should continue until the patient starts shivering. The graduated bath is intended to avoid nervous shock by sudden plunge into the cold water. This bath is often administered every three hours in cases of fever.

It effectively brings down the temperature except in malarial fever. Besides, it also produces a general tonic effect, increases vital resistance and energises the heart.

Neutral Immersion Bath

This bath can be given from 15 to 60 minutes at a temperature ranging from 26°C to 28°C. It can be given for long duration, without any ill-effects, as the water temperature is akin to the body temperature. The neutral bath diminishes the pulse rate without modifying respiration.

This treatment is the best sedative. Since the neutral bath excites activity of both the skin and the kidneys, it is recommended in cases relating to these organs. It is also beneficial for cases of organic diseases of the brain and spinal cord, including chronic inflammatory conditions such as meningitis, rheumatism and arthritis.

A neutral immersion bath taken for 30 to 60 minutes is highly beneficial in general dropsy, due to cardiac or renal diseases. It also helps those suffering from multiple neuritis, alcoholism and other narcotic habits, chronic, diarrhoea, peritonitis and chronic affections of the abdomen. In such cases the bath may be given daily for 15 to 30 minutes. This bath is also useful in the toxemic conditions caused by dyspepsia and pruritus. The neutral bath should not be prescribed in certain cases of eczema and other forms of skin diseases where water-aggravates the symptoms, nor in cases of extreme cardiac weakness.

Hot Immersion Bath

This bath can be taken from two to 15 minutes at a temperature from 36.6°C to 40°C. Generally this bath is started at 37°C and the temperature is then gradually raised to the required level by adding hot water. Before entering the bath, the patient should drink cold water and also wet the head, neck and shoulders with cold water. A cold compress should be applied throughout the treatment. This bath can be advantageously employed in dropsy when there is excessive loss of tone of the heart and blood. This bath also relieves capillary bronchitis and bronchial pneumonia in children. It relieves congestion of the lungs and activates the blood vessels of the skin muscles. The bath should be terminated as soon as the skin becomes red.

In pneumonia and suppressed menstruation, the bath should be administered at 37.7°C to 40°C for about 30 to 45 minutes. This bath should be given when the menstruation is due and may be repeated for two to three days in succession. In dysmenorrhoea, this bath should be given at 38°C to 44.4°C for 15 minutes.

In chronic bronchitis a very hot bath taken for 5 to 7 minutes should be accompanied with rubbing and friction. This relieves congestion of the mucous membrane and provides immediate relief. After the bath, oil should be applied to the skin if necessary.

The hot bath is a valuable treatment in chronic rheumatism and obesity. It gives immediate relief when there is pain due to stones in the gall bladder and the kidneys. The hot bath should not be taken in cases of organic diseases of the brain or spinal cord, nor in cases of cardiac weakness and cardiac hypertrophy.

Epsom Salt Bath

The immersion bath tub should be filled with about 135 litres of hot water at 40°C. One to 1½ kg. of Epsom salt should be dissolved in this water. The patient should drink a glass of cold water, cover the head with a cold towel and then lie down in the tub, completely immersing the trunk, thighs and legs for 15 to 20 minutes. The best time to take this bath is just before retiring to bed. This is useful in cases of sciatica, lumbago, rheumatism, diabetes, neuritis, cold and catarrh, kidney disorders and other uric acid and skin affections.

Precaution

Certain precautions are necessary while taking these therapeutic baths. Full baths should be avoided within three hours after a meal and one hour before it. Local baths like the hip bath and foot bath may, however, be taken two hours after a meal. Clean and pure water must be used for baths and water once used should not be used again. While taking baths, temperature and duration should be strictly observed to obtain the desired effects. A thermometer should always be used to measure the temperature of the bath. Women should not take any of the baths during menstruation. They can take only hip baths during pregnancy till the completion of the third month.

CHAPTER 4

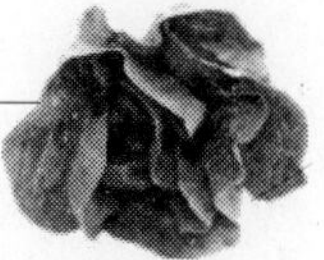

Curative Powers of Earth

Earth was used extensively for remedial purposes in ancient times as well as the middle ages. In modern times, it again came into prominence as a valuable therapeutic agent in the last century through the indefatigable efforts of Emanuel Felke, a German-born Lutheran minister who was nicknamed the 'Clay Pastor'.

Felke found that the forces of earth have remarkable effects upon the human body, especially during the night. These effects are described as refreshing, invigorating and vitalising. Felke believed that for wounds and skin diseases, application of clay or moistened earth was the only true natural bandage. The body is thus repaired with the element from which it is assumed to be made.

Adolf Just (1838-1936), one of the pioneers of nature cure in modern times, believed that all diseases, but especially the serious nervous troubles of our age, would lose their terrors, if only sleeping or lying on the earth at night became customary in the curing of diseases. According to him, by sleeping on the ground, "the entire body is aroused from its lethargy to a new manifestation of vital energy, so that it can now effectively remove old morbid matter and masses of old faeces from the intestines, and receive a sensation of new health, new life and new unthought-of vigour and strength."

Going barefooted all day long, except when it is very cold, is also regarded as a valuable step towards achieving good health and true happiness. Men can draw vital energy and strength out of the earth through their feet. Jesus Christ also attached a great deal of importance to the practice of going barefoot. He himself was barefooted and commanded his disciples likewise. It is advisable to go entirely barefoot as often as possible, especially on the bare ground but in rooms with painted floors it is better to wear chappals, since the painted floor affects the body adversely if one walks on it with bare soles.

The American Indians lay great stress on earth treatment. They believe that healing power is strong in leaves and herbs, powerful in the air, but very powerful in the earth. They have a custom to bury sufferers from all kinds of disease in the earth upto their necks, leave them, there for some hours, and then remove them. They believe that many of them are cured. Presumably the body draws unto itself the healing minerals and some of the earth's magnetism.

Mud Packs

The nature cure practitioners at present are making increasing use of moistened earth in the treatment of diseases. The use of mud packs has been found highly beneficial and effective in the treatment of chronic inflammation caused by internal diseases, bruises, sprains, boils and wounds. This mode of treatment is normally adopted in conjunction with a proper scheme of dietary and other natural therapies.

The advantage of mud treatment is that it is able to retain moisture and coolness for longer periods than cold water packs or compresses. The cold moisture in the mud packs relaxes the pores of the skin, draws the blood into the surface, relieves inner congestion and pain, and promotes heat radiation and elimination of morbid matter.

A mud pack is prepared with clay obtained from about ten

cms. below the surface of the earth, after ensuring that it does not contain any impurities such as compost or pebbles. The clay is then made into a smooth paste with warm water. This is allowed to cool and then spread on a strip of cloth, the size of which may vary according to requirements. The dimensions of the pack meant for application on the abdomen are generally 20 cm. × 10 cm. × 2.5 cm. for adults.

Mud packs have been found to be valuable in treatment of diseases relating to general weakness or nervous disorders. It can also bring down fever and is beneficial in the treatment of scarlet fever, measles and influenza. The mud pack is prescribed for swellings, eye and ear troubles, gout, rheumatism, stomach troubles, kidney and liver malfunctions, diptheria, neuralgia, sexual disorders, headache, toothache and general aches and pains. The mud bandage, after being placed on the body, should be covered with flannel or other protective material. The pack is applied for 10 to 30 minutes.

As the abdomen is the seat of most diseases, mud pack applied to this part of the body can cure many disorders including all forms of indigestion affecting the stomach and bowels. It is most effective in decreasing the external heat and breaking up the morbid matter. It also aids the inactivity of labour pains, and for this purpose, the pack may be renewed every hour or two.

The mud pack is also helpful as an alternate treatment. The area under treatment is first given fomentation for five to 10 minutes until it is well heated. Mud is then applied directly to the skin for five to 15 minutes, depending upon the reaction required.

Hot and cold applications are useful in relieving chronic pains, intestinal cramps and lumbago. Alternate application helps to relieve discomfort caused by flatulence and intestinal obstructions. It is also helpful in amoebiasis, colitis, enteritis and other inflammatory conditions of bacterial origin.

Mud Bath

Mud or clay bath is another mode of treatment. It is applied in the same way as packs, but only on a larger scale on the entire body. In this, mud or clay is first ground and sifted to remove all impurities, and then made into a smooth paste mixed with hot water. The paste is then spread on a sheet which in turn is wrapped round the body. One or two blankets are then wrapped over this, depending on the temperature of the room and that of the pack. A mud both is followed with a cleansing warm water bath and a short cold shower.

The mud bath is found to tone up the skin by increasing the circulation and energising the skin tissues. Frequent mud baths help to improve the complexion, clear spots and patches on the skin following skin disorders or due to smallpox. It is very beneficial in the treatment of skin diseases like psoriasis, leucoderma and even leprosy.

This bath is also valuable in getting relief from rheumatic pain or pain in the joints caused by injuries. The duration of the bath should be from 30 minutes to one hour. Care should also be taken to avoid the patient catching a chill during the bath. Mud applications also form a vital part of natural beauty treatment.

CHAPTER 5

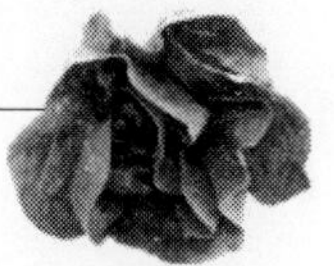

Exercise in Health and Disease

A world famous physical educationist, Eugene Sandow, has very aptly said, "Life is movement, stagnation is death." Physical exercise is essential for the maintenance of normal condition of life. Lack of natural exercise is one of the chief causes of weakness and ill-health.

In recent years, the need for exercise has been recognised even in sickness. Physio and occupational therapy are now standard procedures in medicine to restore the use of muscles and nerves that have been injured by disease or by accident. Patients with organic ailments are now advised to stay in bed for the minimum period considered necessary.

Exercise and Activity

For correct living, it is essential to differentiate between exercise and activity. While both are important as they are involved in vital physical movement, they vary in degree and benefits. Both employ the body in voluntary movement. Activity uses the body to a limited degree and generally to achieve a specific purpose. Exercise employs the body over the widest possible range of movement for the particular purpose of maintaining or acquiring muscle tone and control with maximum joint flexibility. Activity requires less physical effort and often less conscious effort once the routine has been established. Exercise demands considerable physical effort and is more beneficial as mental concentration is simultaneously employed.

Benefits

Systematic physical exercise has many benefits. The more important benefits are mentioned below :

(i) Regular exercise taken properly can achieve the increased use of food by the body, which contributes to health and fitness. The basal metabolic rate and habitual body temperature will slowly rise during several weeks of physical exercise, if the programme is not too hard. The healthy person usually has abundant body heat and a warm radiant glow.

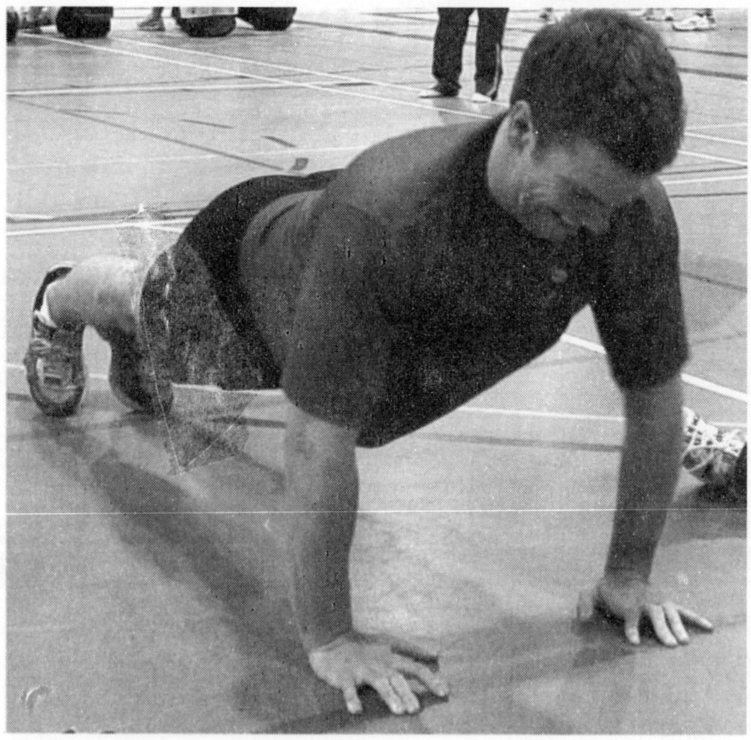

Physical exercise is essential for the maintainance of normal condition of life.

(ii) Regular progressive physical exercise can bring about the balance of autonomic, or involuntary, nervous system. The tone of the vagus nerve, one of the nerves that control sensation and motion, is strengthened. This accounts for stronger pulse waves, higher metabolism and better circulation.

(iii) Exercise can prevent or reduce gravitational ptosis or sag, as it is commonly called. Ptosis results from uneven flow of blood in the feet, legs and lower abdomen.

(iv) Improved capillary action in the working of muscular and brain tissue results from exercise carried to the point of real endurance. This permits greater blood flow and gives the muscles, including the heart, more resistance to fatigue. Massage, heat and moderate exercise are relatively ineffective in producing additional capillary action as compared with vigorous exercise.

(v) The full use of the lungs in vigorous exercise can reduce or prevent lung congestion due to lymph accumulation.

(vi) Gas and intra-intestinal accumulations can be reduced by exercise that acts to knead and squeeze or vibrate the intra-intestinal mass.

(vii) Better respiratory reserve is developed by persistent exercise. This ensures better breath holding, especially after a standard exercise. With greater respiratory reserves, exercise becomes easier.

(viii) Improvement in tone and function of veins can be accomplished by repetitiously squeezing and draining the blood out of them and then allowing them to fill.

(ix) Sweating in exercise aids kidneys by helping to eliminate the waste matter from the body.

(x) Persistent exercise leads to improvement in the quality of blood. Studies have shown improved haemoglobin levels, relatively greater alkalinity, improved total protein content and a greater red cell count.

Systemic exercise promotes physical strength and mental vigour and strengthens will power and self-control leading to harmonious development of the whole system.

Exercise promotes longevity

Medical researchers at Harvard and Stanford Universities who studied the habits and health of 17,000 middle-aged and older men, reported the first scientific evidence that even modest exercise helps prolong life. Dr. Raich S. Paffenbarger, the visiting professor of epidemiology at the Harvard School of Public Health, who is the principal author of the report said, "We have found a direct relationship between the level of physical activity and the length of life in the college men we have studied." He added, "This is the first good evidence that people who are active and fit have a longer life span than those who are not."

A strong connection between a hard and a healthy heart has also been convincingly demonstrated in the same study. The study showed that the less active persons ran three times higher risk of suffering a fatal heart attack than did those who worked the hardest. Review of fatal heart attacks revealed that the less active men were also three times more likely to die unexpectedly and rapidly within an hour after the attack.

A parallel research report from doctors in Dulles also concluded, after a study of the lives and habits of 6,000 men and women, that the physically fit were less likely to develop hypertension. Dr. Steven N. Blair who headed the research group said, "We followed the physical health and habits of these people for an average of four-and-a-half years and the data showed that the lack of physical fitness leads to hypertension."

Exercise increases calorie output. The body fat can be reduced by regular exercise. It is therefore, useful for weight reduction in conjunction with restricted food intake. According to a study by Dr. Peter Wood of Stanford University Medical School, author of 'California Diet and Exercise Programme', very active people eat about 600 more calories daily than their sedentary counterparts but weigh about 20 per cent less. Upto 15 hours after vigorous exercise, the body continues to burn calories at a higher rate than it would have without exercise, moderate physical exercise has been found to be accompanied by less obesity and lower cholesterol levels.

Regular exercise plays an important role in the fight against stress. It provides recreation and mental relaxation besides keeping the body physically and mentally fit. It is nature's best tranquiliser.

Chronic fatigue caused by poor circulation can be remedied by undertaking some exercise on a daily basis. It helps relieve tension and induces sleep. Moderate physical exercise at the end of a trying day can bring a degree of freshness and renewed energy.

Exercise also plays an important role in the treatment of depression. According to Dr. Robert Brown, a clinical associate professor at the University of Virginia School of Medicine, "Exercise produces chemical and psychological changes that improves your mental health. It changes the levels of hormones in blood and may elevate your beta-endorphins (mood-affecting brain chemicals). Exercise also gives a feeling of accomplishment and thereby reduces the sense of helplessness."

Methods of Exercise

Several systems of exercise have been developed over the years, the most popular among them being the Swedish system and yoga asanas, the latter having been practised from ancient times in India. Whichever system you choose to adopt, the exercises should be performed systematically, regularly and under proper guidance.

To be really useful, exercise should be taken in such a manner as to bring into action all the muscles of the body in a natural way. Walking is one such exercise. It is, however, so gentle in character that one must walk several kilometres in a brisk manner to constitute a fair amount of exercise. Other forms of good exercise are swimming, cycling, horse-riding, tennis, etc.

Precautions

Vigorous exercise of any kind should not be taken for an hour and a half after eating, nor immediately before meals. Weak patients and those suffering from serious diseases like cancer, heart trouble, tuberculosis and asthma should not undertake vigorous exercise except under the supervision of a competent physician. If exercising makes you tired, stop immediately. The purpose of exercise should be to make you feel refreshed and relaxed and not tired.

The most important rule about the fitness plan is to start with very light exercise and to increase the effort in gradual and easy stages. The sense of well-being will begin almost immediately. One can start off with a brisk walk for 15 to 20 minutes. A comfortable sense of tiredness should be the aim. It is valueless and possibly harmful to become exhausted or seriously short of breath. Perhaps, one should aim at activities which need about two-thirds of one's maximum ability. One way to assess is to count your own pulse rate.

Counting of pulse is quite easy. Feel the pulse on your left wrist with the middle three fingers of your right hand. Press just firmly enough to feel the beat easily. Now count the number of beats in 15 seconds, with the help of a watch with clear second hand, and calculate your rate by multiplying by four. At rest heart beats 70 to 80 times a minute. This rate increases during exercise. Really vigorous exercise can produce rates as high as 200 beats per minute or more. A reasonable aim is to exercise at about two-thirds of maximum capacity. It follows that heart rate should be about 130 per minute during and just after exercise. Always avoid over-exertion and never allow your pulse go above 190 per minute minus your age.

CHAPTER 6

Therapeutic Value of Massage

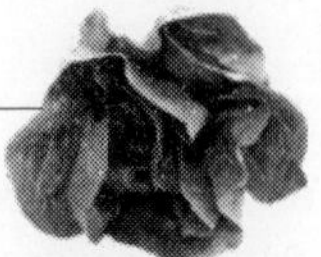

Massage is an excellent form of passive exercise. The word is derived from the Greek word 'massier' which means to knead. It involves the scientific manipulation of the soft tissues of the body. If correctly done on a bare body, it can be highly stimulating and invigorating.

As far back as 400 B.C., the great Hippocrates, the father of medicine, employed massage and manipulation in healing his patients. Since then it has been used as a mode of treatment for many ailments and it has restored many a sufferer to health and vigour.

Benefits

The general massage, dealing with all parts of the body, is highly beneficial in many ways. It tones up the nervous system, influences respiration and quickens the elimination of poisons and waste material from the body through the various eliminative organs such as the lungs, skin, kidneys and bowels. It also boosts blood circulation and metabolic processes. A massage removes facial wrinkles, helps to fill out hollow cheeks and neck and eases stiffness, sore muscles and numbness.

Various Movements

There are five fundamental modes of manipulation in massage and these are: effleurage (stroking), friction (rubbing), petrissage (kneading), tapotement (percussion) and vibration (shaking or trembling).

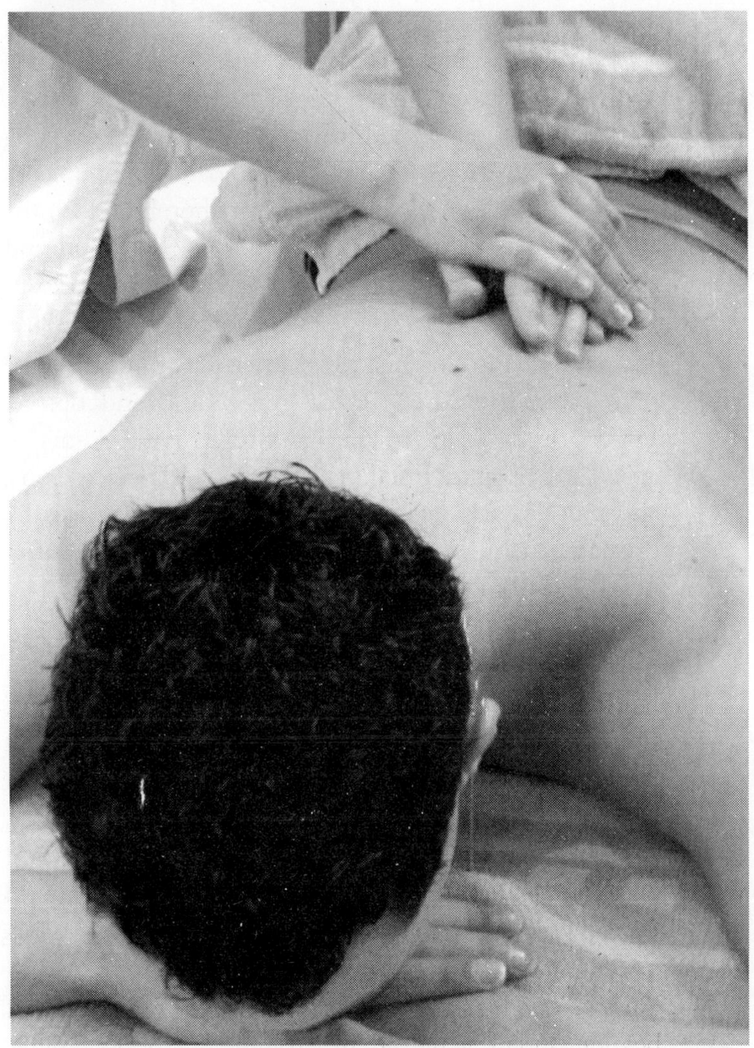

Massage is an important form of therapy.

1. *Effleurage*: This involves sliding with the hands, using long even strokes over the surface of the body. Effleurage is performed in five ways, namely stroking with (i) palms of two hands; (ii) the palm of one hand; (iii) the knuckles; (iv) the ball of the thumb and (v) the finger tips. Effleurage increases blood circulation and soothes the nervous system. It also warms and relaxes. It is very helpful in atrophied condition of the skin.
2. *Friction*: The movements, which are circular in nature are performed with the help of the thumb and tips of fingers or the palm of the hand towards the joints or around the joints. Friction limbers up joints, tendons, and muscles and facilitates the removal of deposits by breaking them. It also helps in reducing swelling after nerve inflammation.
3. *Petrissage*: This is the process of kneading, pressing and rolling of the tissues and is performed with one or both hands, with two thumbs or with thumbs and fingers. One should apply heavy pressure for deep kneading and light pressure for superficial kneading. Petrissage is a treatment of the muscles. It increases nutrition, strengthens muscles, relieves intestinal congestion and helps elimination of poisons. It boosts lung activity and cellular respiration, eliminates fatigue poisons and tones up nerve endings.
4. *Tapotement*: This involves hacking, tapping, clapping and beating and is achieved by striking the body rapidly. Short and quick blows are generally given from the wrist. Tapotement helps in atrophied condition of the muscles. It increases blood supply, soothes nerves and strengthens muscles.
5. *Vibrations*: This is achieved by rapidly shaking the

pressing movements by use of the hand or fingers on the body. Vibrating hand should move constantly. This is beneficial in neuritis and neuralgia after the inflammatory stage is over. It stimulates circulation, glandular activity and nervous plexuses. It also helps in bowel movement.

Another form of massage helpful in most ailments is the vibratory massage. This can be done by trained persons only. The vibratory massage is more efficiently administered by a special, electrically operated machine.

Material for Massage

Cotton seed oil is most commonly used for massaging, but butter is used for filling out cheeks and the neck and also for breast enlargement. If the patient is averse to oil, talcum powder may be used. Oil should not be used by persons with excessive body hair. General body massage may be done for 40 to 45 minutes and local body massage for 10 to 15 minutes. The oil should be washed off completely after massage.

Therapeutic Uses

Massage can be used with advantage as a method of treatment for many common ailments. The various forms of massage and their usefulness in various diseases are described here in brief.

Massage of the Joints: Stiff and swollen joints can be cured by massage combined with mechanical movements. Massage is, however, not recommended in serious inflammatory cases of the joints and in tuberculer joints. It should also be avoided in infectious diseases like diptheria and gonorrhoea which cause formation of pus as massage may spread the pus to the entire system. Sprains and bruises can be cured by massage.

In these cases, affected parts should first be bathed with hot water for 15 to 30 minutes. Next the massage should be done for a few minutes. Gentle stroking and kneading is recommended on and around the injured tissues. Fractures can also be treated through massage.

This form of massage is of great help in atrophy of the muscles which usually follows if the muscles are not used for any length of time. This condition may also be brought about by injuries, diseases of the joints, inflammation of the muscles and nerves, and by too long use of casts, bandages and splints.

A human being carries one-half of the weight of his body in the form of muscular tissues. One-fourth of the blood supply circulates in the muscles. When one gets a good massage treatment, the muscles get regenerated and are then capable of holding half of the blood supply. Massage thus provides additional nourishment to feed the muscular tissues, helping them to grow strong. Tapping, striking and vibrating help the muscle to develop its contractile power. Muscle massage is brought by first effleurage, kneading, followed by tapotement. Later, active and passive movements are given.

Massage is employed for eliminating muscle contraction and for breaking of adhesions. A little moderate kneading, and percussion cause muscles to contract and become stronger. Deep circular kneading and vibration loosens the muscles. Kneading under and round the muscles breaks up adhesions.

Massaging the Nerves: Massage benefits many nerve problems. In case of acute inflammation of the nerves, massage should be done carefully. Light and gentle stroking are recommended. Deep pressure should not be used on swollen nerves for it will increase the inflammation. All that is needed is just a gentle tapotement or beating of the nerve.

Nerve compression is recommended for soothing nerves. Grasp the limb with both hands, and create firm pressure around and down the arm. Start with the shoulder and proceed down to the wrist. As you leave the grip, bring the hands down a little and make another pressure. As a result, blood circulation will increase. Spinal nerve compression is extremely beneficial. It is done by the palm of the hand. Vibration of the fingers stimulate it. Sleeplessness can be cured by long slow and gentle stroking down the spine and entire back.

Abdominal Massage: This form of massage is beneficial in constipation. It stimulates the peristalsis of the small intestines, tones up the muscles of the abdomen walls and mechanically eliminates the contents of both large and small intestines. Abdominal massage should not be done in general, femoral, inguinal and umbilical hernia, inflammation of the uterus, bladder, ovaries and fallopian tubes, kidney stones, bladder or gall bladder, ulcers of the stomach and intestines, and pregnancy.

Abdominal massage should not be done after a heavy meal, but after two hours or so. The bladder should be emptied before the massage. The patient is made to lie on his back with his knees drawn up. This enables the abdomen wall to relax. The masseur should stand at the right side of the patient and use his finger tips for friction round the umbilical region from right to left. He should likewise alternatively knead the walls and roll with both hands, making deep and firm pressure. He should knead with the hand and finger tips and keep clear of any wound or tender places. He should later take up massaging the larger intestines.

The manipulation of the large intestine should begin on the right side. Keep it going upwards and across the transverse colon and move right-down on the left side to the signoid flexure and rectum. Circular kneading should be done with the help of the three middle fingers. At the same time press into the contents of the abdomen, following the course of the larger colon with a crawling motion. Keep kneading by means of a few circular movements in one spot with the help of finger tips. Keep moving the fingers a little further along. Knead repeatedly. Use knuckles of the hand to make deep pressures along the large colon, moving the hands along after each pressure.

Once the kneading of the abdomen is over, follow up by tapotement with both hands cupped or use the knuckles of the hand. Vibration may also be employed. The patient could also be asked to do some gymnastic exercises for strengthening the walls of the abdomen. Since blood pressure increases during abdominal manipulation, patients with hypertension should avoid abdominal massage. Massage should also be avoided in cases where there has been recent bleeding in the lungs, the stomach or the brain.

Chest Massage: Chest massage is helpful in many ways. It strengthens the chest muscles, increases circulation and tones up the nervous system of the chest, heart and lungs. It is especially recommended in weakness of the lungs, palpitation and organic heart disorders. Bust and mammary glands can be developed by proper massage.

The patient is made to lie on the back with the arms at the sides. The masseur starts manipulating the chest by means of strokes with both hands on each side of the breast bone. A circular motion is formed by the movement made up and down, moving down the chest. Next the muscle kneading is done by picking up the skin and muscles with both hands. Treatment is given to both sides of the chest likewise. Circular kneading is next done by placing one hand on each side of the breast bone and making the circular motions outward towards the sides. Tapotement follows by hacking and slapping.

Massage of Back: The purpose of the massage of the back is to stimulate the nerves and circulation for treating backache, rheumatic afflictions of the back muscles, and for soothing the nervous system.

The patient is made to lie down with arms at the sides. The masseur effleurages the back from the shoulders downwards using both hands on each side of the spine. Stroking is done from the sacrum upward. Friction follows with each hand at the sides of the spine going down slowly. Next, kneading by muscle picking is done with squeezing. Alternate rapid pushing and pulling movement of the hands sliding down the spine. Circular kneading should also be done. The treatment should end by slapping, hacking and cupping on each side of the spine. Gentle stroking and light kneading of the back is relieving and soothing. Percussion and vibration result in stimulating experience. Vibration of the end of spine benefits the sacral nerves and pelvic organs. It is recommended in constipation, hemorrhoids, weakness and congestion of the bladder and sexual organs.

Massage of the Throat: This helps to overcome headache, sore throat and catarrh of the throat. The patient is made to throw his head back. The masseur places palms of both hands on sides of neck with thumbs under the chin, and fingers under the ears. A downward stroke is next made towards the chest over the jugular veins. Do not exert heavily on the jugular veins. Repeat several times.

CHAPTER 7

Yoga Therapy

The yoga therapy or 'yoga-chikitsa' refers to the treatment of diseases by means of yogic exercises which may be physical or mental or both. It is a specialised form of yogic culture. This mode of treatment has been practised in India from very ancient times. Many references to yoga have been made in the Upanishads. It was, however, Maharishi Patanjali who in about the first century B.C. gave a systematic account of the traditional yogic teaching.

The term 'Yoga' is derived from the Sanskrit root 'yug' which means "to join". It signifies union between the individual soul (*jivatma*) and the universal soul (*parmatma*). It aims at obtaining relief from pain and suffering. Basically, human evolution takes place on three different planes, namely physical, mental and spiritual. Yoga is a means of attaining perfect health by maintaining harmony and achieving optimum functioning on all three levels through complete self-control.

Yogic kriyas, asanas and pranayama constitute the physical basis of yoga. The practice of kriyas and asanas leads to excellent circulation. It also energises and stimulates major endocrine glands of the body. Yogic exercises promote inner health and harmony, and their regular practice helps prevent and cure many common ailments. They also help eliminate tensions, be they physical, mental or emotional.

Pranayama slows down the ageing process. In ordinary respiration, one breathes roughly 15 times a minute, taking in approximately 20 cubic inches of air. In pranayama the breathing rate is slowed down to once or twice a minute and the breath inhaled is deep and full, taking nearly 100 cubic inches of air.

All yogic exercises should be performed on a clean mat, a carpet or a blanket covered with a cotton sheet. Clothing should be light and loose-fitting to allow free movement of the limbs. The mind should be kept off all disturbances and tensions. Regularity and punctuality in practising yogic exercises is essential. Generally, 5 a.m. to 8 a.m. is the ideal time for yoga practices.

Yoga asanas and pranayama should be practiced only after mastering the techniques with the help of a competent teacher. Asanas should always be practiced on an empty stomach. Shavasana should be practiced for a brief period before starting the rest of the exercises as this will create the right mental condition. Asanas should be performed at a leisurely slow-motion pace, maintaining poise and balance.

Herein are described certain yogic kriyas, asanas and pranayama which have specific therapeutic values and are highly beneficial in the maintenance of health and the healing of diseases.

Kriyas

A disease-free system should be the starting ground for yogasanas and pranayama. There are six specific cleansing techniques, known as Shat Kriyas, which eliminate impurities and help cure many ailments. Of these, the following four can be practised safely.

1. *Jalaneti*: Most diseases of the nose and throat are caused by the accumulation of impurities in the nasal passage. Jalaneti is a process of cleansing the air passage of the nostrils and

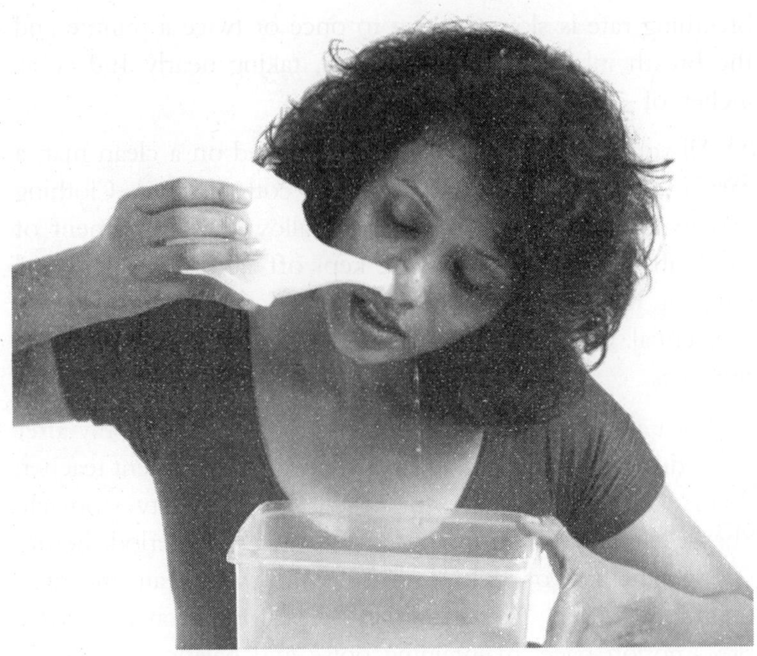

Jalaneti

the throat by washing them with tepid saline water. Take a clean jalaneti pot. Put half a teaspoonful of salt in the pot and fill it with lukewarm drinking water. Stand up and tilt your head slightly to the right. Insert the nozzle of the pot in the left nostril and let the water flow into it. Inhale and exhale through the mouth, allowing the water to flow out through the right nostril. Reverse this process by tilting your head to the left and letting the water flow from the right to the left nostril.

Jalaneti should be practised only in the morning. It will relieve sore throat, cold, cough, sinusitis, migraine, headache and cases of inflammation of the nasal membranes. It keeps the head cool and improves vision.

2. *Vamana Dhouti or Kunjal*: This is a process of cleansing the interior of the stomach. Drink four to six glasses of tepid

water, with a little salt added to it, early in the morning on an empty stomach. Then stand up, bend forward, insert the middle and index fingers of the right hand into the mouth until they touch the uvula. Tickle it until you feel a vomiting sensation. The saline water thus ejected will bring up bile and other toxic matter with it. Repeat the process till all the water is vomited out. This should be done once a week or as and when necessary.

It is beneficial for cleansing the stomach in cases of excessive bile, constipation and gastric troubles. Persons suffering from hyperacidity should perform kunjal with unsalted water. It gives relief from headaches, nervous weakness, chronic cold, cough and asthma. It should not be practised by those suffering from high blood pressure, ulcers and heart trouble.

3. *Kapalabhati*: Kapala means 'skull' and bhati means 'shine'. This is a respiratory exercise for the abdomen and diaphragm. The channels inside the nose and other parts of the respiratory system are purified by this exercise. In the process, the brain is also cleared.

Sit in a comfortable position, preferably in padmasana. Exercise the diaphragm by exhaling suddenly and quickly through both nostrils, producing a hissing sound. Inhaling will be automatic and passive. The air should be exhaled from the lungs with a sudden, vigorous inward stroke of the front abdominal muscles. The abdominal stroke should be complete and the breath should be expelled fully. While inhaling, no wilful expansion is necessary and the abdominal muscles should be relaxed. This exercise should be done in three phases, each consisting of 20 to 30 strokes a minute. A little rest can be taken in between. Throughout, the thoracic muscles should be kept contracted.

Kapalabhati enables the inhalation of a good amount of oxygen which purifies the blood and strengthens the nerve and brain centres. This kriya provides relief in many lung, throat and chest diseases like chronic bronchitis, asthma, pleurisy and tuberculosis.

4. *Trataka*: In Yoga, four exercises have been prescribed for strengthening weak eye muscles, relieving eye strain and curing of eye disease. They are known as 'Trataka' which in Sanskrit means "Winkless gaze at a particular point", or looking at an object with awareness. The four tratakas are: Dakshinayjatru trataka in which, with face forwards, the eyes are fixed on the tip of the right shoulder; Vamajatru trataka, in which the eyes are fixed on the tip of the left shoulder; Namikagra trataka, in which the eyes are focussed on the tip of the nose, and Bhrumadhya trataka, in which the eyes are focussed on the space between the eyebrows. These exercises should be practiced from a meditative position like padmasana or vajrasana. The gaze should be maintained for as long as you are comfortable, gradually increasing the period from 10 to 20 and then to 30 seconds. The eyes should be closed and rested after each exercise. Persons with acute myopia should perform the tratakas with their eyes closed.

Asanas

1. *Shavasana* (Dead body pose): Lie flat on your back, feet comfortably apart, arms and hands extended about six inches from the body, palms upwards and fingers half-folded. Close your eyes. Begin by consciously and gradually relaxing every part and each muscle of the body: feet, legs, calves, knees, thighs, abdomen, hips, back, hands, arms, chest, shoulders, neck, head and face. Relax yourself completely feeling as if your whole body is lifeless. Now concentrate your mind on breathing rhythmically as slowly and effortlessly as possible.

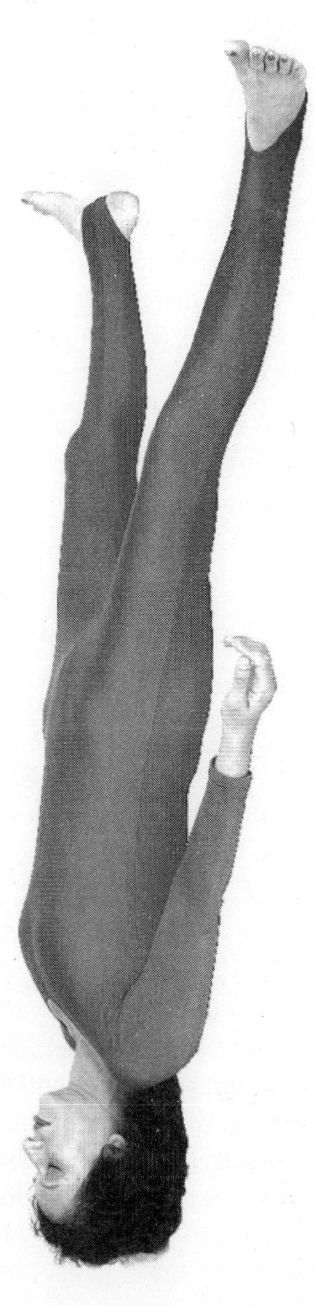

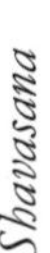

Shavasana

This creates a state of complete relaxation. Remain motionless in this position, relinquishing all responsibilities and worries for 10 to 15 minutes. Discontinue the exercise when your legs grow numb.

This asana helps bring down high blood pressure, and relieves the mind, particularly for those who are engaged in excessive mental activity. This exercise should be done both at the beginning and at the end of the daily round of yogic asanas. During a fast, shavasana soothes the nervous system.

2. *Padmasana* (Lotus pose): Sit erect and stretch your legs out in front of you. Bend one leg to place the foot on the thigh of the other, the sole facing upwards. Similarly, bend the other leg too, so that the heels are opposite each other and placed in such a way that they press down on the other side of the groin. Keep your neck, head and spine straight. Place your palms one upon the other, both turned upward and cupped, and rest them on the upturned heels a little below the navel.

Padmasana is a good pose for doing pranayama and meditation. It helps in the treatment of many heart and lung diseases and digestive disorders. It also calms and refreshes the mind.

3. *Yogamudra*: Sit erect in padmasana. Fold your hands behind your back, holding your left wrist with the right hand. Take a deep breath. While exhaling, bend forward slowly keeping your hands on your back. Bring your face downwards until your nose and forehead touch the floor. While inhaling, slowly rise back to the upright position. The practice of this asana tones up the nervous system, builds up powerful abdominal muscles and strengthens the pelvic organs. It helps pep up digestion, boosts the appetite and removes constipation. It provides relief in gas trouble, flatulence and lumbago. It

tones up and relaxes the nerves of the head and face. It also strengthens the sex glands.

4. *Vajrasana* (Pelvic pose): Sit erect and stretch out your legs. Fold your legs back, placing the feet on the sides of the buttocks with the soles facing back and upwards. Rest your buttocks on the floor between your heels. The toes of both feet should touch. Now, place your hands on your knees and keep the spine, neck and head straight. Vajrasana can be performed even after meals. It improves the digestion and is beneficial in cases of dyspepsia, constipation, colitis, seminal weakness and stiffness of the legs. It strengthens the hips, thighs, knees, calves, ankles and toes.

5. *Shirshasana* (Topsyturvy pose): Shirsha means 'head'. In this asana, one stands on one's head. Kneel on the ground, interlocking the fingers of both hands. Place the 'fingerlock' on the ground in front of you, keeping the elbows apart. Support your head on the fingerlock. Start raising your knees one at a time, to chest level. Then raise your feet slowly so that the calf muscles touch the thighs. Breathe normally. This is the first stage which should be done perfectly as the balance of the final posture depends mainly on this stage. Next, raise your knees first and then slowly raise the feet so that the whole body is straight, like a pillar. This is the final pose. Return to the original position by reversing the order, step by step. This asana should not be done jerkily. The important factor in shirshasana is mastering the balance, which comes through gradual practice. For proper balance, elbows should be placed firmly on the ground, alongside the fingerlock. Initially the asana should be done for 10 seconds only. The duration may be gradually increased by a further 10 seconds each week.

Regular practice of shirshasana will benefit the nervous, circulatory, respiratory, digestive, excretory and endocrine systems. This asana helps cases of dyspepsia, seminal weakness, varicose veins, arteriosclerosis, jaundice, renal colic and congested liver. Those suffering from oozing from the ears, iritis, high blood pressure or a weak heart should not practice this asana.

6. *Viparitakarani* (Inverted action pose): Lie flat on your back, with your feet together and arms by your side. Press your palms down, raising your legs to a perpendicular position without bending the knees. Your palms should touch the waist. Then straighten your legs. The trunk should not make a right angle with the ground but simply an upward slanting position. The chest should not press against the chin but be kept a little away. To return to the ground, bring your legs down slowly, evenly balancing your weight.

Through this asana, the muscles of the neck become stronger and blood circulation is improved. The functioning of the cervical nerves, ganglia and the thyroid also gets improved.

7. *Sarvangasana* (Shoulder stand pose): In Sanskrit 'sarva' means whole and 'anga' means limb. Almost all parts of the body are involved in and benefit from this asana. Lie flat on your back with your arms by the side, palms turned down. Bring your legs up slowly to a 90° angle and then raise the rest of the body by pushing the legs up and resting their weight on the arms. Fix your chin in jugular notch, and use your arms and hands to support the body at the hip region. The weight of the body should rest on your head, back and shoulders, your arms being used merely for balance. The trunk and legs should be in a straight line. The body, legs, hips and trunk should be kept as vertical as possible. Focus your eyes on your big toes. Press your chin against your chest. Hold the pose for one to three minutes. Return to the starting position slowly reversing the procedure.

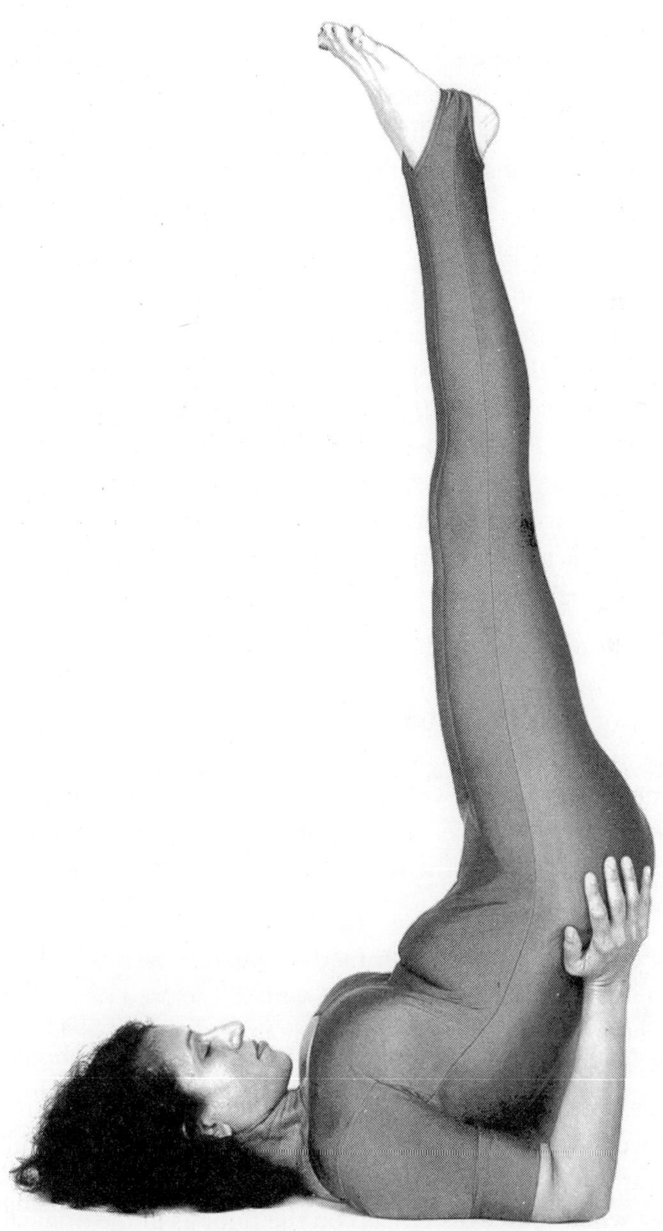

Viparitakarani

Sarvangasana helps relieve bronchitis, dyspepsia, varicose veins and peps up the digestion. It stimulates the thyroid and para-thyroid glands, influences the brain, heart and lungs. It helps lymphatic juices to circulate in the brain and strengthens the mind. This asana should not be done by those suffering from high blood pressure, heart disease and eye trouble.

8. *Matsyasana* (Fish pose): Sit in padmasana. Bend backwards and lie flat on your back without raising your knees. Press your palms beneath the shoulder. Push the hip backwards thus making a bridge-like arch with the spine. Then making hooks of your forefingers, grasp your toes without crossing your arms. Maintain this pose and breath rhythmically and comfortably. Reverse the order and return gradually to the starting position of padmasana. Matsyasana is beneficial in the treatment of acidity, constipation, diabetes, asthma, bronchitis and other lung disorders.

9. *Uttanapadasana* (Leg-lifting pose): Lie on your back with leg and arms straight, feet together, palms facing downwards, on the floor close to the body. Raise your legs about two feet from the floor without bending your knees. Maintain this pose for some time. Then, lower your legs slowly without bending the knees. This asana is helpful for those suffering from constipation. It strengthens the abdominal muscles and intestinal organs.

10. *Halasana* (Plough pose): Lie flat on your back with legs and feet together, arms by your side with fists closed near your thigh keeping your legs straight, slowly raise them to angles of 30°, 60° and 90°, pausing slightly at each point. Gradually, raise your legs above your head without bending your knees and then move them behind until they touch the floor. Stretch your legs as far as possible so that your chin presses tightly against the chest while your arms remain on the floor as in the original

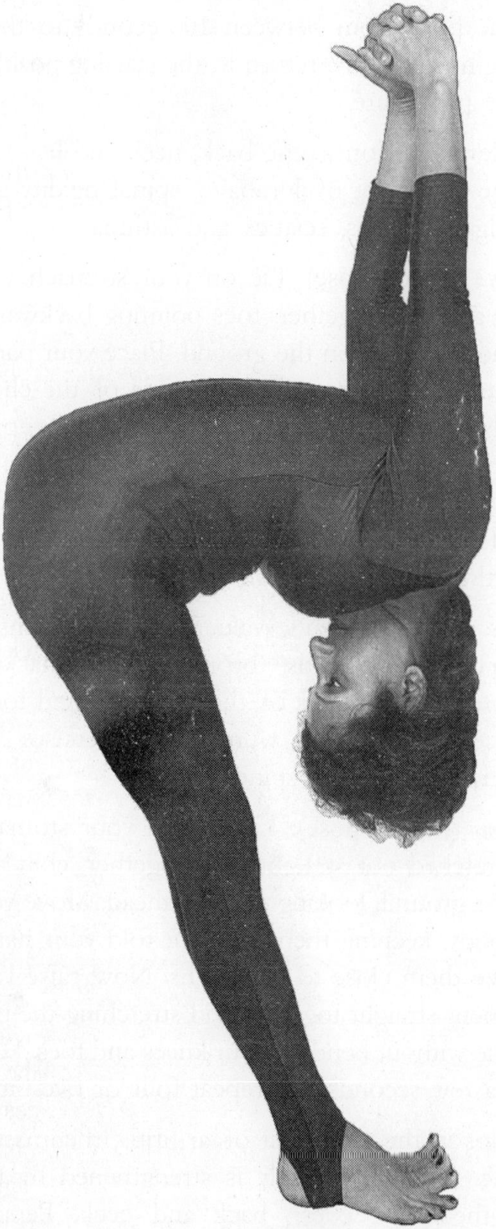

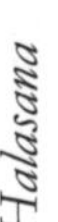

Halasana

position. Hold the pose from between 10 seconds to three minutes, breathing normally. To return to the starting position slowly reverse the procedure.

This asana relieves tension in the back, neck and legs and is beneficial in the treatment of lumbago, spinal rigidity and rheumatism, myalgia, arthritis, sciatica and asthma.

11. *Bhujangasana* (Cobra pose): Lie on your stomach with your legs straight and feet together, toes pointing backwards. Rest your forehead and nose on the ground. Place your palms below the shoulders and your arms by the side of the chest. Inhale and slowly raise your head, neck, chest and upper abdomen from the navel up. Bend your spine back and arch your back as far as you can looking upwards. Maintain this position and hold your breath for a few seconds. Exhale, and slowly return to the original position.

This asana has great therapeutic value in the treatment of diseases like cervical spondylitis, bronchitis, asthma and eosinophilia. It removes weakness of the abdomen and tones up the reproductive system in women. It exercises the vertebrae, back muscles and the spine.

12. *Shalabhasana* (Locust pose): Lie flat on your stomach, with your legs stretched out straight, feet together, chin and nose resting on the ground, looking straight ahead. Move your arms under the body, keeping them straight, fold your hands into fists and place them close to the thighs. Now, raise your legs up keeping them straight together and stretching them as far back as possible without bending your knees and toes. Hold this position for a few seconds and repeat four or five times.

This asana helps in the treatment of arthritis, rheumatism and low backache. The whole body is strengthened by this asana especially the waist, chest, back and neck. Persons

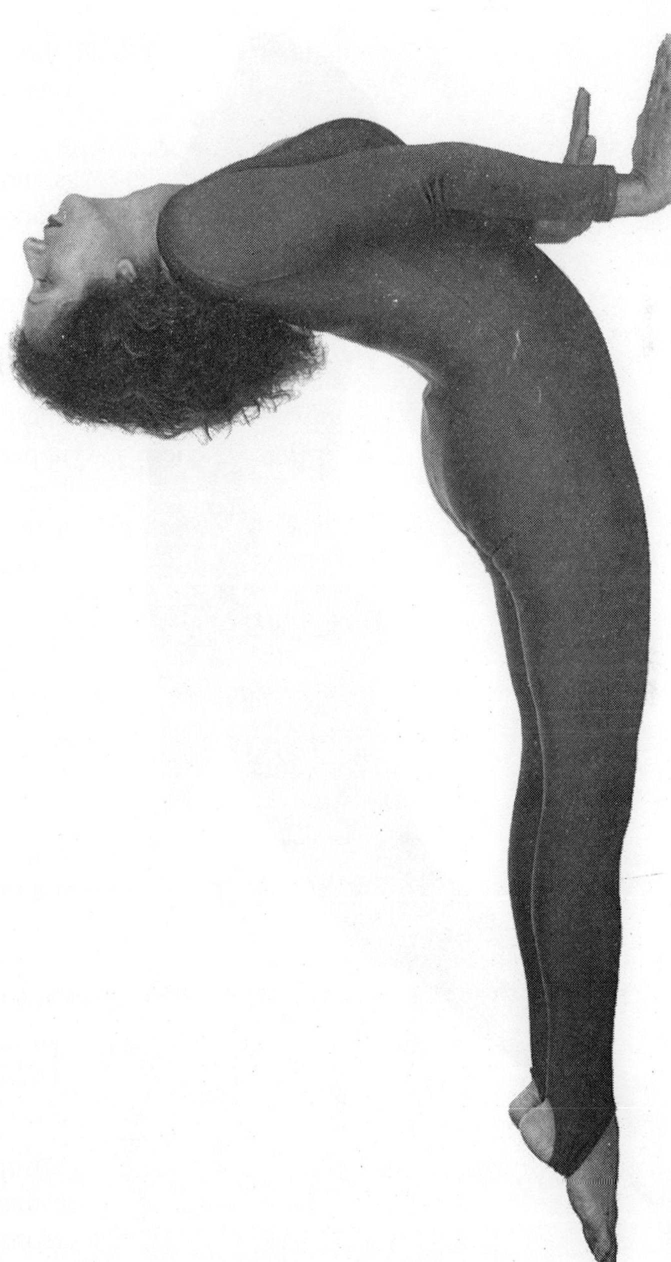

Bhujangasana

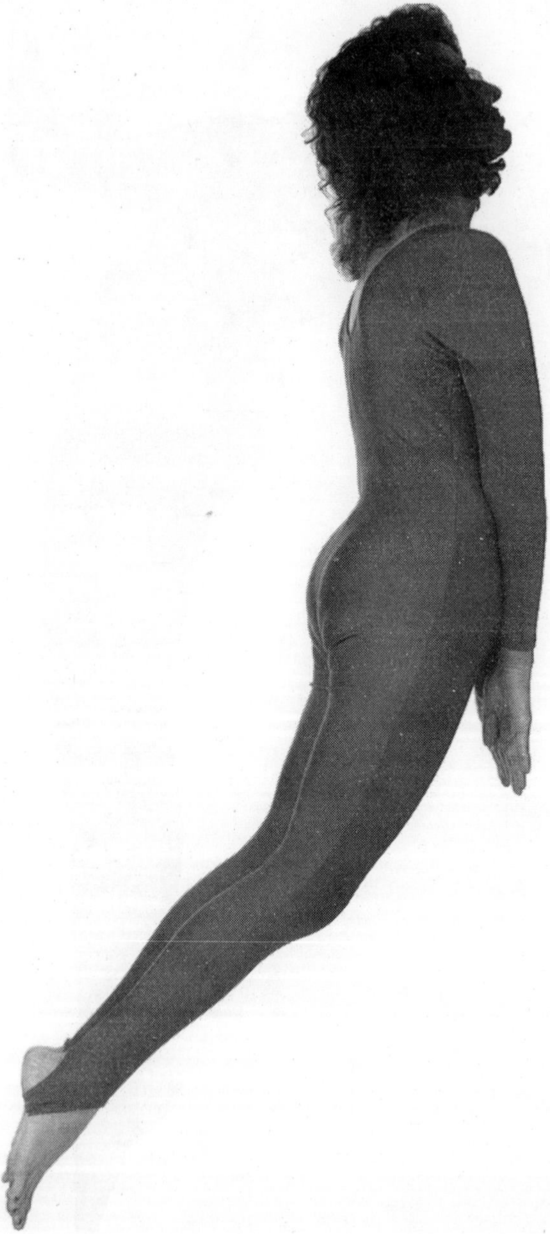

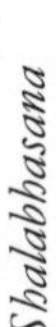

Shalabhasana

suffering from high blood pressure or heart disease should not practise this asana.

13. *Dhanurasana* (Bow pose): Lie on your stomach with your chin resting on the ground, arms extended alongside the body with the legs straight. Bend your legs back towards the hips, bring them forward and grasp your ankles. Inhale and raise your thighs, chest and head at the same time. Keep your hands straight. The weight of the body should rest mainly on the navel region. Therefore, arch your spine as much as possible. Exhale and return slowly to the starting position, by reversing the procedure.

Dhanurasana provides good exercise for the arms, shoulders, legs, ankles, back and neck. It also strengthens the spine. It relieves flatulence and constipation and improves the functioning of the pancreas and the intestines. It should not be done by those with a weak heart, high blood pressure and ulcers of the stomach and bowels.

14. *Makarasana* (Crocodile pose): Lie flat on your abdomen. Spread your legs, with heels pointing towards each other. Bring your left hand under the right shoulder and grasp it. Grasp the left shoulder with your right hand, keeping the elbows together, one upon the other on the ground. Your face should be between your crossed hands. Relax and breathe normally for two or three minutes. Then gradually go back to the sitting position.

This asana completely relaxes both the body and the mind and also rests the muscles. It is beneficial in the treatment of hypertension, heart disease and mental disorders.

15. *Vakrasana*: Sit erect and stretch legs out. Raise your right knee until your foot rests by the side of the left knee. Place your right hand behind your back without twisting the trunk

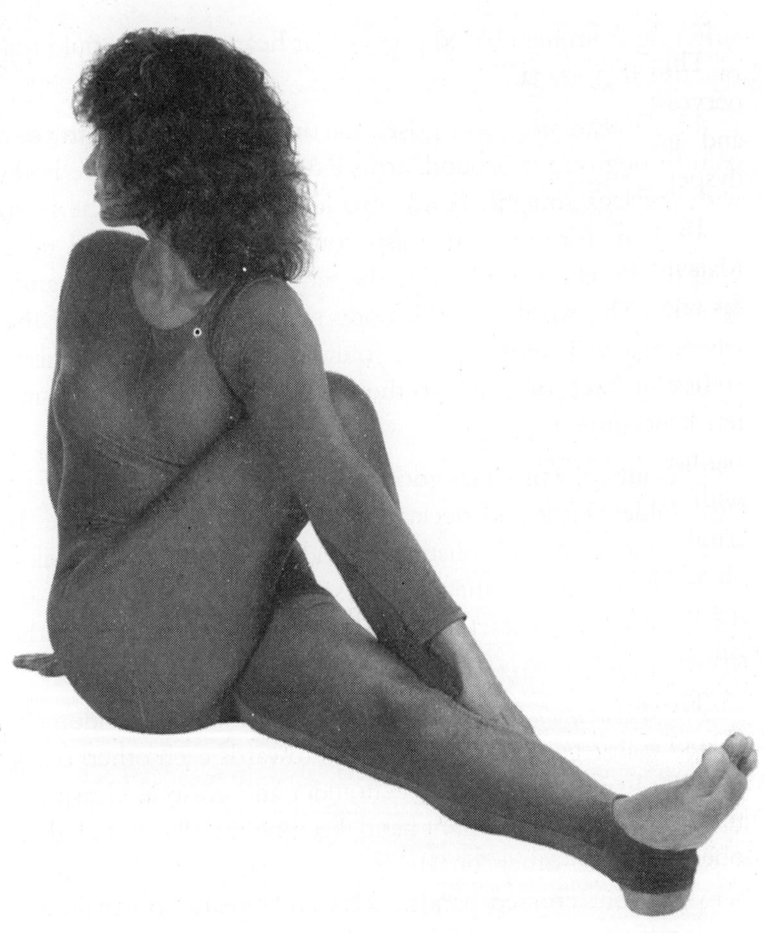

Vakrasana

too much. Then bring your left arm in front of you over the right knee. Place your left palm on the ground near the heel of your right foot. Push your right knee as far to the left arm. Twist your trunk to the right as much as possible. Turn your face to the right over the right shoulder. Release and repeat on the left side.

This asana tones up the spinal and abdominal muscles and nerves and activates the kidneys, intestines, stomach, adrenaline and gonad glands. It relieves cases of constipation and dyspepsia.

16. *Ardhamatsyendrasana*: This is the half position of Matsyendrasana, which is named after the great sage Matsyendra. Sit erect on the ground, stretching your legs in front of you. Insert your left heel in the perineum, keeping the left thigh straight. Place your right foot flat on the floor, crossing the left knee. Pass your left arm over the right knee and grasp the big toe of your right foot. Grasp your left thigh from the rear with your right hand. Turn your head, neck, shoulders and trunk to the right bringing your chin in line with the right shoulder. Maintain this position for a few seconds, gradually increasing the duration to 2 minutes. Repeat the same process on the other side for the same duration.

This asana exercises the vertebrae and keeps them in good shape. It helps the liver, spleen, bladder, pancreas, intestines and other abdominal organs, and also stretches and strengthens the spinal nerves. This asana is beneficial in the treatment of obesity, dyspepsia, asthma and diabetes.

17. *Paschimottanasana* (Posterior stretching pose): Sit erect. Stretch your legs out in front of you, keeping them close to each other. Bend your trunk and head forward from the waist without bending your knees and grasp the big toes with your fingers. Holding your toes, and without bending your knees, rest your forehead on your knees. With practice, the tense muscles become supple enough for this exercise. Old persons and persons whose spine is still should do this asana slowly in the initial stages. The final pose need be maintained only for a few seconds. Return to the starting position gradually.

Paschimottanasana is a good stretching exercise in which the posterior muscles get stretched and relaxed. It relieves sciatica, muscular rheumatism of the back, backache, lumbago and asthmatic attacks. It is also valuable in constipation, dyspepsia and other abdominal disorders.

18. *Gomukhasana* (Cow-face pose): Sit erect on the floor, with your legs outstretched. Fold your left leg back. Place your left foot under the right hip. Similarly, fold back the right leg and cross your right foot over your left thigh. Place your right heel against the left hip. Both soles should face backwards, one

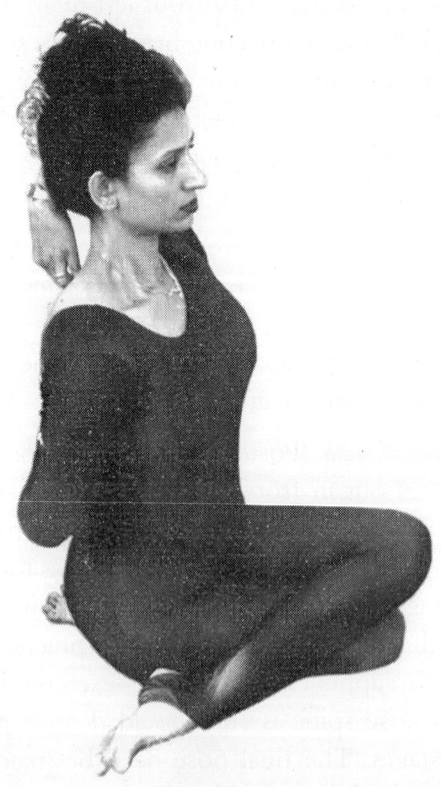

Gomukhasana

over the other. Now interlock your hands behind your back. See to it that if your right leg is over the left, then your right elbow should face upward and the left elbow downward. This position is reversed when the leg position is changed. Hold the pose for 30 seconds and then repeat the procedure reversing the process.

The practice of gomukhasana will strengthen the muscles of the upper arm, shoulder, chest, back, waist and thigh. It is beneficial in the treatment of seminal weakness, piles, urethral disorders and kidney troubles. It also relieves varicose veins and sciatica.

19. *Pavanamuktasana* (Gas-releasing pose): Lie flat on your back, hands by your side. Fold your legs back, placing your feet flat on the floor; make a fingerlock with your hands and place them a little below the knees. Bring your thighs up near your chest. Exhale and raise your head and shoulders and bring your nose between your knees. This is the final position. Maintain this pose for a few seconds and repeat three to five times. Reverse the procedure to get back to the original position.

This asana strengthens the abdominal muscles and internal abdominal organs like the liver, spleen, pancreas and stomach. It helps release excessive gas from the abdomen and relieves flatulence. Persons suffering from constipation should do this exercise in the morning after drinking lukewarm water to help proper evacuation of the bowels.

20. *Chakrasana* (Lateral bending pose): Stand straight with your feet and toes together and arms by your sides, palms facing and touching the thighs. Raise one arm laterally above the head with the palm inwards up to shoulder level and palm upwards when the arm rises above the level of your head. Then, bend your trunk and head sideways with the raised arm

touching the ear, and sliding the palm of the other hand downwards towards the knee. Keep your knees and elbows straight throughout. Maintain the final pose for a few seconds. Then gradually bring your hand back to the normal position. Repeat the exercise on the other side.

This asana induces maximum stretching of the lateral muscles of the body, especially the abdomen. It strengthens the knees, arms and shoulders and increases lung capacity.

21. *Trikonasana* (Triangle pose): Stand erect, with your legs apart. Stretch your arms up to shoulder level. Bend your trunk forwards and twist to the left, looking upwards and keeping your left arm raised at an angle of 90°. Place your right palm on your left foot without bending the knees. Maintain this pose for a few seconds. Then straighten up and return to the normal position. Repeat the procedure on the other side.

Trikonasana is an all-round stretching exercise. It keeps the spinal column flexible and reduces the fat on the lateral sides of the body. Besides, it stimulates the adrenal glands and tones up the abdominal and pelvic organs.

Pranayama

Prana means 'vital force' and Ayama means 'control' in Sanskrit. Thus Pranayama means the control of the vital force through concentration and regulated breathing. By means of controlled breathing that is, inhaling and exhaling by holding the breath for a fixed time and changing the rhythm of inspiration and expiration, it is possible to influence the life-force in the body. Pranayama is the process by which such conscious control is achieved through controlled and rhythmical breathing. Pranayama purifies the channels along which the life stream of 'prana' flows in the body and prevents various disorders. It increases one's resistance to respiratory diseases.

The best position in which to practice pranayama is the padmasan or lotus pose. If for some reason that position is difficult to adopt, it can be done while sitting in any comfortable pose. The important thing is to keep the back, neck and head in a straight line. The body should be in its natural relaxed condition and this can be achieved by resting a few minutes in shavasan. If necessary, use your right finger and thumb on either side of the nose to control the right and left nostrils during inhalation and exhalation. In practising pranayama, a ratio of two to one should be maintained throughout, that is, the exhalation time should be double than required for inhalation. For instance, if inhalation takes 5 seconds, exhalation should take 10 seconds. Both inhalation and exhalation should be smooth and quiet. Some varieties of pranayama beneficial in the treatment of common ailments are as follows:

1. *Anuloma-viloma*: This is also known as Nadishuddhi pranayama. Sit in any comfortable meditative pose, keeping your head, neck and spine erect. Rest your left hand on your left knee. Close your right nostril by pressing the tip of your right thumb against it. Breathe out slowly through the left nostril. Inhale slowly and deeply through the left nostril, keeping the right nostril closed. Close your left nostril with the little finger and ring finger of your right hand and exhale through the right nostril. Then inhale through the right nostril, keeping the left nostril closed and, lastly, exhale through the left nostril, keeping the right nostril closed. This completes one round of anuloma-viloma. Repeat the entire process, inhaling and exhaling should be done very slowly, without making any sound.

This pranayama is a process of purification. It strengthens the lungs and calms the nerves. It helps cure cough and cold, insomnia, chronic headache and asthma.

2. *Ujjayi*: Sit in any comfortable meditative pose. Inhale slowly, deeply and steadily through both nostrils with a low uniform sound through the glottis. Hold your breath for a second or two after inhaling and then exhale noisily only through the left nostril, keeping the right nostril closed. Do this as often as required. This pranayama clears the nasal passage and helps the functioning of the thyroid gland and benefits respiratory disorders, especially bronchitis and asthma. Persons suffering from high blood pressure should not practice ujjayi.

3. *Bhastrika*: 'Bhastrika' means 'bellows'. It is performed by instant and quick expirations of breath. There are many varieties of bhastrika. The simplest technique is as follows: Sit in padmasana. Do 20 strokes of kapalabhati. Inhale and exhale rapidly, making a puffing sound. This is a good exercise for abdominal viscera and lungs.

4. *Sheetali*: Sit in padmasana or any other comfortable posture. Stick your tongue out about an inch from the lips, rolled up at the sides to form a channel like a bird's beak. Suck in air through this channel. After a full inhalation, slowly close your mouth, hold your breath and exhale slowly through both nostrils. This completes the exercise. Repeat as required. This pranayama cools the body and mind, activates the liver and bile and has beneficial effects on the circulation and body temperature.

5. *Sitkari*: In sitkari a sound is produced while inhaling by opening the mouth a little, placing the tip of the tongue against the lower front teeth and then sucking the air in slowly. After holding your breath, exhale through both nostrils. This exercise helps to control thirst, hunger and laziness.

6. *Suryabhedan*: 'Surya-Nadi' is the right nostril and

'Chandra-Nadi' is the left nostril. In this pranayama, one always uses the right nostril for inhalation. Sit in padmasan or any other suitable posture. Keep your head, neck and back straight. Inhale through the right nostril. Hold your breath and then exhale through the left nostril. Repeat as often as required. This pranayama increases gastric juices and helps digestion. It also fortifies the nervous system and clears the sinuses.

7. *Bhramari*: In this pranayama, the buzzing sound of a bee is produced and hence it is called bhramari. Keep your mouth closed while inhaling. Exhale through both nostrils, producing the humming sound of a bee. This pranayama affects the ears, nose, eyes and mouth and makes the complexion glow. It also helps those suffering from insomnia.

CHAPTER 8

Healing Power of Colours

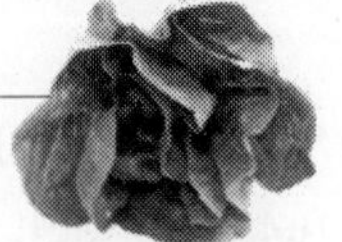

Chromotherapy is a method of treatment of diseases by colour, it is best used as a supportive therapy along with other natural methods of preserving health such as correct diet, adequate rest and relaxation, exercise, yogic asanas and so on.

According to practitioners of chromotherapy, the cause of any disease can be traced to the lack of a particular colour in the human system. Colour therapy is a technique of restoring imbalance by means of applying coloured light to the body. It was a popular method of cure even in ancient times. Some 2,500 years ago, Pythagoras applied colour light therapeutically and 'colour halls' were used for healing in ancient Egypt, China and India.

The pioneer of modern colour therapy was Niels Finsen of Denmark. Following the discovery, in 1877, of the bactericidal action of solar ultra-violet energy, Finsen studied the possibility of assisting the healing of wounds with visible light. He subsequently used red light to inhibit the formation of smallpox scars and, in 1896, founded a Light Institute (now the Finsen Institute of Copenhagen) for the phototreatment of tuberculosis. In 1932, Gerrard and Hessay, two Californian psychologists, scientifically established that blue light had a calming effect and red a stimulating power on human beings.

Blue and red colours are considered as the two extremes with yellow representing the midpoint These are also the three principal colours in a rainbow. A patient is first subjected to an examination to ascertain which colour he lacks. The deficiency is determined by observing the colour of the eyeballs, nails, urine and excrement. In cases of the lack of red the eyes and nails will be bluish, and the urine and excrement white or bluish. If there is a deficiency of the blue colour, the eyes and nails will be reddish, and urine and excrement yellowish or red.

Every substance on earth contains colour. Even the rays cast on earth by celestial bodies contain colour in the form of white light. The rays of the sun contain seven different colours — violet, indigo, blue, green, yellow, orange and red. These are natural colours which are highly beneficial to the maintenance of health and for healing diseases.

According to Dr. Babbit, a well-known authority on chromotherapy, "sunlight is the principal curative agent in nature's laboratory and where light cannot enter, disease does. Chlorosis, anaemia, leukaemia, emaciation, muscular debility, regeneration of heart and liver, dropsical effusion, softening of bones, nervous excitability, physical deformity, stunted growth and consumption are the result of excluding oneself from the beneficial effects of sunlight."

Sunlight plays an important role in the recovery from chronic diseases. Judicious use of sunlight can be part of the curing process in almost every affliction. The rays of the sun improve digestion and nutrition, quicken blood and lymph circulation and increase the elimination of impurities through the skin.

The action and effect of various colours on the body and their healing qualities are as follows:

Red: Symbolic of heat, fire and anger, it is a stimulating and energising colour. It stimulates arterial blood and brings warmth to cool extremities. Used as a general tonic, it is very valuable in the treatment of diseases like low blood pressure, rheumatism, paralysis, anaemia and advanced cases of tuberculosis.

Orange: Symbolic of prosperity and pride, orange is useful for stimulating blood supply and energising the nerves. It is beneficial in the treatment of kidney and gall stones, hernia and appendicitis. It is also used to stimulate the milk producing action of breasts after childbirth.

Violet: Violet is beneficial in the treatment of nervous and emotional disturbances, arthritis, acute cases of consumption and insomnia.

Yellow: Associated with joy and happiness, yellow is laxative and diuretic. It is a stimulant to the brain, the liver and the spleen. It is also effective in the treatment of diabetes, indigestion, kidney and liver disorders, constipation, eye and throat infections, syphilis and impotence.

Purple: Purple or indigo combines the blood-warming red and the cooling antiseptic blue. It is an excellent stimulant without being an irritant. It is beneficial in the treatment of advanced stages of constipation, hydrocele, leucorrhoea, many disorders of the stomach and womb, cataract, migraine and skin disorders. It exerts a soothing effect on the eyes, ears and the nervous system.

Green: Made up of blue and yellow, green is regarded as a colour of harmony. It is a mild sedative. It is useful in the treatment of nervous conditions, hay fever, ulcers, influenza, malaria, colds, sexual disorders and cancer. It preserves and strengthens eyesight. Being highly medicinal and depressive, it is of great help in the treatment of inflammatory conditions.

Blue: Cool, soothing and sedative, blue alleviates pain, reduces bleeding and heals burns. It is beneficial in the treatment of dysentery, colic, asthma, respiratory disorders, high blood pressure and skin aberrations. In a study at the New England State Hospital in the United States, 25 members of staff with normal blood pressure were bathed in blue light for half an hour. It resulted in universal fall in blood pressure. The blood pressure rose when red light was applied.

Methods of Treatment

There are two methods of treating diseases by colour: (i) by the application of light through different coloured glasses; and (ii) by external or internal use of colour-charged water.

In the first method, sheets of glass, 30 cms × 36 cms, of the required colours are needed. These are placed at the window frames or any other convenient place in such a way that the sun's rays can pass through them and fall directly on the patient's body. The usual duration of the colour treatment is 30 minutes. In case of local application, a pane of glass can be placed in front of the diseased part so that the light passing through the glass falls on the afflicted area. At night lanterns can be used for the purpose. A single lantern can have glass panes of four different colours and the required colour can be focussed on the patient or the affected parts.

In the second method, coloured bottles are needed. These bottles should be cleaned and filled up to three-fourths level with fresh well water, distilled water or rain water. The bottles should be corked and then placed in bright sunlight for three to four hours. After this exposure, the water is said to acquire medicinal properties and this colour-charged water can be used both internally and for external applications. Wounds and ulcers can be washed with this water and it can also be used to massage the affected parts or applied as compress on them. For internal use, an adult can take 30 ml. of colour-charged water as a single dose. The dose can be repeated as required.

Diet

A correct and balanced diet is essential during the treatment of diseases through chromotherapy. The patients should take food items with analogous colouring. The various colours contained in different food items are:

Red: Beets, radish, red cabbage, tomatoes, watercress, most red-skinned fruits, red berries and water melon.

Orange: Orange-skinned vegetables and fruits such as carrot, orange, apricot, mango, peach and papaya.

Violet: Egg plant, berries, black carrot and purple grapes.

Yellow: Lime and lemon, sweet lime, grapes, pumpkin, melon, banana, mango, yellow apple and guava.

Purple: Foods having both blue and violet colouring.

Green: Most of the green vegetables and fruits such as gourds, spinach, plantain, lettuce, pea, green mango, gooseberry, pears, beans, etc.

Blue: Blue plum, blue beans, blue grapes, etc.

Contraindications

There are some important contraindications to colour treatment which should be borne in mind while adopting this mode of cure. For instance, the red colour would be injurious in a naturally inflammatory condition of the system, and in case of persons with feverish and excitable temperament. If the red light is employed for too long and frequently, it may produce dangerous fevers. The danger can be obviated by using the red light for a few minutes at a time or by placing a wet bandage over the head.

Similarly, yellow should not be used when the nerves are very active or irritable. Yellow or orange reddish tones may prove injurious in fevers, acute inflammations, delirium, diarrhoea, neuralgia, palpitation of the heart and any condition of over-excitement.

In cases of paralysis, chronic rheumatism, gout, and in all cold, pale and dormant conditions of the system, blue, indigo and violet may prove too cooling and constricting and should be avoided.

CHAPTER 9

Sleep: Restorative of Tired Body and Mind

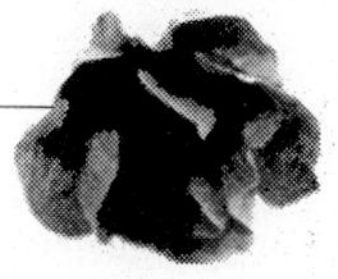

Sleep is one of nature's greatest inventions and blessings of life. It is a periodic rest of the body which is absolutely essential for its efficient functioning. It has been called "most cheering restorative of tired bodies."

Sleep is the indispensable condition to the recuperation of energy. We go to bed fatigued and get up refreshed. Sleep repairs the wear and tear of the body and mind incurred during waking hours. Nothing is so restorative to the nerves as sound and uninterrupted sleep. Sleep is thus a vital element in a total way of life. It is a basic need in man's mental as well as physical life.

During sleep most of the functions of the body are carried on at the lowest level possible in health. Heat production is from 10 to 15 per cent below the basal level. The mechanism regulating the body temperature are less sensitive than in the waking state and are depressed by 0.5 to 1.0 degree F. The rate of the heart is reduced by 10 to 30 beats per minute and a decline in blood pressure of about 20 mm occurs in quiet restful sleep. The urine volume is considerably reduced, but its concentration in solids is increased. The tone of all the skeletal muscles is lessened. The eyes are usually rolled upward and the pupils constricted.

Loss of sleep exerts seriously detrimental effects upon the nervous system. Long periods of wakefulness may cause profound psychological changes such as loss of memory, irritability, hallucination and even schizophrenic manifestations.

During the last World War, prisoners in Nazi concentration camps who kept awake for days by strong lights and blaring wireless sets, collapsed.

Sleep versus Rest

For correct living, it is essential to differentiate between sleep and rest. At rest the body is disturbed by all exterior noises; but in sleep it is screened from them by partial loss of consciousness and also by what is called "dream protection". One useful purpose of the dream is to convert outside noises that might awake the sleeping person, into fantasies that do not disturb him.

During rest the limbs are normal, but in sleep they swell. Blood flows from the brain, distends the arteries, and makes the limbs bigger. In sleep more muscles are relaxed than in rest, though the sleeping person changes his position about 35 times in one night, without knowing it. Many organs which work during rest suspend their activities in sleep. Thus the recouping value of sleep is much more than that of rest or simple lying down.

Theories of Sleep

Many theories of sleep have been advanced to explain the temporary loss of consciousness which we know as sleep. The oldest theory is that sleep is induced by a reduction in the blood supply to the brain or at least to conscious centres. This is known as ischemic theory. Even the ancient Greek physicians were aware that the carotid artery was in a way concerned with the onset of sleep. The name itself expresses this belief. The Greek word 'Karotides' for carotid arteries is derived from karoo which means 'put to sleep'. In modern times, the drowsiness after a meal, presumably due to the diversion of blood from the brain to the digestive organs, is cited in support of the ischemic theory.

Another important theory about sleep is the chemical theory. As a result of experiments in the metabolism of sleeping subjects, it is considered that the fatigue inducing sleep may be a mild form of blood poisoning or toxaemia. This "poisoning" is believed to be brought on by the expenditure of energy during the waking hours.

According to this theory, every contraction of a muscle and every impulse passing through the brain or the nerves breaks down a certain amount of tissue. The debris from broken down tissue is then thrown into the bloodstream. In the waking state, much of the waste from broken down tissue is got rid of through the natural eliminating processes of lungs, kidneys, bowels and skin. But there comes a saturation point when there is such an accumulation of waste that it cannot be disposed of by these processes and it then invades the grey matter of the brain. In such an eventuality, mental and physical alertness are impaired. It is nature's warning that the waste product must be reduced to replenish the lost energy. So we get tired and the urge to get sleep becomes irresistible.

During sleep, the cells and tissues that break down to produce toxic waste become less active and the production of toxic waste is vastly reduced. Simultaneously, constructive activities take place within the body during sleep, which rebuild the broken down tissue.

Another theory places a sleeping centre in the hypothalamus. Many of the bodily changes in sleep such as constriction of pupils, reduced frequency of heart beat, increased gastric tone and secretion are manifestations of the activity of hypothalamus nuclei, especially parasympathetic centres. Perhaps some of the sleeping pills affect this centre in the brain.

Although the various theories have certain amounts of experimental evidence to support them, none has really solved what is the most mysterious process in our lives. All we know is that sleep substitutes constructive measures for the destructive processes of our waking hours. We cannot live without sleep.

Duration

Another mystery about sleep is that no two persons need the same amount of sleep. Dr. Nathaniel Kleitman, Associate Professor of Physiology at the University of Chicago, who conducted years of extensive experiments at the University's 'Sleeping laboratory' says that there is no more a normal duration of sleep than there is normal height and weight. A study of 25 subjects spread over thousands of nights showed that the average amount of sleep needed to feel well rested is seven-and-a-half hours, though individuals varied from six to nine hours. According to Dr. Demmis Williams, a noted authority on sleep, the amount of sleep needed for an individual's well-being, is determined by what he feels he needs, not by what other people, including the doctor, thinks is reasonable.

On the whole, women sleep from 45 minutes to one hour more than men. The amount of sleep required varies at different ages as follows:

New born	18 to 20 hours
Growing children	10 to 12 hours
Adults	6 to 9 hours
Aged persons	5 to 7 hours

The depth of ordinary restful sleep fluctuates throughout the sleep. In most adults, sleep deepens through the first hour, after which it lightens rather sharply and then more gradually until morning or until the usual time of wakening. In growing children, however, sleep deepens a second time for a little while. According to Dr. Lindlahr, a famous naturopath, two hours before and two hours after midnight are the most valuable for sleep of all the twenty-four hours of the day. In these four hours, mental and physical vigour are at their lowest ebb and sleep is soundest and most natural.

It is believed that three-quarters of our sleep consists of what is called 'slow wave sleep'. The restorative processes occur during this time. The remaining quarter is taken by what is called 'rapid eye movement (REM) sleep'. It is also called paradoxical or dreaming sleep and it comes in episodes of about 20 minutes duration about five times in a night. It involves dreaming, irregular heart rates, raised blood pressure and erection of the penis. It is in this phase of sleep that normal healthy young men may have wet dreams. Both forms of sleep are considered equally important, being normal sleeping rhythms.

Sleeping Positions

There are many theories about good and bad sleeping positions. Practically everyone changes positions several times during sleep. Hence how one starts out is of no consequence. It is a good thing we do turn about in our beds. If we did not, we would awaken in the morning stiff, having maintained the same position all night. For proper sleep, however, one should not sleep on one's back but on the side with one or both legs brought well up and the head and the shoulder slightly forward.

Sleeping pills are no remedy for sleeplessness. They are habit-forming and become less effective when taken continuously. They lower the I.Q., dull the brain and can prove fatal if taken in excess or before or after alcohol. The side-effect of sleeping pills include indigestion, skin rashes, lowered resistance to infection, circulatory and respiratory problems, poor appetite, high blood pressure, kidney and liver problems and mental confusion.

Sleeping well is an art. It needs a perfect blend of healthy habits and control of mind. A clean body and mind, relaxed mood, physical exercises, and perfect dietary control are some of the basic sleep-inducing methods.

Unpleasant situations at bed time such as arguments, quarrels, watching a horror movie, listening to loud music which would create anxiety, fear, excitement and worries should be avoided. Such situations stimulate the cerebral cortex and tend to keep one awake.

The sleeping place should be well ventilated, with balanced temperature and free from noises. The bed should be neither too hard nor too soft, but comfortable, the pillow should not be too hard or too high. The bed clothes should be loose-fitting and light coloured. Another important rule is not to eat heavy food shortly before bed time.

Part II

Health Through Nutrition

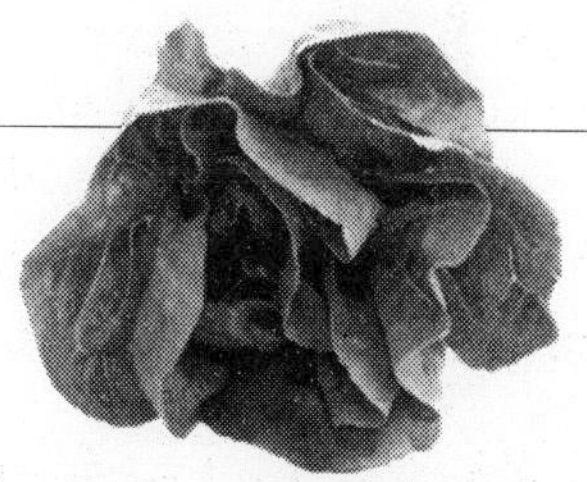

CHAPTER 10

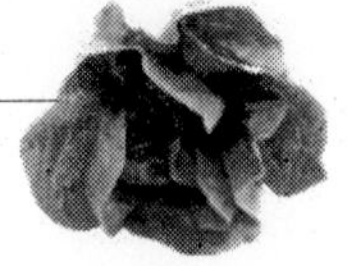

Optimum Nutrition for Vigour and Vitality

Your food shall be your medicine
—Hippocrates

Diet plays a vital role in the maintenance of good health and in the prevention and cure of disease. In the words of Sir Robert McCarrison, one of the best known nutritionists, "The right kind of food is the most important single factor in the promotion of health; and the wrong kind of food is the most important single factor in the promotion of disease."

The human body builds up and maintains healthy cells, tissues, glands and organs only with the help of various nutrients. The body cannot perform any of its functions, be they metabolic, hormonal, mental, physical or chemical, without specific nutrients. The food which provides these nutrients is thus one of the most essential factors in building and maintaining health.

Nutrition, which depends on food, is also of utmost importance in the cure of disease. The primary cause of disease is a weakened organism or lowered resistance in the body, arising from the adoption of a faulty nutritional pattern. There is an elaborate healing mechanism within the body but it can perform its function only if it is abundantly supplied with all the essential nutritional factors.

It is believed that at least 45 chemical components and elements are needed by human cells. Each of these 45 substances, called essential nutrients, must be present in adequate diets. The list of these nutrients, include oxygen and water. The other 43 essential nutrients are classified into five main groups, namely carbohydrates, fats, proteins, minerals and vitamins. All 45 of these nutrients are vitally important and they work together. Therefore, the absence of any of them will result in disease and eventually in death.

Research has shown that almost all varieties of disease can be produced by an under-supply of various nutrients. These nutritional deficiencies occur on account of various factors, including the intense processing and refining of foods, the time lag between the harvesting and consumption of vegetables and fruits, the chemicals used in bleaching, flavouring, colouring and preserving foods and the chemical fertilisers, fungicides insecticides and sprays used for treating the soil. Therefore, as a first principle of nutrition, one should insist upon whole meal flour and whole meal bread and avoid the white stuff.

Research has also shown that diseases produced by combinations of deficiencies can be corrected when all the nutrients are supplied, provided irreparable damage has not been done. A well-balanced and correct diet is thus of utmost importance for the maintenance of good health and the healing of diseases. Such a diet, obviously should be made up of foods, which in combination would supply all the essential nutrients.

It has been found that a diet which contains liberal quantities of (i) seeds, nuts, and grains, (ii) vegetables and (iii) fruits, would provide adequate amounts of all the essential nutrients. These foods have, therefore, been aptly called basic food groups and the diet containing these food groups as optimum diet for vigour and vitality. It is described, in brief, below:

(i) *Seeds, nuts and grains*: These are the most important and the most potent of all foods and contain all the important nutrients needed for human growth. They contain the germ, the reproductive power which is of vital importance for the lives of human beings and their health. Millet, wheat, oats, barley, brown rice, beans and peas are all highly valuable in building health. Wheat, mung beans, alfalfa seeds and soya beans make excellent sprouts. Sunflower seeds, pumpkin seeds, almonds, peanuts and soya beans contain complete proteins of high biological value.

Seeds, nuts and grains are also excellent natural sources of essential unsaturated fatty acids necessary for health. They are also good sources of lecithin and most of the B vitamins. They are the best natural sources of vitamin C, which is perhaps the most important vitamin for the preservation of health and prevention of premature ageing. Besides, they are rich sources of minerals and supply necessary bulk in the diet. They also contain auxones, the natural substances that play an important role in the rejuvenation of cells and prevention of premature ageing.

(ii) *Vegetables*: They are extremely rich source of minerals, enzymes and vitamins. Faulty cooking and prolonged careless storage, however, destroy these valuable nutrients. Most of the vegetables are, therefore, best consumed in their natural raw state in the form of salads.

There are different kinds of vegetables. They may be edible roots, stems, leaves, fruits and seeds. Each group contributes to the diet in its own way. Fleshy roots have high energy value and good sources of vitamin B. Seeds are relatively high in carbohydrates and proteins and yellow ones are rich in vitamin A. Leaves, stems and fruits are excellent sources of minerals, vitamins, water and roughage.

To prevent loss of nutrients in vegetables, it would be advisable to steam or boil vegetables in their juices on a slow fire and the water or while cooking liquid should not be drained off. No vegetable should be peeled unless it is so old that the peel is tough and unpalatable. In most root vegetables, the largest amount of mineral is directly under the skin and these are lost if vegetables are peeled. Soaking of vegetables should also be avoided if taste and nutritive value are to be preserved.

(iii) *Fruits*: Like vegetables, fruits are an excellent source of minerals, vitamins and enzymes. They are easily digested and exercise a cleansing effect on the blood and digestive tract. They contain high alkaline properties, a high percentage of water and a low percentage of proteins and fats. Their organic acid and high sugar content have immediate refreshing effects. Apart from seasonal fresh fruits, dry fruits, such as raisins, prunes and figs are also beneficial.

Fruits are at their best when eaten in the raw and ripe states. In cooking, they lose portions of the nutrient salts and carbohydrates. They are most beneficial when taken as a separate meal by themselves, preferably for breakfast in the morning. If it becomes necessary to take fruits with regular food, they should form a larger proportion of the meals. Fruits, however, make better combination with milk than with meals. It is also desirable to take one kind of fruit at a time. For the maintenance of good health, at least one pound of uncooked fruits should form part of the daily diet. In case of sickness, it will be advisable to take fruits in the form of juices.

The three basic health-building foods mentioned above should be supplemented with certain special foods such as milk, vegetable oils and honey. Milk is an excellent food. It is considered as 'Nature's most nearly perfect food'. The best way to take milk is in its soured form—that is, yogurt and cottage cheese. Soured milk is superior to sweet milk as it is in a predigested form and more easily assimilated. Milk helps maintain a healthy intestinal flora and prevents intestinal putrefaction and constipation.

High quality unrefined vegetable oils should be added to the diet. They are rich in unsaturated fatty acids, Vitamin C and F and lecithin. The average daily amount should not exceed two tablespoons. Honey too, is an ideal food. It helps increase calcium retention in the system, prevents nutritional anaemia besides being beneficial in kidney and liver disorders, colds, poor circulation and complexion problems. It is one of nature's finest energy-giving food.

A diet of the three basic food groups, supplemented with the special foods mentioned above, will ensure a complete and adequate supply of all the vital nutrients needed for health, vitality and prevention of diseases. It is not necessary to include animal protein like egg, fish or meat in this basic diet, as animal protein, especially meat, always has a detrimental effect on the healing processes. High animal protein is harmful to health and may cause many of our common ailments.

Daily menu

Based on what has been stated above, the daily menu of a health-building and vitalising diet should be on the following lines:

Upon arising — A glass of luke-warm water mixed with the juice of half a lime and a teaspoon of honey, or a glass of freshly squeezed juice of any available seasonal fruit such as apple, pineapple, orange, sweet lime and grapes.

Breakfast — Fresh fruits such as apple, orange, banana, grapes, or any available seasonal fruits, a cup of butter-milk or unpasteurised milk and a handful of raw nuts or a couple of tablespoons of sunflower and pumpkin seeds.

Mid-morning snack — One apple or a banana or any other fruit.

Lunch — A bowl of freshly prepared steamed vegetables using salt, vegetable oil and butter for seasoning, one or two slices of whole grain bread or chappatis and a glass of butter-milk.

Mid-afternoon — A glass of fresh fruit or vegetable juice or any available fruit.

Dinner — A large bowl of fresh salad made up of green vegetables such as tomatoes, carrot, cabbage, cucumber, red beet and onion with lime juice dressing, any available sprouts such as alfalfa seeds and mung beans, a warm vegetable course, if desired, one tablespoon of fresh butter, cottage cheese or a glass of butter-milk.

The above menu is a general outline around which an individual diet can be built. It can be modified and changed to adopt to specific requirements and conditions. The menu for lunch and dinner is interchangeable.

Do not drink liquids with meals. The water should be taken half an hour before meals or an hour after meals. Milk, butter-milk and vegetable soups are foods and can be taken with meals.

CHAPTER 11

Miracles of Alkalizing Diet

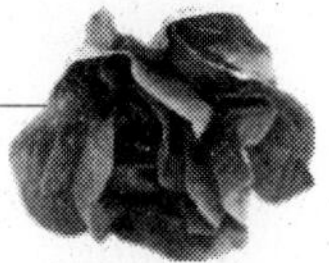

The human body is composed of various organs and parts, which are made up of tissues and cells. These tissues and cells are composed of 16 chemical elements.

The balance or equilibrium of these chemical elements in the body is an essential factor in the maintenance of health and healing of disease. The acid-alkaline balance plays a vital role in this balanced body chemistry. All foods, after digestion and absorption leave either an acid or alkaline ash in the body depending on their mineral composition. The normal body chemistry is approximately 20 per cent acid and 80 per cent alkaline. This is the acid-alkaline balance.

In normal health, the reaction of the blood is alkaline and that is essential for our physical and mental well-being. The preponderence of alkalis in the blood is due to the fact that the products of the vital combustions taking place in the body are mostly acid in character. Carbohydrates and fats form about nine-tenths of the normal fuel of the body. In normal health, this great mass of material is converted into carbon dioxide gas and water. Half of the remaining one-tenth fuel is also converted into the same gas and water. This huge amount of acid is transported by the blood to the various points of discharge, mainly the lungs. By virtue of its alkalinity, the blood is able to transport the acid from the tissues to the discharge points.

Acidosis

Whenever the alkalinity of the blood is reduced, even slightly, its ability to transport the carbon dioxide gets reduced. This results in the accumulation of acid in the tissues. This condition is known as acidosis or hypo-alkalinity of the blood. Its symptoms are hunger, indigestion, burning sensation and pain in the pharynx, nausea, vomiting, headache, various nervous disorders and drowsiness. Acidosis is the breeding ground for most diseases. Nepthritis or Bright's disease, rheumatism, premature old age, arteriosclerosis, high blood pressure, skin disorders and various degenerative diseases are traceable to this condition. It seriously interferes with the functions of the glands and organs of the body. It also lowers the vitality of the system, thereby increasing the danger of infectious diseases.

The main cause of acidosis or hypo-alkalinity of the blood is faulty diet, in which too many acid-forming foods have been consumed. In the normal process of metabolism or converting the food into energy by the body, various acids are formed in the system and in addition, other acids are introduced in food. Whenever there is substantial increase in the formation of acids in the system and these acids are not properly eliminated through the lungs, the kidneys and the bowels, the alkalinity of the blood is reduced, resulting in acidosis.

Other causes of acidosis are depletion of alkali reserve due to diarrhoea, dysentery, cholera etc., accumulation of carbon dioxide in asphyxia and anoxia as in circulatory and pulmonary diseases and accumulation of acetone bodies resulting from starvation, vomiting and diabetes millitus.

Acidosis can be prevented by maintaining a proper ratio between acid and alkaline foods in the diet. Certain foods leave alkaline ash and help in maintaining the alkalinity of the blood, while others leave acid ash which reduce the blood alkalinity. All flesh foods leave highly acid ash and lower the alkali reserve of the blood and tissue fluids to a very large extent. Eggs do the same but less strongly than meats. Cereals of all kinds, including all sorts of breads are also acid-forming foods, though much less than meats. All fruits, with exceptions like plums and prunes and all green and root vegetables are highly alkaline foods and help to alkalinize the blood and other tissue fluids.

Thus, our daily diet should consist of four-fifths of alkaline-forming foods such as juicy fruits, tubers, legumes, ripe fruits, leafy and root vegetables and one-fifth of acid-forming foods containing concentrated proteins and starches such as meat, fish, bread and cereals. Eating sensibly in this manner will ensure the necessary alkalinity of the blood, which will keep the body in perfect health.

Whenever a person has acidosis, the higher the ratio of alkaline forming foods in his diet, the quicker will be the recovery. Acids are neutralised by alkalis. It is, therefore, imperative that persons suffering from various ailments are given adequate alkaline ash foods to offset the effects of acid-forming foods and leave a safe margin of alkalinity.

The most agreeable and convenient means of alkalizing the blood are citrus fruits and fruit juices. The alkalizing value of citrus fruits are due to the large percentage of alkaline salts, mainly potash, which they contain. Each pint of orange juice contains 12 grains of potassium, one of the most potent of alkalis. Lemon juice contains nine grains of the alkali to the pint and grape seven grains.

Diet in Disease

Breakfast may consist of fresh fruits, lunch may comprise

raw vegetables with acid and sub-acid fruits, and for dinner raw and cooked green vegetables, or light starchy vegetables like beet, carrot, cauliflower, egg-plant and squashes may be taken. Sweet fruits may be added to this diet after seven days.

Foods are classified as acid-producing or alkaline-producing depending on their reaction on the urine. Calcium, magnesium, sodium and potassium present in foods contribute to the alkaline effect, while sulphur, phosphorus and chlorine contribute to the acidic effect. Depending on the predominating constituents in a particular food, it is classified as acid-forming or alkaline-forming.

The effect of foodstuffs upon the alkalinity of the blood depends upon their residues which they leave behind after undergoing oxidation in the body. It is an error to presume that because a food tastes acid, it has an acidic reaction in the blood. For instance, fruits and vegetables have organic acids in combination with the soda and potash in the form of acid salts. When the acids are burnt or utilised in the body, the alkaline soda or potash is left behind. Hence the effect of the natural fruit acids is to increase the alkalinity of the blood rather than reduce it.

Based on the above observations, the following charts show the common foods with acid and alkaline ash:

A—Foods Leaving An Acid Ash
(One-fifth class)

Barley	Eggs
Bananas (unripe)	Grain Foods
Beans	Lentils
Bread	Meats
Cereals	Nuts except almonds

Cakes
Chicken
Confections
Corn
Chocolate
Coffee
Oatmeal
Peas
Rice
Sugar
Sea Foods
Tea

B—Foods Leaving An Alkaline Ash
(Four-fifths class)

Almonds
Apples
Apricots
Bananas (ripe)
Beets
Cabbage
Carrots
Cauliflower
Celery
Coconuts
Cottage Cheese
Cucumbers
Dates
Figs (Fresh and dry)
Grapes
Lemons
Lettuce
Melons
Milk
Onions
Oranges
Parsley
Peaches
Pears
Pineapple
Potatoes
Pumpkins
Radishes
Raisins
Spinach
Soyabeans
Tomatoes
Turnips

CHAPTER 12

Vitamins and Their Importance in Health and Disease

The word 'Vitamine', meaning a vital amine was proposed by a Polish researcher, Dr. Cacimir Funk, in 1911 to designate a new food substance which cured beri-beri. Other terms were proposed as new factors were discovered, but the word vitamin, with the final 'e' dropped, met with popular favour.

Vitamins are potent organic compounds which are found in small concentrations in foods. They perform specific and vital functions in the body chemistry. They are like electric sparks which help to run human motors. Except for a few exceptions, they cannot be manufactured or synthesized by the organism and their absence or improper absorption results in specific deficiency disease. It is not possible to sustain life without all the essential vitamins. In their natural state they are found in minute quantities in organic foods. We must obtain them from these foods or in dietary supplements.

Vitamins, which are of several kinds, differ from each other in physiological function, in chemical structure and in their distribution in food. They are broadly divided into two categories, namely fat soluble and water soluble. Vitamins A, D, E and K are all soluble in fat and fat solvents and are therefore, known as fat soluble. They are not easily lost by ordinary cooking methods and they can be stored in the body to some extent, mostly in the liver. They are measured in international units. Vitamin B Complex and C are water soluble. They are dissolved easily in cooking water. A portion of these vitamins may actually be destroyed by heating.

They cannot be stored in the body and hence they have to be taken daily in foods. Any extra quantity taken in any one day is eliminated as waste. Their values are given in milligrams and micrograms, whichever is appropriate.

Vitamins, used therapeutically, can be of immense help in fighting disease and speeding recovery. They can be used in two ways, namely, correcting deficiencies and treating disease in place of drugs. Latest researches indicate that many vitamins taken in large doses, far above the actual nutritional needs, can have a miraculous healing effect in a wide range of common complaints and illnesses. Vitamin therapy has a distinct advantage over drug therapy. While drugs are always toxic and have many undesirable side effects, vitamins, as a rule are non-toxic and safe.

The various functions of common vitamins, their deficiency symptoms, natural sources, daily requirements and their therapeutic uses are discussed in brief as follows:

Vitamin A

Known as anti-opathalmic, vitamin A is essential for growth and vitality. It builds up resistance to respiratory and other infections and works mainly on the eyes, lungs, stomach and intestines. It prevents eye diseases and plays a vital role in nourishing the skin and hair. It helps to prevent premature ageing and senility, increases life expectancy and extends youthfulness. The main sources of this vitamin are fish liver oil, liver, whole milk, curds, pure ghee, butter, cheese, cream and egg yolk, green leafy and certain yellow root vegetables such as spinach, lettuce, turnip, beets, carrot, cabbage and tomato and ripe fruits such as prunes, mangoes, papaya, apricots, peaches, almonds and other dry fruits. A prolonged deficiency of vitamin A may result in inflammation of the eyes, poor vision, frequent colds, night blindness and increased susceptibility to infections, lack of appetite and vigour, defective teeth and gums and skin disorders.

The recommended daily allowance of vitamin A is 5,000 international units for adults and 2,600 to 4,000 international units for children. When taken in large therapeutic doses, which are usually 25,000 to 50,000 units a day, it is highly beneficial in the treatment of head and chest colds, sinus trouble, influenza and other infectious diseases. It is also valuable in curing night blindness and other eye diseases as well as many stubborn skin disorders. This vitamin can be given upto 1,00,000 units a day for a limited period of four weeks under doctor's supervision.

In a recent year-long study, huge doses of vitamin A given twice a year reduced death by about 30 per cent among Indonesian children. This has raised hope in the fight against a significant cause of childhood mortality in developing countries.

B Complex Vitamins

There are a large variety of vitamins in the B group, the more important being B_1 or thiamine, B_2 or riboflavin, B_3 or niacin or nicotinic acid, B_6 or pyridoxine, B_9 or folic acid. B_{12} and B_5 or pantothenic acid. B vitamins are synergistic. They are more potent together than when used separately.

Thiamine

Known as anti-beriberi, anti-neuritic and anti-ageing vitamin, thiamine plays an important role in the normal functioning of the nervous system, the regulation of carbohydrates and good digestion. It protects heart muscle, stimulates brain action and helps prevent constipation. It has a mild diuretic effect.

Valuable sources of this vitamin are wheat germ, yeast, the outer layer of whole grains, cereals, pulses, nuts, peas, legumes, dark green leafy vegetables, milk, egg, banana and apple. The deficiency of thiamine can cause serious impairment of the digestive system and chronic constipation, loss of weight, diabetes, mental depression, nervous exhaustion and weakness of the heart.

The recommended daily allowance for this vitamin is about two milligrams for adults and 1.2 mg for children. The need for this vitamin increases during illness, stress and surgery as well as during pregnancy and lactation. When taken in a large quantity, say upto 50 mg, it is beneficial in the treatment of digestive disorders, neuritis and other nervous troubles as well as mental depression. For best results, all other vitamins of B group should be administered simultaneously. Prolonged ingestion of large doses of any one of the isolated B complex vitamins may result in high urinary losses of other B-vitamins and lead to deficiencies of these vitamins.

Riboflavin

Vitamin B_2 or riboflavin, also known as vitamin G, is essential for growth and general health as also for healthy eyes, skin, nails and hair. It helps eliminate sore mouth, lips and tongue. It also functions with other substances to metabolise carbohydrates, fats, and protein. The main sources of this vitamin are green leafy vegetables, milk, cheese, wheat germ, egg, almonds, sunflower, seeds, citrus fruits and tomato. Its deficiency can cause a burning sensation in the legs, lips and tongue, oily skin, premature wrinkles on face and arm and eczema.

The recommended daily allowance for this vitamin is 1.6 to 2.6 mg for adults and 0.6 to one mg for children. Its use in larger quantities, say from 25 to 50 mg, is beneficial in the treatment of nutritional cataracts and other eye ailments, digestive disturbances, nervous depression, general debility and certain types of high blood pressure.

Niacin

Vitamin B_3 or niacin or nicotinic acid is essential for proper circulation, healthy functioning of the nervous system and proper protein and carbohydrate metabolism. It is essential for synthesis of sex hormones, cartisone, thyroxin and insulin. It is contained in liver, fish, poultry, peanut, whole wheat, green leafy vegetables, dates, figs, prunes and tomato. A deficiency can lead to skin eruptions, frequent stools, mental depression, insomnia, chronic headaches, digestive disorders and anaemia.

The recommended daily allowance is 12 to 20 mg for adults and 4.8 to 12 mg for children. Large doses of this vitamin say upto 100 mg with each meal, preferably together with other B group vitamins, affords relief in case of migraine and high blood pressure caused by nervousness, high cholesterol and arteriosclerosis.

Pyridoxine

Vitamin B_6 or pyridoxine is actually a group of substances—pyridoxine, pyridoxinal and pyridoxamine—that are closely related and function together. It helps in the absorption of fats and proteins, prevents nervous and skin disorders and protects against degenerative diseases. The main sources of this vitamin are yeast, wheat, bran, wheat germ, pulses, cereals, banana, walnuts, soyabeans, milk, egg, liver, meat and fresh vegetables. Deficiency can lead to dermatitis, conjunctivitis, anaemia, depression, skin disorders, nervousness, insomnia, migraine headaches and heart diseases.

The recommended daily requirement is 2.0 mg for adults and 0.2 mg for children. This vitamin used therapeutically from 100 to 150 mg daily can relieve painful joints and the discomforts of pregnancy and pre-menstrual symptoms. Vitamin B_6 is now the most intensively studied of all vitamins. Researchers are on the threshold of a number of promising developments involving treatments of various ailments with this vitamin. They include hyperactivity in children, asthma, arthritis, kidney stones', blood clots in heart attack victims and nervous disorders.

Folic Acid

Vitamin B_9 or folic acid, along with Vitamin B_{12} is necessary for the formation of red blood cells. It is essential for the growth and division of all body cells for healing processes. It aids protein metabolism and helps prevent premature greying. Valuable sources of this vitamin are deep green leafy vegetables such as spinach, lettuce, brewers yeast, mushrooms, nuts, peanuts and liver. A deficiency can result in certain types of anaemia, serious skin disorders, loss of hair, impaired circulation, fatigue and mental depression.

The minimum daily requirement of this vitamin is 0.4 mg. To correct anaemia and deficiencies 5 mg or more are needed daily. Some authorities believe that folic acid is contraindicated in leukemia and cancer.

Pantothenic Acid

Vitamin B_5 or pantothenic acid helps in cell building, maintaining normal growth and development of the central nervous system. It stimulates the adrenal glands and increases the production of cortisone and other adrenal hormones. It is essential for conversion of fat and sugar to energy. It also helps guard against most physical and mental stresses and toxins and increases vitality. The main sources of this vitamin are whole grain bread and cereals, green vegetables, peas, beans, peanuts and egg yolk. It can be synthesised in the body by intestinal bacteria. A deficiency can cause chronic fatigue, hypoglycemia, greying and loss of hair, mental depression, stomach disorders, blood and skin disorders.

The minimum daily requirement of this vitamin has not been established, but is estimated to be between 30 and 50 mg a day. The usual therapeutic doses are 50 to 200 mg. In some studies 1,000 mg or more were given daily for six months without side effects. It is useful in the treatment of insomnia, low blood pressure and hypoglycemia or low blood sugar.

Vitamin B 12

Vitamin B 12 or cobolamin, commonly known as 'red vitamin', is the only vitamin that contains essential mineral elements. It is essential for proper functioning of the central nervous system, production and regeneration of red blood cells and proper utilisation of fat, carbohydrates and protein for body building. It also improves concentration, memory and balance. Valuable sources of this vitamin are kidney, liver, meat, milk, eggs, bananas and peanuts. Its deficiency can lead to certain types of anaemia, poor appetite and loss of energy and mental disorders.

The recommended daily allowance of this vitamin is 3 mcg. Taken in large therapeutic doses from 50 to 100 mcg., it is beneficial in the treatment of lack of concentration, fatigue, depression, insomnia and poor memory.

Vitamin C

Vitamin C or ascorbic acid is essential for normal growth

and the maintenance of practically all the body tissues, especially those of the joints, bones, teeth and gums. It protects one against infections and acts as a harmless antibiotic. It promotes healing and serves as protection against all forms of stress and harmful effects of toxic chemicals. It helps prevent and cure the common cold. It also helps in decreasing blood cholesterol. This vitamin is found in citrus fruits, berries, green and leafy vegetables, tomatoes, potatoes, sprouted Bengal and green grams. A deficiency can cause scurvy marked by weakness, anaemia, bleeding gums and painful and swollen parts, slow healing of sores and wounds, premature ageing and lowered resistance to all infections.

The recommended daily allowance is 50 to 75 mg for adults and 30 to 50 mg for children. Smokers and older persons have greater need for vitamin C. It is used therapeutically in huge doses from 100 to 10,000 mg a day. It prevents and cures colds and infections effectively, neutralises various toxins in the system, speeds healing processes in virtually all cases of ill health, increases sexual vitality and prevents premature ageing. According to Dr. Linus Pauling, a world famous chemist and nutrition expert, "because vitamin C is one of the least toxic vitamins, it is very safe to use in high doses". Your body will take exactly what it needs and excrete any excess naturally.

Vitamin D

Vitamin D is necessary for proper bone and teeth formation, and for the healthy functioning of the thyroid gland. It assists in the assimilation of calcium, phosphorus and other minerals from the digestive tract . This vitamin is found in the rays of the sun, fish, milk, eggs, butter and sprouted seeds. A deficiency can cause gross deformation of bones and severe tooth decay.

The recommended daily allowance of this vitamin for both adults and children is 400 to 500 international units. Therapeutically, upto 4,000 to 5,000 units a day for adults or half of this for children, is a safe dose, if taken for not longer than one month. It is beneficial in the treatment of muscular fatigue, constipation and nervousness. It can be toxic if taken in excessive doses, especially for children. Signs of toxicity are unusual thirst, sore eyes, itching skin, vomiting, diarrhoea, urinary urgency, abnormal calcium deposits in blood vessel walls, liver, lungs, kidneys and stomach.

Vitamin E

Vitamin E is essential for normal reproductory functions, fertility, and physical vigour. It prevents unsaturated fatty acids, sex hormones and fat soluble vitamins from being destroyed in the body by oxygen. It dilutes blood vessels and improves circulation. It is essential for the prevention of heart diseases, asthma, arthritis and many other conditions. It is available in wheat or cereals germ, whole grain products, green leafy vegetables, milk, eggs, all whole, raw or sprouted seeds and nuts. Its deficiency can lead to sterility in men and repeated abortions in women, degenerative developments in the coronary system, strokes and heart disease.

The official estimated requirement of this vitamin is 15 international units. Expert nutritionists estimate the actual requirement at 100 to 200 I.U. a day. The therapeutic doses are from 200 to 2400 I.U. daily. It is beneficial in the treatment of various forms of paralysis, diseases of the muscles, artheriosclerosic heart disease by diluting blood vessels. It prevents formation of scars in burns and post-operation healing. It protects against many environmental poisons in air, water and food. It also has a dramatic effect on the reproductive organs and prevents miscarriage, increases male and female fertility and helps to restore male potency.

Vitamin K

Vitamin K is necessary for the proper clotting of blood, prevention of bleeding and normal liver functions. It aids in reducing excessive menstrual flow. This vitamin is contained in egg yolk, cow's milk, yogurt, alfalfa, green and leafy vegetables, spinach, cauliflower, cabbage and tomato. Its deficiency can lead to insufficient bile salts in the intestines, colitis, lowered vitality and premature ageing.

CHAPTER 13

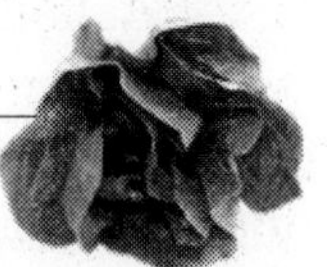

Minerals and Their Importance in Nutrition

The term "minerals" refers to elements in their simple inorganic form. In nutrition they are commonly referred to as mineral elements or inorganic nutrients.

Minerals are vital to health. Like vitamins and amino acids, minerals are essential for regulating and building the trillions of living cells which make up the body. Body cells receive the essential food elements through the bloodstream. They must, therefore, be properly nourished with an adequate supply of all the essential minerals for the efficient functioning of the body.

Minerals help maintain the volume of water necessary to life processes in the body. They help draw chemical substances into and out of the cells and they keep the blood and tissue fluid from becoming either too acidic or too alkaline. The importance of minerals, like vitamins, is illustrated by the fact that there are over 50,000 enzymes in the body which direct growth and energy and each enzyme has minerals and vitamins associated with it. Each of the essential food minerals does a specific job in the body and some of them do extra work, in teams, to keep body cells healthy. The mineral elements which are needed by the body in substantial amounts are calcium, phosphorus, iron, sulphur, magnesium, sodium, potassium and chlorine. In addition, the body needs minute (trace) amounts of iodine, copper, cobalt, manganese, zinc, selenium, silicon, fluorine and some others.

Calcium

The human body needs calcium more than any other mineral. A man weighing 70 kg. contains one kg. of calcium. About 99 per cent of the quantity in the body is used for building strong bones and teeth and the remaining one per cent is used by the blood, muscles and nerves.

Calcium performs many important functions. Without this mineral, the contractions of the heart would be faulty, the muscles would not contract properly to make the limbs move and blood would not clot. Calcium stimulates enzymes in the digestive process and coordinates the functions of all other minerals in the body. Calcium is found in milk and milk products, whole wheat, leafy vegetables such as lettuce, spinach and cabbage; carrots, watercress, oranges, lemons, almonds, figs and walnuts. A daily intake of about 0.4 to 0.6 grams of calcium is considered desirable for an adult. The requirement is larger for growing children and pregnant and lactating women. Deficiency may cause porous and fragile bones, tooth decay, heart palpitations, muscle cramps, insomnia and irritability.

A large increase in the dietary supply of calcium is needed in tetany and when the bones are decalcified due to poor calcium absorption, as in rickets, osteomalacia and the malabsorption syndrome. Liberal quantity of calcium is also necessary when excessive calcium has been lost from the body, as in hyperparathyroidism or chronic renal disease.

Phosphorus

It combines with calcium to create the calcium-phosphorus balance necessary for the growth of bones and teeth and in the formation of nerve cells. This mineral is also essential for the assimilation of carbohydrates and fats. It is a stimulant to the nerves and brain.

Phosphorus is found in abundance in cereals, pulses, nuts, egg yolk, fruit juices, milk and legumes. Usually about one gram of phosphorus is considered necessary in the daily diet. A phosphorus deficiency may bring about loss of weight, retarded growth, reduced sexual powers and general weakness. It may result in poor mineralisation of bones, deficient nerve and brain function.

While taking calcium in therapeutic doses for calcium deficiency conditions or for treating certain ailments, it is advisable to take the calcium supplement in which phosphorus has been added in the correct proportions. This is necessary as calcium cannot achieve its objectives unless phosphorus is present in a proper balance.

Iron

Iron is an important mineral which enters into the vital activity of the blood and glands. Iron exists chiefly as haemoglobin in the blood. It distributes the oxygen inhaled into the lungs to all the cells. It is the master mineral which creates warmth, vitality and stamina. It is required for a healthy complexion and for building up resistance in the body.

The chief sources of iron are grapes, raisins, spinach, all green vegetables, whole grain, cereals, dried beans, dark coloured fruits, beets, dates, liver and egg yolk. The Indian Council of Medical Research has recommended an allowance of 20 to 30 mg. of iron in a balanced diet for an adult. Iron deficiency is generally caused by severe blood loss, malnutrition, infections and by excessive use of drugs and chemicals. Deficiency of dietary iron may cause nutritional-anaemia, lowered resistance to disease, a general run down condition, pale complexion, shortness of breath on manual exertion and loss of interest in sex.

Iron is the classic remedy for anaemia. However, there are several forms of anaemia, and iron deficiency anaemia is only one. If one is taking iron pills due to insufficient intake of iron in the normal diet, one should also take at least 400 mg. of folic acid or folate every day, along with 10 to 25 mg. of vitamin B_{12}. Both these vitamins are essential in building healthy blood cells.

Sulphur

All living matter contains some sulphur; this element is therefore essential for life. The greater part of the sulphur in the human body is present in the two sulphur-containing amino acids, methionine and cysteine, or in the double form of the latter cystine. The main purpose of sulphur is to dissolve waste materials. It helps to eject some of the waste and poisons from the system. It helps keep the skin clear of blemishes and makes hair glossy. It is also valuable in rheumatic conditions.

The main sulphur-containing foods are radishes, carrots, cabbage, cheese, dried beans, fish and eggs. There is no recommended dietary allowance. But a diet sufficient in protein will generally be adequate in sulphur. Deficiency of sulphur may cause eczema and imperfect development of hair and nails. Sulphur creams and ointments have been remarkably successful in treating a variety of skin problems.

Magnesium

All human tissues contain small amounts of magnesium. The adult human body contains about 25 gms. of this mineral. The greater part of this amount is present in bones in combination with phosphate and carbonate. Bone ashes contain less than one per cent magnesium. About one-fifth of the total magnesium in the body is present in the soft tissues, where it is mainly bound to protein. Next to potassium, magnesium is the predominant metallic cation in living cells. The bones seem to provide a reserve supply of this mineral in case of shortage elsewhere in the body.

Biochemists call magnesium the "coll, alkaline, refreshing, sleep-promoting mineral." Magnesium helps one keep calm and cool during the sweltering summer months. It aids in keeping nerves relaxed and normally balanced. It is necessary for all muscular activity. This mineral is an activator for most of the enzyme systems involving carbohydrate, fat and protein in energy-producing reactions. It is involved in the production of lecithin which prevents building up of cholesterol and consequent atherosclerosis. Magnesium promotes a healthier cardiovascular system and aids in fighting depression. It helps prevent calcium deposits in kidneys and gallstones and also brings relief from indigestion.

Magnesium is widely distributed in foods. It is a part of the chlorophyll in green vegetables. Other good sources of this mineral are nuts, soyabeans, alfalfa, apples, figs, lemons, peaches, almonds, whole grains, brown rice, sunflower seeds and sesame seeds. The recommended dietary allowances for magnesium are 350 mg. per day for adult man, 300 mg. for women and 450 mg. during pregnancy and lactation. Deficiency can lead to kidney damage and kidney stones, muscle cramps, arteriosclerosis, heart attack, epileptic seizures, nervous irritability, marked depression and confusion, impaired protein metabolism and premature wrinkles.

Chronic alcoholics often show a low plasma magnesium concentration and a high urinary output. They may, therefore, require magnesium therapy especially in an acute attack of delirium tremens. Magnesium has also proved useful in bladder and urinary problems and in epileptic seizures. This mineral together with vitamin B_6 or pyridoxine has also been found effective in the prevention and treatment of kidney stones. Magnesium can be taken in therapeutic doses up to 700 mg. a day.

Sodium

Sodium chloride, the chemical name for common salt, contains 39 per cent of sodium, an element which never occurs in free form in nature. It is found in an associated form with many minerals especially in plentiful amounts with chlorine. The body of a healthy person weighing about 65 kg. contains 256 g. of sodium chloride. Of this the major part, just over half, is in the extra-cellular fluid. About 96 g. is in bone and less than 32 g. in the cells.

Sodium is the most abundant chemical in the extra-cellular fluid of the body. It acts with other electrolytes, especially potassium, in the intracellular fluid, to regulate the osmotic pressure and maintain a proper water balance within the body. It is a major factor in maintaining acid-base equilibrium, in transmitting nerve impulses, and in relaxing muscles. It is also required for glucose absorption and for the transport of other nutrients across cell membranes. Sodium can help prevent catarrh. It promotes a clear brain, resulting in a better disposition and less mental fatigue. Because of its influence on calcium, sodium can also help dissolve any stones forming within the body. It is also essential for the production of hydrochloric acid in the stomach and plays a part in many other glandular secretions.

There is some natural salt in every food we eat. Vegetable foods rich in sodium are celery, cucumbers, watermelon, lemons, oranges, grapefruit, beet-tops, cabbage, lettuce, corn, lady's fingers, apple, berries, pears, squash, pumpkin, peaches, lentils, almonds and walnuts. Animal food sources include shell fish, lean beef, kidney, bacon and cheese. The sodium chloride requirements for persons living in the tropics have been estimated at 10 to 15 g. per day for adults who are engaged in light work and 15 to 20 g. for those engaged in hard work. The requirements of children are from five to 10 g. and those for adolescent boys and girls from 10 to 25 g.

Both deficiency and excess of salt may produce adverse effects on the human body. Deficiencies of sodium however, are and may be caused by excessive sweating, prolonged use of diuretics, or chronic diarrhoea. Deficiency may lead to nausea, muscular weakness, heat exhaustion, mental apathy and respiratory failure. Over-supply of sodium is a more common problem because of overuse of dietary sodium chloride or common salt. Too much sodium may lead to water retention, high blood pressure, stomach ulcers, stomach cancer, hardening of arteries and heart disease.

In case of mild deficiency of sodium chloride, taking a teaspoon of common salt in one half litre of water or any fruit juice quickly restores the health. In severe conditions, however, administration of sodium chloride in the form of normal saline by intravenous drip may be resorted to. The adverse effects of excessive use of sodium chloride can be rectified by avoiding the use of common salt.

Potassium

Potassium is essential to the life of every cell of a living being and is among the most generously and widely distributed of all the tissue minerals. It is found principally in the intracellular fluid where it plays an important role as a catalyst in energy metabolism and in the synthesis of glycogen and protein. The average adult human body contains 120 g. as potassium and 245 g. as potassium chloride. Out of this body potassium, 117 g. is found in the cells and 3 g. in the extracellular compartment.

Potassium is important as an alkalizing agent in keeping a proper acid-alkaline balance in the blood and tissues. It is essential for muscle contraction and therefore important for proper heart function. It promotes the secretion of hormones and helps the kidneys in detoxification of blood. Potassium prevents female disorders by stimulating the endocrine hormone production. It is involved in the proper functioning of the nervous system and helps overcome fatigue. It also aids in clear thinking by sending oxygen to the brain and assists in reducing blood pressure.

Potassium is widely distributed in foods. All vegetables, especially green leafy vegetables, grapes, oranges, lemons, raisins, whole grains, lentils, sunflower seeds, nuts, milk, cottage cheese and butter-milk are rich sources. Potatoes, especially potato peelings, and bananas are especially good sources. Potassium requirements have not been established but an intake of 0.8 to 1.3 g. per day is estimated as approximately the minimum need. Potassium deficiency may occur during gastrointestinal disturbances with severe vomiting and diarrhoea, diabetic acidosis and potassium-losing nephritis. It causes undue nervous and body tiredness, palpitation of the heart, cloudiness of the mind, nervous shaking of the hands and feet, great sensitivity of the nerves to cold, and excessive perspiration of the feet and hands.

In simple cases of potassium deficiency, drinking plenty of tender coconut water daily, can make up for it. It is advisable to consume plenty of figs, apricots, prunes, almonds and tomatoes during the use of oral diuretics. Potassium-rich foods should be restricted during acute renal failure and Addison's disease.

Chlorine

In the human body, chlorine is liberated by the interaction of common salt, taken, along with food, and hydrochloric acid liberated in the stomach during the process of digestion. It is essential for the proper distribution of carbon dioxide and the maintenance of osmotic pressure in the tissues.

This food element is necessary for the manufacture of glandular hormone secretions. It prevents building of excessive fat and auto-intoxication. Chlorine regulates the blood's alkaline-acid balance and works with Potassium in a compound form. It aids in the cleaning out of body waste by helping the liver to function.

Chlorine is found in cheese and other milk products, green leafy vegetables, tomatoes, all berries, rice, radishes, lentils, coconuts and egg yolk. No dietary allowance has been established, but an average intake of daily salt will ensure adequate quantity of chlorine. Deficiency of this mineral can cause loss of hair and teeth.

Iodine

The chief store-house of iodine in the body is the thyroid gland. The essential thyroxine, which is secreted by this gland, is made by the circulating iodine. Thyroxine is a wonder chemical which controls the basic metabolism and oxygen consumption of tissues. It increases the heart rate as well as urinary calcium excretion. Iodine regulates the rate of energy production and body weight and promotes proper growth. It improves mental alacrity and promotes healthy hair, nails, skin and teeth.

The best dietary sources of iodine are kelp and other seaweeds. Other good sources are turnip greens, garlic, watercress, pineapples, pears, artichokes, citrus fruits, egg yolk and seafoods and fish liver oils. The recommended dietary allowances are 130 mcg. per day for adult males and 100 mcg. per day for adult females. An increase to 125 mcg. per day during pregnancy and to 150 mcg. per day during lactation has been recommended. Deficiency can cause goitre and enlargement of the thyroid gland.

Small doses of iodine are of great value in the prevention of goitre in areas where it is endemic and are of value in treatments, at least in the early stages. Larger doses have a temporary value in the preparation of patients with hyperthyroidism for surgical operation.

Copper

There are approximately 75 to 150 mg. of copper in the adult human body. Newborn infants have higher concentrations than adults. Liver, brain, kidney, heart, and hair contain relatively high concentration. Average serum copper levels are higher in adult females than in males. Serum copper levels also increase significantly in women both during pregnancy and when taking oral contraceptives.

This mineral helps in the conversion of iron into haemoglobin. It stimulates the growth of red blood cells. It is also an integral part of certain digestive enzymes. It makes the amino acid tyrosine usable, enabling it to work as the pigmenting factor for hair and skin. It is also essential for the utilisation of vitamin C. Copper is found in most foods containing iron, especially in almonds, dried beans, peas, lentils, whole wheat, prunes and egg yolk. The recommended dietary allowance has not been established but 2 mg is considered adequate for adults. A copper deficiency may result in bodily weakness, digestive disturbances and impaired respiration.

Cobalt

Cobalt is a component of vitamin B_{12}, a nutritional factor necessary for the formation of red blood cells. Recent research in vitamin B_{12} has shown that its pink colour is attributed to the presence of cobalt in it. The presence of this mineral in foods helps the synthesis of haemoglobin and the absorption of food-iron. The best dietary sources of cobalt are meat, kidney and liver. All green leafy vegetables contain some amount of this mineral. No daily allowance has been set. Only a very small amount up to 8 mcg is considered necessary.

Manganese

The human body contains 30 to 35 mg. of manganese, widely distributed throughout the tissues. It is found in the liver, pancreas, kidney, pituitary gland.

This mineral helps nourish the nerves and brain and aids in the coordination of nerve impulses and muscular actions. It helps eliminate fatigue and reduces nervous irritability. Manganese is found in citrus fruits, the outer covering of nuts, grains, in the green leaves of edible plants, fish and raw egg yolk. No official daily allowance of manganese has been established, but 2.5 to 7 mg. is generally accepted to be the average adult requirement. A deficiency of this mineral can lead to dizziness, poor elasticity in the muscles, confused thinking and poor memory.

Zinc

There are about 2 g. of zinc in the body where it is highly concentrated in the hair, skin, eyes, nails, and testes. It is a constituent of many enzymes involved in metabolism.

Zinc is a precious mineral. Our need for this mineral is small, but its role in growth and well-being is enormous, starting before birth. It is needed for healthy skin and hair, proper healing of wounds, successful pregnancies and male virility. It plays a vital role in guarding against disease and infection. It is needed to transport vitamin A to the retina. There are 156 enzymes that require zinc for their functioning. It has long been known that growth and sexual maturity depend on zinc.

The main dietary sources of zinc are milk, liver, beans, meat, whole grains, nuts and seeds. The recommended dietary allowance of zinc is 15 mg daily. Deficiency can result in weight loss, skin diseases, loss of hair, poor appetite, diarrhoea and frequent infection. Those suffering from rheumatoid arthritis may have a zinc deficiency. Heavy drinkers lose a lot of zinc in their urine.

Selenium

Selenium and vitamin E are synergistic and the two together are stronger than the sum of the equal parts. Selenium slows down ageing and hardening of tissues through oxidation. Males seem to have a greater need for this mineral. Nearly half of the total supply in the body is concentrated in the testicles and in the seminal ducts adjacent to the prostate gland.

Selenium is useful in keeping youthful elasticity in tissues. It alleviates hot flushes and menopausal distress. It also helps in the prevention and treatment of dandruff. This mineral is found in Brewer's yeast, garlic, onions, tomatoes, eggs, milk and sea food. There is no official dietary allowance for selenium but, 50 to 100 mcg. is considered adequate. Deficiency of this mineral can cause premature loss of stamina.

Silicon

This is known as the "beauty mineral" as it is essential for the growth of skin, hair shafts, nails and other outer coverings of the body. It also makes the eyes bright and assists in hardening the enamel of the teeth. It is beneficial in all healing processes and protects body against many diseases such as tuberculosis, irritations in mucous membranes and skin disorders.

Silicon is found in apples, cherries, grapes, asparagus, beets, onions, almonds, honey, peanuts and the juices of the green leaves of most other vegetables. No official dietary allowance has been established for this mineral. Deficiency can lead to soft brittle nails, ageing symptoms of skin such as wrinkles, thinning or loss of hair, poor bone development, insomnia, osteoporosis.

Fluorine

Fluorine is the element that prevents diseases from decaying the body. It is a germicide, and acts as an antidote to poison, sickness and disease. There is a strong affinity between calcium and fluorine. These two elements, when combined, work particularly in the outer parts of bones. They are found in the enamel of the teeth and the shiny, highly polished bone surface. Fluorine is found in goat's milk, cauliflower, watercress, garlic, beets, cabbage, spinach and pistachio nuts.

Minerals thus play an important role in every bodily function and are present in every human cell. Although the amount needed may be small, without even that trace of the mineral, dysfunction is bound to occur at some level in the body. A zinc deficiency may show up in ridged fingernails with white spots. Lack of sulphur can cause lack-lustre hair and dull-looking skin. Less obvious deficiencies may surface as fatigue, irritability, loss of memory, nervousness, depression and weakness. Minerals also interact with vitamins. Magnesium, for instance, must be present in the body for utilisation of B-complex, C and E vitamins. Sulphur also works with the B-complex vitamins. The body needs all the trace minerals in proper balance. Coffee, tea, alcohol, excess salt and many drugs can rob the body of minerals or make them ineffective. Industrial pollutants cause toxic minerals to enter the body. Minerals at toxic levels also have the effect of destroying the usefulness of other vitamins and minerals. Exercise improves the activity of certain vitamins and minerals while stress and fatigue work against them.

A well-balanced diet provides as abundance of minerals and vitamins. In refining cereals, grains and sugar, we have robbed them of their natural vitamins and minerals. The dietary sources of these nutrients are whole grains, cereals, bran and germ. It is the bran and germ which are removed in processing. To obtain a balance of nutrients, it is, therefore, necessary to avoid refined and processed foods but an intake of adequate green leafy vegetables which are an excellent source of many nutrients should be ensured.

CHAPTER 14

Amazing Power of Amino-Acids

In 1838, a Dutch chemist, G.J. Mulder, described a certain organic material as "unquestionably the most important of all known substances in the organic kingdom. Without it, no life appears possible on our planet. Through its means the chief phenomena of life are produced." This complex nitrogen-bearing substance was called protein from the Greek word meaning "take the first place." Protein is now a group name signifying the principal nitrogenous constituents of the protoplasm of all plant and animal tissues.

Proteins are extremely complex organic compounds of the elements carbon, hydrogen, oxygen, nitrogen and, with some exceptions, sulphur. Most proteins also contain phosphorus, and some specialised proteins contain iron, iodine, copper and other inorganic elements. The presence of nitrogen distinguishes proteins from carbohydrates and fats.

Proteins are thus vital substances, which form important constituents of muscles, tissues and the blood. Proteins supply the building material for the body and make good the wear and tear of tissues. Several substances concerned with vital life processes such as enzymes which help in the digestion of food, are chiefly protein in nature.

There are several varieties of protein. Each type contains a specific number of "building blocks" known as amino-acids. Before they can be absorbed by the body, all proteins must first be broken down into amino-acids. When food stuffs are ingested, the nutrients and amino-acids do not immediately diffuse into all the different tissues. There are a series of biochemical reactions in the digestive tract which collect these proteins, break them down and then utilise them as needed. Any interference with the normal digestive process causes incomplete protein digestion resulting in gas, bloating, etc.

There are about 22 amino acids needed for the normal functioning of the body. The body can manufacture many amino acids if it has an adequate nitrogen source, but it cannot produce certain others in sufficient amounts to meet its needs. The amino acids that the body cannot synthesise in adequate amounts are called essential or indispensable because they must be supplied by the diet in proper proportions and amounts to meet the requirements for maintenance and growth of tissue. Non-essential or dispensable amino acids are those that the body can synthesise in sufficient amounts to meet its needs if the total amount of nitrogen supplied by protein is adequate. The essential and non-essential amino acids are listed in table A.

TABLE A

Classification of amino acids with respect to their essentiality

Essential	Non-essential
Histidine*	Alanine
Isoleucine	Arginine
Leucine	Asparagine
Lysine	Aspartic acid
Methionine	Cysteine
Phenylalanine	Cystine
Threonine	Glutamic acid

* Histidine is required for infants but its essentiality for adults has not been clearly established.

Tryptophan	Glutamine
Valine	Glycine
	Hydroxyproline
	Proline
	Serine
	Tyrosine

It will be seen from this statement that nine amino acids are essential for maintenance of nitrogen equilibrium in human bodies. The estimated requirements of essential amino acids for infants, children and adults are given in table B (see next page). Men in the older age group appear to differ in their requirements. Studies seem to suggest an increased need for methionine and lysine for them. Infants and children have proportionally greater demands for essential amino acids than adults. In addition, infants require histidine as an essential amino acid.

Factors in addition to the age, sex and physiological condition of an individual influence the requirements for specific amino acids. If total protein intake is low, small surpluses of certain amino acids can increase the need for others.

The non-essential amino acids in protein also affect the quality of the protein. For example, the amount of the sulphur-containing essential amino acid methionine required may be somewhat reduced if cystine, a sulphur-containing non-essential amino acid, is supplied in the diet. Likewise, the presence in the diet of tyrosine, a non-essential amino acid similar in structure to phenylalanine, may reduce the requirement for phenylalanine.

Much research has been done on amino acids in recent

TABLE B

Estimated amino acid requirements of man*

	Requirement (mg./kg. of body weight/day)			**Amino acid pattern for high quality proteins. mg/g. of proteins****
	Infant	**Child**	**Adult**	
AMINO ACID	**(3-6 mths.)**	**(10-12 yr)**		
Histidine	33	?	?	17
Isoleucine	80	28	12	42
Leucine	128	42	16	70
Lysine	97	44	12	51
Total sulphur containing amino acids	45	22	10	26
Total aromatic amino acids	132	22	16	73
Threonine	63	28	8	35
Tryptophan	19	4	3	11
Valine	89	25	14	48

* From Food and Nutrition Board, National Research Council : Improvement of Protein Nutriture. Washington, D.C., National Academy of Sciences, 1973.

** 2 g. per kg. of body weight per day of protein of the quality listed in column 4 would meet the amino acid needs of the infant.

times and this has paved the way for dramatic treatments and cure of different problems by their judicious use. They are now dubbed as 'the nutrients of the 80's' and 'medical foods'.

The various functions of the essential and frequently investigated non-essential amino acids, their deficiency symptoms and their therapeutic uses are discussed below:

Tryptophan

Of all the essential amino acids, tryptophan is the one that is most investigated by nutrition researchers. It is essential to blood clotting, digestive juices and the optic system. It induces sleep and quietens the nervous system. It wards off signs of premature old age—cataracts of the eyes, baldness, deterioration of sex glands and malformation of teeth enamel. It is also necessary to the female reproductive organs and for proper utilisation of vitamin A by the body. Major sources of this amino acid are seeds, nuts and most vegetables. Lack of tryptophan causes symptoms similar to those of vitamin A deficiency.

A number of scientists feel that it can be used as a safe and effective food remedy for insomnia and pain. Under experimental conditions, tryptophan in doses of one gram or more has been shown to be most effective for persons who suffer from mild insomnia and for those who take a long time to fall asleep. Tryptophan may also be a natural painkiller. Researches at Temple University in Philadelphia have indicated that it worked without causing the side effects associated with other anesthesia or analgesics.

Tryptophan as a food medicine should be taken between meals with a low-protein food such as fruit juice or bread. One to three grams a day seems to be the range favoured by most researchers.

Methionine

This is a vital sulphur-bearing compound which helps dissolve cholesterol and assimilates fat. It is required by haemoglobin, the pancreas, the lymph and the spleen. It is necessary to maintain normal body weight and also helps maintain the proper nitrogen balance in the body. Rich sources of methionine are Brazil nut, hazel nut, and other nuts. It is also found in Brussel sprouts, cabbage, cauliflower, pineapples and apples. Its deficiency can lead to chronic rheumatic fever in children, hardening of the liver (cirrhosis) and nephritis of the kidneys. Studies show that methionine and choline prevent tumours and proliferation.

Lysine

Lysine inhibits viruses. Its use along with vitamin C, zinc and vitamin A helps eliminate virus infections. Vitamin C protects this amino acid while in the body so that lysine plus vitamin C has a much stronger anti-virus effect than if either is used separately. Lysine also influences the female reproductive cycle. Lack of adequate lysine in the diet may cause headaches, dizziness, nausea and incipient anaemia. The main sources of this amino acid are most kinds of nuts, seeds, vegetables and sub-acid fruits. Lysine upsets in the body have also been associated with pneumonia, nephrosis and acidosis as well as malnutrition and rickets in children.

It is considered a natural remedy for cold, sores, shingles and genital herpes. In a study published in 1983, a group of researchers polled over 1,500 people whose daily intake of lysine was over 900 mg. 88 per cent said that lysine seemed to reduce the severity of their attacks of herpes virus and accelerated the healing time. These results have, however, been disputed by some scientists.

Valine

Valine is an essential body growth factor, particularly for mammary glands and ovaries. Valine is directly linked with the nervous system. It is essential for the prevention of nervous and digestive disorders. Major sources are almonds, apples and most vegetables. Lack of this amino acid makes a person sensitive to touch and sound.

Isoleucine

This amino acid is essential for maintaining the nitrogen balance vital to all body functions. It also regulates metabolism of the thymus, spleen and pituitary glands. Rich sources are sunflower seeds, all nuts, except cashew nuts, avacados and olives.

Leucine

It is the complement of isoleucine, with a similar chemical composition although in different arrangement. Its functions and sources are also similar.

Phenylalanine

This is essential to the production of hormone adrenaline; to the production of the thyroid secretion and the hair and skin pigment, melanin. It is effective in weight control because of its effect on the thyroid. Its use before meals suppresses the appetite substantially. Patients taking half a teaspoon of the powder 30 minutes before each meal, lose from a quarter to half a pound a day. It is also essential for the efficient functioning of kidneys and bladder. Major sources are nuts, seeds, carrots, parsley and tomatoes. An important recently discussed therapeutic use of phenylalanine is its ability to overcome most conditions of lethargy through stimulation of adrenaline.

Threonine

This amino acid is found in various types of milk and is a major constituent in cow's milk. Other sources are nuts, seeds, carrots and green vegetables. Without threonine, a child's development will be incomplete and there will be malfunctioning of the brain. This amino acid has a powerful anti-convulsive effect.

Histidine

This helps tissue growth and repair. It is active in producing normal blood supply. It is also vital to the formation of glycogen in the liver. It is found in root vegetables and all green vegetables. Studies indicate that the free form of histidine in the blood is low in cases of rheumatoid arthritis and if taken orally, may possibly depress the symptoms of this ailment. Oral histidine has, however, a tendency to stimulate hydrochloric acid secretion in the stomach and persons who are susceptible to an overabundance of acid and also those who have ulcers should avoid taking pure histidine. Orthopaedic and joint pains are caused by a lack of histidine.

Arginine

This is called the "fatherhood" amino acid as it comprises 80 per cent of all male reproductive cells. It is essential for normal growth. Serious lack of this amino acid reduces the sex instinct causing impotence. It is found in most vegetables, especially, green and root vegetables.

Cystine

It provides resistance by building up white-cell activity. It is an indispensable amino acid. It is one of the mainstays of health as it is essential for the proper formation of skin and helps one recover from surgery. It promotes the formation of [illegible]rolene which helps hair growth. It is used in the treatment [illegible] skin diseases, for low white blood-cell counts and for some [illegible]ases of anaemia.

Tyrosine

This can be called an anti-stress amino acid. Dr. Richard Wurtman who recently conducted experiments on the use of this amino acid says: "Supplemented tyrosine may be useful therapeutically in persons exposed chronically to stress."

Tyrosine is also beneficial for depression, nervousness, irritability and despondency. Research has established this amino acid to be effective in the management and control of depression in conjunction with glutamine, tryptophan, niacin and vitamin B_6. It is also helpful in the treatment of allergies and high blood pressure.

Although individual need may vary. Dr. Wurtman considers 100 mg. per kilogram of body weight per day an optional dose. This works out to about 5.4 grams of tyrosine a day for a person weighing 120 pounds. The supplement may be divided into three separate doses each day. When tyrosine is taken, a supplement of valine, another essential amino acid should not be taken as valine may block tyrosine's entry to the brain.

Glutamine

This little known non-essential amino acid is known as "sobriety nutrient". It is considered beneficial in the treatment of alcoholism. According to Roger J. Williams, a world-known nutritionist, glutamine reduces the usually irresistible craving for alcohol that recovering drinkers almost inevitably encounter.

Cysteine

There is some evidence that cysteine (not to be confused with cystine) has certain therapeutic value as a nutritional supplement. Dr. H. Ghadimi, chairman of the nutri[illegible] committee at Nassau country, (New York) medical centre u[illegible] cysteine supplements to treat his patients suffering from obesity. He considers that there is link between obesity and over-production of insulin and that cysteine supplements taken along with vitamin C at the end of meals somehow neutralises some of the excess insulin, which is responsible for fat production. He regards this amino acid as 'anti-cancer and anti-ageing' and claims that like vitamin C, cysteine protects the body from damage by oxidants.

When one or more of the essential amino acids are left out of the diet, symptoms similar to those of vitamin deficiencies may be experienced such as low blood pressure, anaemia, poor muscle tone, slow healing of wounds, loss of weight, poor resistance to infections and bloodshot eyes. Children who do not get the required amounts of amino acids in their daily diet suffer from stunted growth and permanent damage to the glands. On the other hand, those getting the full quota of amino acids in their diet will be rewarded with vigour, vitality and long life. The best food proteins with all the essential amino acids are found in almonds, cheese and eggs.

Amino acids are being increasingly and successfully used in the treatment of several diseases such as stomach ulcers, burns, kidney diseases and liver diseases. It has also been observed that the diseases of old age can be largely prevented if elderly persons obtain the proper food supplements of amino acids, vitamins and minerals. Amino acids are needed at every stage from infancy to old age—to repair worn out tissues and to create new ones.

CHAPTER 15

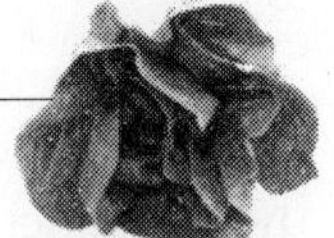

Secrets of Food Combining

The observance of rules of food combining is neither faddish nor eccentric. It is a simple, scientifically-based system of selecting foods, from among many different types, which are compatible. This facilitates easy and efficient digestion and ensures after-meal comfort.

Digestion is not merely a chemical or physical process, but also a physiological one. When food enters the body, it undergoes several changes before it is broken down into its constituent parts and assimilated. But no food can be assimilated by the system and used by various organs unless it has first been digested and then absorbed in the digestive system known as the alimentary canal, while the residue, unfit for absorption is eliminated from the system.

The chemical part of digestion is accomplished by a series of juices and their enzymes. The juices alternate between alkalies and acids, and their character is determined by the requirement of the enzymes they contain. These enzymes remain active in suitable media of well defined acid-alkaline ranges and are destroyed in unsuitable media.

For instance, the salivary amylase (ptyalin) or starch-splitting enzyme of the mouth is active only in an alkaline medium and is destroyed by a mild acid. The gastric enzyme, pepsin, which initiates protein digestion, is active only in the acid medium and is destroyed by alkalies.

A noteworthy feature of the digestive secretions is that the body suits its fluids and enzymes to the character of the food eaten. There are, however, severe limitations in this process. It is possible to suit the juices to a particular food, however, complex it may be, but not to a variety of foods taken together. It is the combining of many varieties and incompatible foods at a meal that causes 90 per cent of digestive disorders.

There is a marked tendency to gastro-intestinal fermentation with certain combinations of foods. There is no fermentation and digestion will be much more satisfactory when the foods comprising a meal are of the same type. This generally means eating similar foods at one time in order to accomplish the most complete digestion.

The most important rule for combining foods is to avoid mixing protein and carbohydrate concentrated foods. Although every food contains some protein, those regarded as protein concentrated foods demand the longest digestive time. They are held in the stomach for some hours until the gastric juice has performed its task. This may vary from two-and-a-half to six hours, depending upon the complexity of the protein in the food, if a protein food is mixed with starch-concentrated or sugar-concentrated foods, it will usually result in fermentation. This may lead to indigestion and gas in the stomach.

Animal-food proteins, such as meats, fish and cheese, require very high concentration of hydrochloric acid. Their gastric digestion will be greatly inhibited by carbohydrate fermentation in the stomach. This will produce more gas and increased discomfort. Eating meat, potatoes, bread and sweets should, therefore, be especially avoided.

Protein foods are best digested when eaten with fresh vegetable salad. Primary protein foods such as nuts, seeds and soyabeans also combine very well with acid fruits like oranges, pineapple, grapefruit and lemons, and fairly well with sub-acid fruits, like grapes, pears, apples, berries, apricots and peaches. These vegetables and fruits are rich natural sources of vitamin C which aids protein digestion.

The second important rule for food combining is to avoid mixing proteins and fats at the same meal. Fat in foods inhibits the secretion of gastric juice through the small wall. Thus when fat-concentrated foods are taken with protein foods, gastric catabolism will decrease by the degree of lipid concentration in the stomach. Fat will remain undigested in the stomach until gastric juices complete their work on the complex protein molecules.

Although all primary protein foods contain high concentration of fat, such lipids will be held in suspension, awaiting catabolism in the intestine, without impeding gastric action. Free fats like oil, butter and milk tend to coat the gastric mucosa, thereby inhibiting its effort to secrete gastric juice. Fat surrounding fried foods is also regarded as free fat and it interferes with gastric catabolism.

Another important rule for food combining is to avoid mixing carbohydrates and acid fruits in the same meal. The starch-splitting enzyme ptyalin in the saliva plays an important role as the food is chewed. It converts the complex starch molecules into simpler sugars. Ptyalin requires a neutral or slightly alkaline medium for proper functioning and this is the normal condition of the saliva in the mouth. However, when acid foods are taken, the action of ptyalin is halted. It is, therefore, necessary to avoid acid fruits in the same meal as sweet fruits or starches. Thus tomatoes should not be eaten with starches especially potatoes or bread.

Refined sugar products are also acidic, both in the mouth and in the bloodstream. The acidifying of the saliva by sucrose is one of the main causes of tooth decay. It can also cause severe damage to the digestion.

Food combining is designed to facilitate easier digestion. The chart in Table I, represents diagramatically food combining rules in an easy-to-follow method. Accompanying this chart are the lists of food in their correct classification.

TABLE 1

Food Combining Chart

Food Groups	Proteins	Fats	Starches	Vege-tables	Sweet Fruits	Sub-acid Fruits	Acid Fruits
Proteins	Good	Poor	Poor	Good	Poor	Fair	Good
Fats	Poor	Good	Fair	Good	Fair	Fair	Fair
Starches	Poor	Fair	Good	Good	Fair	Fair	Poor
Vege-tables	Good	Good	Good	Good	Poor	Poor	Poor
Sweet Fruits	Poor	Fair	Fair	Poor	Good	Good	Poor
Sub-acid Fruits	Fair	Fair	Fair	Poor	Good	Good	Good
Acid Fruits	Good	Fair	Poor	Poor	Poor	Good	Good

Proteins: Nuts, seeds, soyabeans, cheese, eggs, poultry*, meat*, fish*, yogurt.

Fats: Oils, olives, butter, margarine.

Starches: Whole cereals, peas, beans, lentils.

Vegetables: Leafy green vegetables, sprouted seeds, cabbage, cauliflower, broccoli, green peas, celery, tomatoes, onions.

Sweet fruits: Bananas, figs, custard apples, all-dried fruits, dates.

Sub-acid-fruits: Grapes, pears, apples, peaches, apricots, plums, guavas, raspberries.

Acid fruits: Grapefruit, lemons, oranges, limes, pineapple, strawberries.

* Not recommended for good nutrition.

In a nutshell, starches, fats, green vegetables and sugars may be eaten together as they require either an alkaline or neutral medium for their digestion. Similarly, proteins, green vegetables and acid fruits may be eaten together as they require an acid or neutral medium for their digestion. But starches and proteins, fats and proteins and starches and acid fruits should not be eaten together as a general rule, if the best results are required from the ingestion of the food eaten. This in brief is the whole basis for successful food combination.

An important point to remember about meals is that the smaller the number of courses they consist of, the better it will be. They should approximate to a one-course meal as much as possible. Simple meals in every way are more conducive to health, than more elaborate ones, no matter how well they may be combined.

A meal consisting of proteins, carbohydrates and fats may remain in the stomach for six to seven hours before the stomach is emptied. If carbohydrates are eaten without proteins, they remain in the stomach for a relatively short period. A fruit meal remains in the stomach for even shorter time. It is advisable to eat these different foods at different meals—a fruit meal, a starch meal and a protein meal. The ideal practice is a fruit meal for breakfast, a starch meal with salad and non starchy vegetables for lunch, and a protein meal with a salad and non starchy vegetables for dinner.

CHAPTER 16

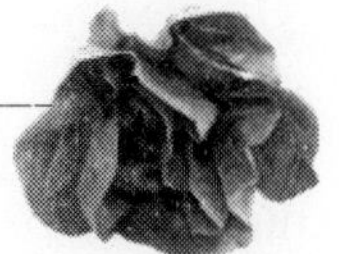

Health Promotion the Vegetarian Way

The word "vegetarian" was coined by the Vegetarian Society of the United Kingdom in about 1847. The word does not come from vegetable as is generally assumed; it is a derivation of the Latin word 'vegetari' which means to enliven.

The practice of vegetarianism, however, goes far back in history. Many noted philosophers and religious teachers urged their followers to avoid a flesh diet. Brahminism, Jainism, Zoroastrianism and Buddhism acknowledged the sacredness of life and the need to live without causing suffering; so did many of the early Christians.

There are various types of vegetarians. "Vagans" are the strictest vegetarians who eat only plant foods and exclude all animal by-products such as eggs, milk, cheese, curd, butter, ghee and even honey. There are "lacto vegetarians" who eat plant foods as well as dairy products and "lacto-avo vegetarians" who eat eggs besides plant foods and dairy products. There are even fish-eating vegetarians. The common factor among them is that they do not eat the flesh of warm-blooded animals.

Meat seems to have assumed an exaggerated importance nutritionally. It is generally mistakenly believed that nutritional deficiencies, especially of proteins and vitamin B_{12} and poor health may result if animal foods are eliminated. Studies, however, have indicated no health problems or deficiency diseases for those on a vegetarian diet.

Of the 22 amino-acids—the essential components of

proteins—needed by the body for its normal functioning, only nine need be supplied by the diet as the body synthesises the remaining 13. The body can use 100 per cent of this protein if all ten amino-acids are in ideal proportions. If, however, one or more of the essential amino acids are present in less than the ideal amount, the value of the entire protein is reduced in the same proportions. On a quality rating scale of 1 to 100, egg protein is 95, milk is 82, meat and poultry are 67, fish 80, grains are between 50 to 70 and legumes, nuts and seeds are between 40 and 60.

The so-called protein deficiency in a vegetarian diet is in fact more imaginary than real as the contribution of the protein value of green vegetables has been ignored and the true protein requirement is less than that assumed. Green vegetable protein is as high in quality as milk protein and thus makes a very valuable contribution to the vegetarian's protein nutrition. The high quality of this protein balances the lower quality of other vegetarian proteins such as nuts and beans. The recommended daily allowance of 70 value proteins is 44 grams per day for women and 56 for men. Researchers have now discovered that the actual protein requirement is much less, being 15 grams per day of 100 value protein or 21.5 grams of 70 value protein or 30 grams of 50 value protein. A wholesome vegetarian diet can, therefore, easily meet the body's protein needs.

Moreover, it is possible to combine two low-value plant proteins to get a protein of higher quality. Thus, wheat which has a deficiency in the amino-acid lysine but an abundance of sulpur-containing amino-acids can be combined with beans which have the opposite enrichment combination. Taken together, they complement each other to form a complete protein.

As regards the adequacy of B_{12} nutrition, lacto-avo

vegetarians and lacto vegetarians should not feel concerned on this score, as the B_{12} needs can be easily supplied by dairy products and eggs. A quarter litre of milk or hundred gms. of cheese or one egg per day will supply the recommended daily allowance. This vitamin once eaten is stored in the liver. Vagans, however, do not get this vitamin in their food, yet reliable scientific studies have found no evidence of B_{12} deficiency diseases. It is therefore, presumed that this vitamin can be synthesised in the body.

Auto-intoxication

Most diseases of the human body are caused by auto-intoxication or self-poisoning. The flesh of animals increases the burden of the organs of elimination and overloads the system with animal waste matter and poisons. Chemical analysis has proved that uric acid and other uremic poisons contained in the animal body are almost identical to caffeine, thein and nicotine, the poisonous stimulating principles of coffee, tea and tobacco. This explains why meat stimulates the animal passions and creates a craving for liquor, tobacco and other stronger stimulants. Excessive uric acid resulting from meat-eating also causes diseases such as rheumatism, Bright's disease, kidney stones, gout and gall stones. Meat proteins cause putrefication twice as rapidly as do vegetable proteins.

The morbid matter of the dead animal body is foreign and uncongenial to the excretory organs of man. It is much harder for them to eliminate the waste matter of an animal carcass than that of the human body. Moreover, the formation of ptomaines or corpse poisons begins immediately after the death of the animal and meat and poultry are usually kept in cold storage for many days and even months before they reach the kitchen.

Another powerful influence tends to poison the flesh of slaughtered animals. As is well known, emotions of worry, fear and anger actually poison blood and tissues. Imagine the excitable condition of animals after many days of travel, closely packed in shaking vehicles—hungry, thirsty, scared enroute to the slaughter-houses. Many die even before the end of their journey. Others are driven half dead with fear and exhaustion to the slaughter pans, their instinctive fear of death augmented by the sight and odour of the bloody shambles.

Flesh is often a carrier of disease germs. Diseases of many kinds are on the increase in animals, making flesh foods more and more unsafe. People are continually eating flesh that may contain tuberculosis and cancerous germs. Often animals are taken to the market and sold for food when they are so diseased that their owners do not wish to keep them any longer. And some of the processes of fattening them to increase their weight and consequently their market value, produce disease. Shut away from light and pure air, breathing the atmosphere of filthy stables, perhaps fattening on decaying food, the entire body now becomes contaminated with foul matter.

Benefits of Vegetarianism

A vegetarian diet can have many nutritional benefits, if it is rich in fruits and vegetables, and contains moderate amounts of seeds, nuts, whole grains and legumes. One of the main benefits of a proper vegetarian diet is its low caloric content in relation to the bulk supplied, which helps maintain ideal weight.

Another benefit of the vegetarian diet is the much lower intake of fat, if dairy products, seeds and nuts are eaten sparingly. This accounts for lower serium cholesterol levels found in vegetarians, which considerably reduces the risk of developing heart diseases and breast and colon cancer.

A third nutritional advantage of the vegetarian diet is its high fibre content. Fibre, being indigestible, increases the bulk of the faeces, keeps them soft and makes them easy to expel. One study has indicated that lacto-avo vegetarians consume twice as much and vagans four times as much fibre as non-vegetarians. High fibre intake has been associated with decreased risks of diseases of the colon, appendicitis, cancer of the colon and rectum, hiatus hernia, piles and varicose veins.

McCarrison, one of the greatest authorities on food, has outlined a perfect diet. According to him, "a perfectly constituted diet is one in which the principal ingredients are milk, milk products, any whole cereal grain or mixture of cereal grains, green leafy vegetables and fruits. These are the protective foods. They make good the defects of other constituents of the diet, protect the body against infection and disease of various kinds, and their use in sufficient quantity ensures physical efficiency."

Vegetarianism is thus a system based on scientific principles and has proved adequate for the best nutrition free from the poisons and bacteria of diseased animals. It is the best diet for man's optimum physical, mental and spiritual development.

CHAPTER 17

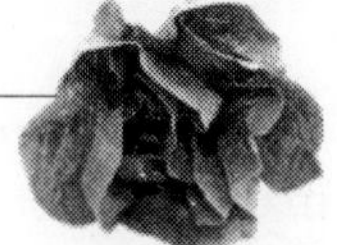

Importance of Dietary Fibre

Fibre forms the skeletal system of plants. Without it no plant or tree would be able to stand upright. Dietary fibre, the roughage of yesteryears, consists of those parts of the plant foods that cannot be digested by enzymes or other digestive secretions in the alimentary canal.

Dietary fibre plays an important role in the maintenance of health and prevention of disease. There is sufficient evidence to suggest that an artificial depletion of fibre as in case of refined cereals and sugar has over the last 100 years contributed to several degenerative diseases. Recent studies in this area indicate that sufficient intake of fibre-rich diet may help prevent obesity, colon cancer, heart disease, gallstones, irritable bowel syndrome, diverticulosis and diabetic conditions.

Studies have also established that dietary fibre is a collection of elements with a variety of functions rather than a single substance with single function as was assumed earlier. This new insight into the true nature of fibre has given the lie to old beliefs that bran is synonymous with fibre, that all fibre is fibrous or stringy and that all fibre tastes the same.

Physiological Effects

Fibre in the diet promotes more frequent bowel movements and softer stools having increased weight. The softness of stools is largely due to the presence of emulsified gas which is produced by the bacterial action on the fibre. A high fibre intake results in greater efficiency in the peristaltic movement of the colon. This helps in relieving constipation which is the main cause of several acute and chronic diseases.

Recent studies suggest that increasing the dietary fibre intake may be beneficial for patients with irritated bowel syndrome who have diarrhoea and rapid colonic transit, as well as to those who have constipation and slow transit. The high fibre diet, like bran, thus regulates the condition inside the colon so as to avoid both extremes—constipation and diarrhoea.

Investigations have shown that several potential carcinogens are produced in the faeces. Their production is related to the acidity of the gut content. The greater the acidity in the bowel content, the less is the production of these carcinogens. The breaking down of the fibre by bacteria renders the faeces more acidic. This reduces the amount of possible carcinogenic substances. Fibre also reduces the possibility of formation of harmful toxins in the large intestine by reducing the intestinal transit time of the food contents.

Dietary fibre increases the bacteria in the large intestines which require nitrogen for their growth. This in turn reduces the chances of cancerous changes in cells by reducing the amount of ammonia in the large bowel. Fibre reduces the absorption of cholesterol in the diet. It also slows down the rate of absorption of sugars from the food in the digestive system. Certain types of fibre increase the viscosity of the food content. This increased viscosity indirectly reduces the need for insulin secreted by the pancreas. Thus a fibre-rich diet can help in diabetes mellitus.

Sources of Fibre

The most significant food sources of fibre are unprocessed wheat bran, whole cereals such as wheat, rice, barley, rye, millets; legumes such as potato, carrots, beet, turnip and sweet potato; fruits like mango and guava and leafy vegetables such as cabbage, lettuce and celery. The percentage of fibre content per 100 gms. of some foods are: bran 10.5–13.5, whole grain cereals 1.0–2.0, nuts 2.0–5.0, legumes 1.5–1.7, vegetables 0.5–1.5, fresh fruits 0.5–1.5 and dried fruits 1.0–3.0. The foods which are completely devoid of fibre are meat, fish, eggs, milk, cheese, fats and sugars.

Bran, the outer coverings of grains, is one of the richest sources of dietary fibre. And it contains several types of fibre including cellulose, hemicellulose and pectin. Wheat and corn bran are highly beneficial in relieving constipation. Experiments show that oat bran can reduce cholesterol levels substantially. Corn bran is considered more versatile. It relieves constipation and also lowers LDL cholesterol, which is one of the more harmful kinds. Besides being rich in fibre, bran has a real food value being rich in lime, iron and vitamins and containing a considerable amount of protein.

Dr. Dennis P. Burkitt, a noted British physician remarks, "Grain roughages, such as rice bran and wheat bran, are an essential part of a healthy diet, and are preventive against diseases like piles, constipation, bowel cancer, varicose veins and even coronary thrombosis." Dr. Burkitt worked for many years in Africa and found after a series of observations that rural Africans who eat bulk of fibrous foods rarely suffer from any of these diseases.

Legumes have high fibre content. Much of this fibre is water-soluble, which makes legumes likely agents for lowering cholesterol. Soyabeans, besides this, can also help control glucose levels.

The types of fibre contained in vegetables and fruits contribute greatly towards good health. The vegetables with the biggest fibre ratings include sweet corn, carrots, potatoes, parsnips and peas. And among the high ranking fruits are raspberries, pears, strawberries and guavas.

Types of Fibres

There are six classes of fibre. They are cellulose, hemicellulose, pectin, gums, mucilages and legnin. They differ in physical properties and chemical interactions in the gut, though all except legnin are poly-saccharides. The facts known so far about these forms of fibre as a result of various studies are discussed below.

Cellulose: It is the most prevalent fibre. It is fibrous and softens the stool. It abounds in fruits, vegetables, bran, whole-meal bread and beans. It is also present in nuts and seeds. It increases the bulk of intestinal waste and eases it quickly through the colon. Investigations indicate that these actions may dilute and flush cancer-causing toxins out of the intestinal tract. They also suggest that cellulose may help level out glucose in the blood and curb weight gain.

Hemicellulose: It is usually present wherever cellulose is and shares some of its traits. Like cellulose, it helps relieve constipation, waters down carcinogens in the bowel and aids in weight reduction. Both cellulose and hemicellulose undergo some bacterial breakdown in the large intestine and this produces gas.

Pectin: This form of fibre is highly beneficial in reducing serum cholesterol levels. It however, does not have influence on the stool and does nothing to prevent constipation. Researches are being conducted to ascertain if pectin can help eliminate bile acids through the intestinal tract thereby preventing gallstones and colon cancer. It is found in apples, grapes, berries, citrus fruits, guava, raw papaya and bran.

Gums and Mucilages: They are the sticky fibres found in dried beans, oat bran and oatmeal. Investigations have shown that they are useful in the dietary control of diabetes and cholesterol.

Legnin: The main function of legnin is to escort bile acid and cholesterol out of the intestines. There is some evidence that it may prevent the formation of gallstones. It is contained in cereals, bran, whole meal flour, raspberries, strawberries, cabbage, spinach, parsley and tomatoes.

The best way to increase fibre content in the diet is to increase the consumption of wholemeal bread, brown rice, peas, beans, lentils, root vegetables and sugar-containing fruits, such as dates, apples, pears and bananas. The intake of sugar, refined cereals, meat, eggs and dairy products should be reduced. Candies, pastries, cakes which are rich in both sugar and fat, should be taken sparingly. White processed bread should be completely eliminated from the diet.

Requirement

There are divergent views as to the requirement of dietary fibre for good health. There is no recommended daily dietary allowance for it and hardly any data about optimum amounts. Some Africans known for lower incidence of degenerative diseases take about 150 grams of fibre a day. In Europe and North America, where there is a high incidence of such diseases, people take 25 grams or less a day. Dr. John H. Cummings, a noted fibre expert in England, considers that a fibre intake of 30 grams (about one ounce) per day is sufficient for good health.

Excessive consumption of fibre, especially bran, should however, be avoided. Due to its content of crude fibre, bran is relatively harsh and it may irritate the delicate functioning of the digestive system, especially in the sick and the weak. Excessive use of fibre may also result in loss of valuable minerals like calcium, phosphorus, magnesium and potassium from the body through excretion due to quick passage of food from the intestine.

CHAPTER 18

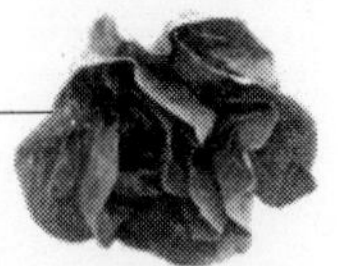

Lecithin—An Amazing Youth Element

Lecithin is the most abundant of the phospholipids. It is a fatty food substance, which serves as a structural material for every cell in the body. It is an essential constituent of the human brain and nervous system. It forms 30 per cent of the dry weight of the brain and 17 per cent of the nervous system.

Lecithin is also an important component of the endocrine glands and the muscles of the heart and kidneys. It makes up 73 per cent of the total liver fat. Nervous, mental or glandular overactivity can consume lecithin faster than its replacement. This may render a person irritable and exhausted. It is, therefore, of utmost importance to add lecithin to the diet, if the body's own supply decreases as in old age or working under stress.

Rich Sources

Lecithin is derived from the Greek Word, *likithos,* meaning egg yolk. Egg yolk is a rich source of lecithin, and also a rich source of cholesterol. This combination makes it possible for the lecithin to emulsify the cholesterol. Vegetable oils, whole grain cereals, soyabeans, liver and milk are other rich sources of lecithin. The cells of the body are also capable of synthesizing it as needed, B vitamins are present in it. Since these B vitamins are generally removed when grains are refined, people who eat exclusively white flour products are lacking them.

Benefits

The action of lecithin on the heart is the most important of all its proved benefits. It achieved its popularity initially in this area. Cholesterol is a fatty substance that tends to collect in the walls of the arteries and veins, thus narrowing them. This may eventually lead to a fatal blood clot. Scientific studies have shown that lecithin has the ability to break up cholesterol into small particles which can be easily handled by the system. With sufficient intake of lecithin, cholesterol cannot build up against the walls of the arteries and veins.

Like cholesterol, lecithin is continuously produced in the liver, passes into the intestine with bile and is absorbed in the blood. It helps in the transportation of fats. It also helps the cells to remove fats and cholesterol from the blood and to utilise them. It increases the production of bile acids made from cholesterol, thereby reducing the amount in the blood. It will thus be seen that cholesterol can cause trouble only if lecithin is lacking in the system.

All atheroscleroses or changes in the arterial walls are characterised by an increase of the blood cholesterol and a decrease in lecithin. It has been shown that experimental heart disease, produced by feeding cholesterol, could be prevented merely by giving a small quantity of lecithin. Atherosclerosis has been produced in various species of animals by increasing the blood cholesterol or decreasing the lecithin.

In normal health, when a diet high in fat is taken, there is tremendous increase in the production of lecithin. This helps in changing the fat in the blood from large particles to smaller and smaller ones. In case of atherosclerosis, however, the lecithin in the blood remains very low regardless of the quantity of fat entering the blood. The result is that, the fat particles remain too large to be able to pass through the arterial walls. A more serious situation can develop if there is lack of lecithin in cells also.

Besides reducing the cholesterol level in the blood, there is mounting scientific evidence to suggest several other benefits from lecithin. It has been suggested that its intake in sufficient amounts can help rebuild those cells and organs which need it. Lecithin helps to maintain their health once they are repaired. It may mean that a deficiency of lecithin in the diet may be one of the causes of ageing and that its use may be beneficial in retarding the ageing process.

Edward R. Hewith in his book, *The Years Between 75 and 90* says, "with older people the fats remain high in the blood for from five to seven hours and in some cases as long as 20 hours, thus giving the fats more time to become located in the tissues. If lecithin is given to older people before a fatty meal, it has been found that the fats in the blood return to normal in a short time, in the same way they do in younger people."

In some cases, the cosmetic effect of lecithin does as much for the mental outlook of persons as it does for their physical well-being. It has been found to eliminate the yellow or yellow-brown plaques on the skin or around the eyes caused by fatty deposits. It is a natural tranquilliser which is beneficial in nervous exhaustion. It can produce great alertness in elderly people.

Some studies have indicated that lecithin increases the gamma globulin in the blood. This helps fight infection. It provides an increased immunity against pneumonia. It has also been found to lower blood pressure in some people. In combination with vitamin E, it has proved helpful in lowering the requirements of insulin in diabetics. It has also proved valuable in the treatment of certain skin ailments, including acne, eczema and psoriasis.

Lecithin has been suggested as a sexual aid. It was used in Germany 30 years ago as a restorative of sexual powers, for glandular exhaustion and nervous and mental disorders. Seminal fluid is rich in lecithin. Because of its loss from the body, its need for men is regarded as specially great. Its use is also considered valuable in minimising pre-menstrual and menopausal tension.

Dr. N.A. Ferri, an eminent physician remarks—"Lecithin has a versatile function in life. It is an extremely important factor in the digestion and oxidation of fats, thus creating more muscle and glandular activity, resulting in greater body exertion and less fat accumulations. Lecithin is essential not only for tissue integrity of the nervous and glandular system in all living cells, but has been regarded as also the most effective generator and regenerator of great physical, mental and glandular activity. Shattered nerves, depleted brain power, waning activity of vital glands, find in lecithin, especially in the cellular structure of the nervous system and endocrine glands a source of dynamic energy."

The best way to increase lecithin is to eat the same amount of fat as usual, but reduce animal fat except that from fish. Oil may be used for cooking, seasoning and salad dressing. All hydrogenated fats such as margarines, cooking fats, hydrogenated peanut butter and processed cheese should be avoided as also foods prepared with them.

CHAPTER 19

Role of Enzymes in Nutrition

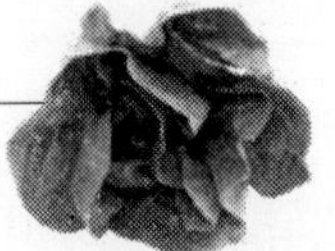

Enzymes are chemical substances produced in the living organism. They are marvellous organic catalysts which are essential to life as they control all the chemical reactions that take place in a living system. Enzymes are part of all living cells, including those of plants and animals.

The term enzyme, which literally means in yeast, was coined following the demonstration of catalytic properties of yeast and yeast juices. Although enzymes are produced in the living cell, they are not dependent upon the vital processes of the cell and work outside the cell. Certain enzymes of yeast, for instance, when expressed from the yeast cells are capable of exerting their usual effect, that is, the conversion of sugar to alcohol.

A striking feature of enzymes is that while they enter into chemical reaction, they remain intact in the process. They however, act with maximum efficiency at a certain temperature. Lowering the temperature below or raising it above this level slows the reaction. A high degree of heat, that is above 60°C, permanently destroys their action.

It has been estimated that there are over 20,000 enzymes in the human body. This estimate is based on the number of bodily processes that seem to require action. However, so far only about 1,000 enzymes have been identified. But their great role in nutrition and other living processes has been firmly established. They are protein molecules made up of chains of amino acids. They play a vital role and work more efficiently than any reagent concocted by chemists. Thus for instance, a chemist can separate proteins into their component amino acids by boiling them at 166°C for over 18 hours in a strong solution of hydrochloric acid, but the enzymes of the small intestines can do so in less than three hours at body temperature in a neutral medium.

A feature which distinguishes enzymes from inorganic catalysts is that they are absolutely specific in their actions. This means that a particular enzyme can cause reactions involving only a particular type of substance or a group of closely related substances. The substance on which the enzyme acts is known as "substrate". The specificity of an enzyme is, however, related to the formation of the enzyme-substrate complex which requires that the appropriate groupings of both substrate and enzyme should be in correct relative position. The substrate must fit the enzyme like a key fits its lock.

Enzymes which are used in the cells which make them are called intracellular enzymes. Enzymes which are produced in cells which secrete them to other parts of the body are known as extracellular enzymes. Digestive juices are an example of the latter type.

Nomenclature

There are few enzymes whose names have been established by long usage such as ptyalin, pepsin, trypsin and erepsin. Apart from these, enzymes are usually named by adding the suffixes to the main part of the name of the substrate upon which they act. Thus amylases act upon starch (amylum), lactase acts upon lactose, lipases act upon lipids, maltase acts upon maltose and protesses act upon proteins. There are, however, several enzymes which act upon many substances in different ways. These enzymes are named by their functions rather than substrates. Thus, an enzyme which causes deaminations is called a deaminase and oxidising enzyme an oxidase.

Some enzymes work efficiently only if some other specific substance is present in addition to substrate. This other substance is known as an "activator" or a "conenzyme". "Activators" are usually inorganic ions. They increase the activity of a complete enzyme and may take part in the formation of the enzyme-substrate complex. Many of the conenzymes are related to vitamins. This explains why vitamin deficiencies profoundly alter metabolism. Thus, for instance, thiamine, as thiamine pyrophosphate, functions as a conenzyme in at least 14 enzyme systems. Conenzymes, like enzymes, are being continuously regenerated in the cells.

Enzymes play a decisive role in the digestion of food as they are responsible for the chemical changes which the food undergoes during digestion. The chemical changes comprise the breaking up of the large molecules of carbohydrates, fats and proteins into smaller ones or conversion of complex substances into simple ones which can be absorbed by the intestines. They also control the numerous reactions by which these simple substances are utilized in the body for building up new tissues and producing energy. The enzymes themselves are not broken down or changed in the process. They remain as powerful at the end of a reaction as they were at the beginning. Moreover, very small amounts can convert large amounts of material. They are thus true catalysts.

The process of digestion begins in the mouth. The saliva in the mouth, besides helping to masticate the food, carries an enzyme called ptyalin which begins the chemical action of digestion. It initiates the catabolism (breakdown) of carbohydrates by converting starches into simple sugars. This explains the need for thorough mastication of starchy food in the mouth. If this is not done the ptyalin cannot carry out its functions as it is active in an alkaline, neutral or slightly acid medium and is inactivated by the highly acid gastric juices in the stomach.

Although enzymatic action starts while food is being chewed, digestion moves into high gear only when the chewed food has passed the esophagus and reached the stomach. While the physical action of peristalsis churns and kneads solid food into a semi-solid amorphous mixture called chyme, this mixture undergoes chemical changes initiated by gastric juices secreted by the walls of the stomach. These juices include mucus for lubricating the stomach, hydrochloric acid and gastric juice. The enzyme or active principle of the gastric juice is pepsin. This enzyme in combination with hydrochloric acid starts the breakdown of proteins into absorbable amino acids called polypeptides. An additional enzyme, rennin, plays an important role in the stomach of the infant. It curdles milk and allows the pepsin to work upon it. The gastric juice has no effect upon starches or fats.

When the chyme leaves the stomach and enters the small intestine through the pylorus—the lower escape valve, it still contains much food which is in the form of raw material not yet ready for absorption in the body. Digestion is completed inside the small intestine by several juices. From liver comes a liquid called bile which converts fat globules into a smooth emulsion.

The pancreas contributes various enzymes which continue the breakdown of proteins, help to divide starch into sugars and work with bile in digesting fats. The small intestine itself secretes enzymes from its inner wall to complete the reactions. When all the enzymes have done their work, the food is digested and rendered fit for absorption by the system.

The following table briefly summarizes the chemical digestion of carbohydrates, fats and proteins by various enzymes:

Source of Enzyme	Enzyme	Substrate	Products
Mouth Salivary glands	Salivary amylase (ptyalin)	Starch	Dextrins and maltose
Stomach Gastric mucosa	Gastric protease pepsin rennin Gastric lipase	 Proteins casein Short chain and medium chain triglycerides	 Polypeptides Insoluble casein Fatty acids and glycerol
Small Intestine	Pancreatic Proteases trypsin chymotrypsin carboxypeptidases	Proteins and polypeptides	Smaller polypeptides and amino acids
	Pancreatic lipase (steapsin)	Fats	Mono and diglycerides, fatty acids and glycerol
	Pancreatic amylase (amylopsin)	Amylase and amylopectin	Maltose, maltotriose and a-limit dextrins
Intestinal mucosa Brushborder	Intestinal peptidases aminopeptideses dipeptideses	Polypeptides Dipeptides	Smaller polypeptides and amino acids
	Intestinal saccharidases a-dextrinase (isomaltase)	 a-limit dextrins	 Glucose
	Sucrase	Sucrase	Glucose and fructose
	Maltase	Maltase	Glucose (2 molecules)
	Lactose	Lactose	Glucose and galactose

Enzymes form part of the food we eat. Raw foods contain enzymes in abundance; cooking, pasteurising, pickling, smoking and other processings denature enzymes. It is, therefore, essential to include in our diet, substantial amount of raw foods in the form of fruits, raw salads and sprouts. Studies have revealed that the body without sufficient raw materials from raw foods, may tire and produce fewer enzymes year after year. This may lead to wearing out of body processes and consequent worn out looks.

CHAPTER 20

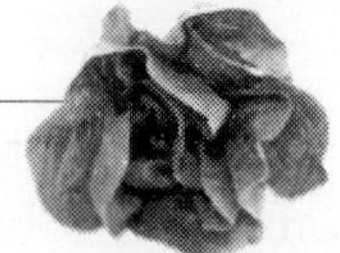

Raw Juice Therapy

Raw juice therapy is a method of treatment of disease through an exclusive diet of juices of fruits and vegetables. It is also known as juice fasting. It is the most effective way to restore health and rejuvenate the body.

During raw juice therapy, the eliminative and cleansing capacity of the organs of elimination, namely lungs, liver, kidneys and the skin, is greatly increased and masses of accumulated metabolic waste and toxins are quickly eliminated. It affords physiological rest to the digestive and assimilative organs. After the juice fasting or raw juice therapy, the digestion of food and the utilisation of nutrients is vastly improved.

An exclusive diet of raw juices of fruits and vegetables results in much faster recovery from diseases and more effective cleansing and regeneration of the tissues than the fasting on pure water. Dr. Ragnar Berg, a world-renowned authority on nutrition and biochemistry observes: "During fasting the body burns up and excretes huge amounts of accumulated wastes. We can help this cleansing process by drinking alkaline juices instead of water while fasting. I have supervised many fasts and made extensive examinations and tests of fasting patients, and I am convinced that drinking alkali-forming fruit and vegetable juices, instead of water, during fasting will increase the healing effect of fasting. Elimination of uric acid and other inorganic acids will be accelerated. And sugars in juices will strengthen the heart. Juice fasting is, therefore, the best form of fasting."

As juices are extracted from plants and fruits, they posess definite medicinal properties. Specific juices are beneficial in specific conditions. Besides specific medicinal virtues, raw fruit and vegetable juices have an extraordinary revitalising and rejuvenative effect on all the organs, glands and functions of the body.

Favourable Effects

The favourable effect of raw juices in the treatment of disease is attributed to the following facts:

(1) Raw juices of fruits and vegetables are extremely rich in vitamins, minerals, trace elements, enzymes and natural sugars. They exercise beneficial effect in normalising all the body functions. They supply needed elements for the body's own healing activity and cell regeneration, thereby speeding the recovery.

(2) The juices extracted from raw fruits and vegetables require no digestion and almost all their vital nutrients are assimilated directly in the bloodstream.

(3) Raw juices are extremely rich in alkaline elements. This is highly beneficial in normalising acid-alkaline balance in the blood and tissues as there is over-acidity in most conditions of ill-health.

(4) Generous amounts of easily assimilable organic minerals in raw juices especially calcium, potassium and silicon help in restoring biochemical and mineral balance in the tissues and cells, thereby preventing premature ageing of cells and disease.

(5) Raw juices contain certain natural medicines, vegetal hormones and antibiotics. For instance, string beans are said to contain insulin-like substance. Certain hormones needed by the pancreas to produce insulin are present

in cucumber and onion juices. Fresh juices of garlic, onions, radish and tomatoes contain antibiotic substances.

Precautions

Certain precautions are, however, necessary in adopting an exclusive diet of raw juices. Firstly, all juices should be made fresh immediately before drinking. Canned and frozen juices should not be used. It will be advisable that one should have one's own juicer for extracting fresh juices. Secondly, only fresh ripe fruits and vegetables, preferably organically grown, should be used for extraction of juices. Thirdly, only as much juice as needed for immediate consumption should be extracted. Raw juices oxidise rapidly and lose their medicinal value in storage, even under refrigeration. Fourthly, the quality of the juices has a distinct bearing on the results obtained. In case of incomplete extraction of juices, their effective power is proportionately reduced due to the absence of the vitamins and enzymes which are left behind in fibre and the pulp. Finally, if juices are too sweet they should be diluted in water on 50 : 50 basis or mixed with other less sweet juices. This is especially important in some specific conditions such as diabetes, hypoglycemia, arthritis and high blood pressure.

Fruit and vegetable juices may be divided into six main types. These are: (i) Juices from sweet fruits such as prunes and grapes. (ii) Juices from sub-acid fruits like apple, plum, pear, peach, apricot and cherry, (iii) Juices from acid fruits like apple, orange, lemon, grapefruit, strawberry and pineapple, (iv) Juices from vegetable fruits, namely, tomato and cucumber. (v) Juices from green leafy vegetables like cabbage, celery, lettuce, spinach, parsley and watercress, (vi) Juices from root vegetables like beetroot, carrot, onion, potato and radish.

Generally speaking, fruit juices stir up toxins and acids in the body, thereby stimulating the eliminative processes. Vegetable juices, on the other hand, soothe the jaded nerves and work in a much milder manner. They carry away toxic matter in a gentle way. Owing to their differing actions fruit and vegetable juices should not be used at the same time or mixed together.

It is desirable to use juices individually. In any case not more than three juices should be used in any one mixture. The following broad rules apply when using mixtures of juices:

1. Juices from sweet fruits may be combined with juices of sub-acid fruits, but not with those of acid fruits, vegetable fruits or vegetables.
2. Juices from sub-acid fruits may be combined with juices of sweet fruits, or acid fruits, but not with other juices.
3. Juices from acid fruits may be combined with those of sub-acid fruits or vegetable fruits, but not with other juices.
4. Juices from vegetable fruits may be combined with those of acid fruits or of green leafy vegetables, but not with other juices.
5. Juices from green leafy vegetables may be combined with those of vegetable fruits or of the root vegetable, but not with other juices.
6. Juices from root vegetables may be combined with those of green leafy vegetables, but not with other juices.

A proper selection of juices in treating a particular ailment is very essential. Thus, for instance, juices of carrot, cucumber, cabbage and other vegetables are very valuable in asthma, arthritis and skin disease, but juices of orange and mosambi aggravate their symptoms by increasing the amount of mucus.

Treatment of Diseases

Some common ailments and fruit and vegetable juices found beneficial in their treatment are mentioned below:

Acidity: Grapes, orange, mosambi, carrot and spinach.

Acne: Grapes, pear, plum, tomato, cucumber, carrot, potato and spinach.

Allergies: Apricot, grapes, carrot, beet and spinach.

Arteriosclerosis: Grapefruit, pineapple, lemon, celery, carrot, lettuce and spinach.

Anaemia: Apricot, prune, strawberry, red grape, beet, celery, carrot and spinach.

Arthritis: Sour cherry, pineapple, sour apple, lemon, grapefruit, cucumber, beet, carrot, lettuce and spinach.

Asthma: Apricot, lemon, pineapple, peach, carrot, radish and celery.

Bronchitis: Apricot, lemon, pineapple, peach, tomato, carrot, onion and spinach.

Bladder Ailments: Apple, apricot, lemon, cucumber, carrot, celery, parsley and watercress.

Colds: Lemon, orange, grapefruit, pineapple, carrot, onion, celery and spinach.

Constipation: Apple, pear, grapes, lemon, carrot, beet, spinach and watercress.

Colitis: Apple, apricot, pear, peach, pineapple, papaya, carrot, beet, cucumber and spinach.

Diabetes: Citrus fruits, carrot, celery, lettuce and spinach.

Diarrhoea: Papaya, lemon, pineapple, carrot and celery.

Eczema:	Red grapes, carrot, spinach, cucumber and beet.
Epilepsy:	Red grapes, figs, carrot, celery and spinach.
Eye Disorders:	Apricot, tomato, carrot, celery, parsley and spinach.
Gout:	Red sour cherries, pineapple, tomato, cucumber, beet, carrot, celery and spinach.
Halitosis:	Apple, grapefruit, lemon, pineapple, tomato, carrot, celery and spinach.
Headache:	Grapes, lemon, carrot, lettuce and spinach.
Heart Disease:	Red grapes, lemon, cucumber, carrot, beet and spinach.
High blood pressure:	Grapes, orange, cucumber, carrot, and beet.
Influenza:	Apricot, orange, lemon, grapefruit, pineapple, carrot, onion and spinach.
Insomnia:	Apple, grapes, lemon, lettuce, carrot and celery.
Jaundice:	Lemon, grapes, pear, carrot, celery, spinach, beet and cucumber.
Kidney Disorders:	Apple, orange, lemon, cucumber, carrot, celery, parsley and beet.
Liver Ailments:	Lemon, papaya, grapes, carrot, tomato, beet and cucumber.
Menstrual Disorders:	Grapes, prunes, cherry, spinach, lettuce, turnips and beet.
Menopausal Symptoms:	Fruits and Vegetables in season.
Neuritis.	Orange, pineapple, apple, carrot and beet.
Obesity:	Lemon, grapefruit, orange, cherry,

	pineapple, papaya, tomato, beet, cabbage, lettuce, spinach and carrot.
Piles:	Lemon, orange, papaya, pineapple, carrot, spinach, turnip and watercress.
Prostate Troubles:	All fruit juices in season, carrot, asparagus, lettuce and spinach.
Psoriasis:	Grapes, carrot, beet, and cucumber.
Rheumatism:	Grapes, orange, lemon, grapefruit, tomato, cucumber, beet, carrot and spinach.
Stomach Ulcers:	Apricot, grapes, cabbage and carrot.
Sinus Trouble:	Apricot, lemon, tomato, carrot, onion and radish.
Sore Throat:	Apricot, grapes, lemon, pineapple, prune, tomato, carrot and parsley.
Tonsilitis:	Apricot, lemon, orange, grapefruit, pineapple, carrot, spinach and radish.
Varicose Veins:	Grapes, orange, plum, tomato, beetroot, carrot and watercress.

When on a raw juice therapy, the prescribed juice should be drunk every three hours. One can thus take juices five to six times a day. A glass of water mixed with lemon juice and 20 to 30 grams of honey may be taken first thing in the morning on arising. Thereafter, the prescribed juice may be taken at three-hourly intervals. The quantity of juice on each occasion may be 250 ml on the first day. This quantity may be increased by 50 ml each succeeding day till one takes 600 ml on each occasion. The juice diet can be continued for 30 to 40 days without any ill-effects. The patient should take adequate rest during the raw juice therapy.

Raw juices act as a cleansing agent and start eliminating toxins and morbid matter from the system immediately. This often results in symptoms such as pain in the abdomen, diarrhoea, loss of weight, headache, fever, weakness, sleeplessness and bad breath. These reactions, which are part of the cleansing process, should not be suppressed by the use of drugs. They will cease when the body is able to expel all toxins.

After the raw juice therapy, the return to normal balanced diet should be gradual, and in stages. In the beginning, two juice meals may be replaced by milk and fruits. Then gradually juice meals may be substituted by a balanced-diet.

CHAPTER 21

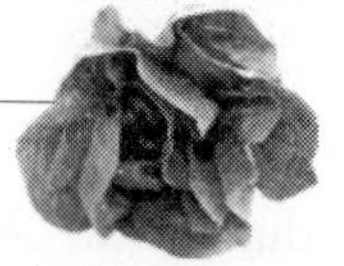

Sprouts for Optimum Nutrition

Sprouts are considered as wonder foods. They rank as the freshest and most nutritious of all vegetables available to the human diet. By a process of natural transmutation, sprouted food acquires vastly improved digestibility and nutritional qualities when compared to non-sprouted embryo from which it derives.

Sprouted foods have been part of the diet of many ancient races for thousands of years. Even to this day, the Chinese retain their fame for delicious mung bean sprouts. Sprouts provide all the essential vitamins and minerals. They should form a vital component of our diet. Sprouting requires no constant care but only an occasional sprinkling of water.

All edible grains, seeds and legumes can be sprouted. Generally the following are used for sprouting:

(i) *Grains*: Wheat, maize, ragi, bajra and barley.

(ii) *Seeds*: Alfalfa seeds, radish seeds, fenugreek seeds, carrot seeds, coriander seeds, pumpkin seeds and muskmelon seeds.

(iii) *Legumes*: Mung, Bengal gram, groundnut and peas.

Alfalfa, as the name in Arabic signifies, is the king of all sprouts. Grown as a plant, its roots are known to burrow as much as 12 metres into the subsoil to bring up valuable trace minerals of which manganese is especially important to health and digestion; it is a vital component of human insulin. Apart from minerals, alfalfa is also a rich source of vitamins A, B,

C, E and K and amino acids. Sesame seeds are another good source of nourishment. They contain all the essential amino acids in their 20 per cent protein content and higher concentration of calcium than does milk. They are high in lecithin, unsaturated fats, vitamin E and vitamin B complex, besides other live nutrients.

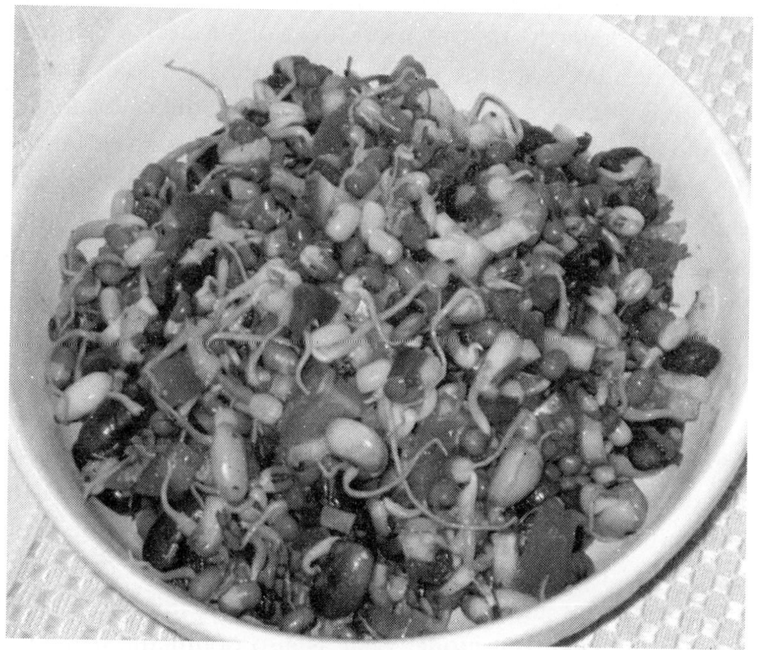

Sprouts are the freshest and most nutritious of all vegetables.

How to Sprout

As a first step, a good variety of seeds should be used for sprouting. It should be ensured that the seeds, legumes or grains are of the sproutable type. Soyabeans do not sprout well as they often become sour. Wheat has to be grown in soil. It is advisable to use seeds which are not chemically treated as this slows down the germination rate. The seeds should be washed thoroughly and then soaked overnight in a jar of pure water. The jar should be covered with cheesecloth or wire screening. The duration of soaking will depend upon the size of the seed. Small seeds are soaked for five hours, medium size for eight hours and beans and grains for 10 to 12 hours.

On the following morning, the seeds should be rinsed and the water drained off. Not more than one-fourth of the jar should be filled with the seeds for sprouting. Soaking makes the seeds grains or legumes fatty, pulpy and full of water. It should, therefore, be ensured that the jar has enough room for the seeds to expand during sprouting. They will expand about eight times their original size. The jar should be kept at a place which is exposed neither to chill nor hot winds. It should also be ensured that the mouth of the jar is not completely covered so as to allow air in. The seeds should be rinsed and water drained off three times every day till they are ready to eat.

The seeds will germinate and become sprouts in two or three days from commencement of soaking, depending on temperature and humidity. Care should always be taken to ensure that sprouts do not lie in water. They should be kept well drained to prevent souring. Sprouts are at their optimum level of flavour and tenderness when tiny green leaves appear at the tips. Their nutritional value is also optimum. To retain their freshness and nutritional value, they should be placed in a refrigerator, if they cannot be consumed immediately after reaching suitable maturity. Sprouts can be kept for several days in this way.

Some caution is necessary in sprouting. Soaking for a longer period than required makes the seeds rot or ferment. The main factors for germination are water, air, heat and darkness. There may be poor germination or no germination at all if any of these factors are not present such as insufficient water, or too much water, lack of sufficient heat, lack of fresh air, either too cold or too hot surroundings and too much light.

Benefits

There is an amazing increase in nutrients in sprouted foods when compared to their dried embryo. In the process of sprouting, the vitamins, minerals and protein increase substantially with corresponding decrease in calories and carbohydrate content. These comparisons are based on an equivalent water content in the foods measured. Analysis of dried seeds, grains and legumes shows a very low water content. But this increases upto tenfold when the same food is converted into sprouts. For accurate comparison each must be brought to a common denomination of equal water content to assess the exact change brought in nutritional value.

Sprouted mung beans, for instance, have an 8.3 increase of water content over dried beans. Hence the nutritional value of sprouted and dried mung beans can be compared by multiplying the analysed nutrients of sprouted mung beans by the factor of 8.3. Based on this criterion, the changes found in sprouted mung beans when compared with the figures for the beans in the dried state are as follows:

Energy content—calories	Decrease 15 per cent
Total carbohydrate content	Decrease 9 per cent
Protein availability	Increase 30 per cent
Calcium content	Increase 34 per cent
Potassium content	Increase 80 per cent
Sodium content	Increase 690 per cent
Iron content	Increase 40 per cent
Phosphorus content	Increase 56 per cent

Vitamin A content	Increase 285 per cent
Thiamine or Vitamin B_1 content	Increase 208 per cent
Riboflavin or Vitamin B_2 content	Increase 515 per cent
Niacin or Vitamin B_3 content	Increase 256 per cent
Ascorbic acid or Vitamin C content	An infinite increase

The increase in protein availability is of great significance. It is a valuable indicator of the enhanced nutritional value of a food when sprouted. The simultaneous reduction in carbohydrate content indicates that many carbohydrate molecules are broken down during sprouting to allow an absorption of atmospheric nitrogen and reforming into amino-acids. The resultant protein is the most easily digestible of all proteins available in foods.

The remarkable increase in sodium content supports the view that sprouted foods offer nutritional qualities. Sodium is essential to the digestive process within the gastro-intestinal tract and also to the elimination of carbon dioxide. Together with the remarkable increase in vitamins, sodium materially contributes to the easy digestibility of sprouts.

Dried seeds, grains and legumes do not contain discernible traces of ascorbic acid, yet when sprouted, they reveal quite significant quantities which are important in the body's ability to metabolise proteins. The infinite increase in ascorbic acid derives from their absorption of atmospheric elements during growth.

Sprouts have several other benefits. They supply food in predigested form, that is, the food which has already been acted upon by the enzymes and made to digest easily. During sprouting, much of the starch is broken down into simple sugars such as glucose and sucrose by the action of the enzyme 'amylase'. Proteins are converted into amino acids and amides.

Fats and oils are converted into more simple fatty acids by the action of the enzyme lipase.

During sprouting, the beans lose their objectionable gas producing quality. Research has shown that oligosaccharides are responsible for gas formation, For maintenance of health, some amount of gas production is necessary but it should be within safe limits. As the process of germination ends and sprouting begins, the percentage of oligosaccharides is reduced by 90. Sprouts contain a lot of fibre and water and, therefore, are helpful in overcoming constipation.

Sprouts are an extremely inexpensive method of obtaining a concentration of vitamins, minerals and enzymes. They have in them all the constituent nutrients of fruits and vegetables and are 'live' foods. Eating sprouts is the safest and best way of getting the advantage of both fruits and vegetables without contamination and harmful insecticides.

It should, however, be ensured that seeds and dried beans are purchased from a store where they are fresh, unsprayed and packaged as food. Seeds that are packaged for planting purposes may contain mercury compounds or other toxic chemicals.

CHAPTER 22

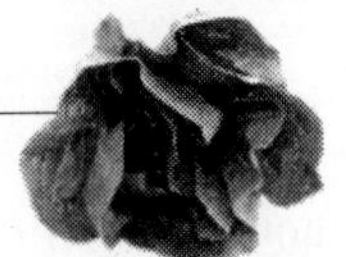

Role of Water in Nutrition

Water is one of the most precious gifts of nature. It is an essential and major component of all living things on earth. Water is one of the essential nutrients. Though not a food, it carries nutrients throughout the body. In fact, it is more essential to human life than food; for a person may live for weeks without food but only for days without water.

The most important property of water is its versatility. It can be used effectively both inside and outside the body. It can be used in any form be it liquid, solid or steam. It can be used hot, cold or lukewarm, depending on the need.

Water is the largest constituent of human body. About 60 to 70 per cent of the total body weight consists of water. Thus, the body of a 65-kg person contains approximately 40 litres of water. Of this, about 25 litres are within the cells and the remaining 15 litres in the extracellular fluids.

Functions

Water is essential to the composition of the body for the smooth functioning of the different processes. It helps absorption of the food materials through the intestinal tract. It keeps blood in a liquid state thus enabling easy circulation even in the tiniest blood vessels. Water maintains body temperature constantly at 98.4 F in all weathers and keeps the skin moist and cold. It always keeps the mucus membrane moist and helps to secret different fluids in various glands of the body.

Water helps the kidneys to remove unwanted body waste like urea and salt in the form of urine. It also helps removal of body wastes through lungs as water vapour, through skin as perspiration and sweat and, to a small extent, through the large intestine as faeces. It is estimated that as much as 37 gallons of fluids are daily filtered off from the blood and restored to the body by the kidneys, only when there is proper proportion of water in the blood.

Water Intake

The water consumption is mainly through drinking water, other fluids and the water content in the food consumed. Some of our common vegetables contain as much water as milk and even more. Thus, 100 grams of melon, tomato, and radish contain over 90 per cent of water against only 87 per cent of water contained in milk. Besides taking water through drink and in foods, the body itself generates water by the combustion going on in the system.

The rate at which water is eliminated from the body must be replaced by its intake so as to maintain the balance in the system. On occasions, water content of the body suffers considerable fluctuation. Running and other strenuous exercises cause a great loss by perspiration and through the lungs. This loss has to be replaced by a drink or food.

Any great variation in the normal quantity of water in the body interferes with the vital processes and causes acute distress. Death may occur within three days of abstention from water. Loss of water takes place, no matter whether we drink or not. So if we do not drink sufficient water, blood thickens and the kidneys fail to deal with it efficiently. This may result in the accumulation of poisons and lead to death. Some persons unconsciously form a habit of living on less than optimum quantity of water. This may lead to ill heath and symptoms like headache, nervousness, loss of appetite, digestive disturbances and lack of concentration in work. These symptoms will rapidly disappear with proper intake of water.

For the maintenance of good health, an adult should take eight to 10 glasses of pure, fresh water daily, whether one feels thirsty or not. This quantity is enough to flush the body and meet all internal needs. However, it is bad to drink excess of water also since it weakens the kidneys and stomach.

Drinking water along with meals is not healthy, for it dilutes the gastric juices and hampers digestion. Water should be drunk half an hour before or one hour after a meal. Drinking a glass of water early in the morning after a mouthwash, is good for health. It prevents stomach disorders and constipation. Scientifically, drinking water early in the morning helps, saliva formation which together with some useful enzymes helps in effective cleaning of the intestinal tract. The age old practice of drinking water in a copper vessel early morning is one of the oldest methods with the same principle.

Bathing

Invisible perspiration carries noxious substances with it and while the water evaporates, the poisonous substances remain on the surface of the skin, sometimes on the pores themselves. A bath is very necessary not only to wash off these poisonous matter from the skin, but also for keeping the skin in a healthy condition. Cold water or water at body temperature should be used for bathing. The application of cold water followed by friction facilitates rush of blood to the skin. This gives the skin its necessary exercise and keeps it healthy and capable of normal functioning for the rest of the day.

Any water, however, is not good. Water used for drinking, cooking and bathing should be free from bacteria, dissolved mineral impurities and suspended matters. Rain water is best for drinking purpose. However, purified water from a river, spring, well or a lake is equally good. The clear water must be further treated. If the water is from open sources like river or large over-flooded tanks, there is always the risk of it being contaminated by bacteria of diseases like dysentry, typhoid and cholera. In such a case, water should be rendered harmless by boiling. Constant use of hard water for drinking may cause stomach disorders. It is therefore necessary to remove hardness by boiling.

CHAPTER 23

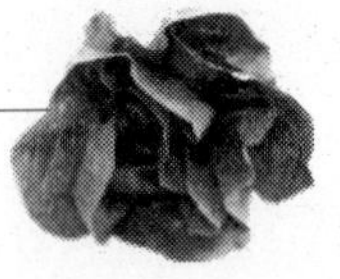

Raw Foods for Good Health and Longevity

Eating should not be considered as a trivial affair. Serious thought should be given in planning our daily diet. For, what we eat has a profound effect on our health and longevity. Latest researches show that food can provide health, vigour and vitality, and free us from various diseases, or it can make us unhealthy and miserable.

Before the discovery of fire, man's evolution and development depended on the consumption of natural, raw foods, as provided by nature. After fire came into existence, man started cooking natural foods without much thought. Cooking of natural foods led to their debasement and destruction of most of their essential nutrients needed for the maintenance of good health. Further loss of nutrients took place when man started refining and processing of natural foods. This has inevitably led to ill-health and vast varieties of diseases from which modern man suffers. He can get rid of these diseases and regain health, if he discards unnatural refined, processed and too much dependence on cooked foods.

Benefits of Raw Foods

Raw foods differ in nature from cooked foods, irrespective of their degree of cooking. They have certain distinctive advantage. These advantages are described herein in brief.

Normal Functioning of the Body

Raw foods contain certain vital ingredients which are essential for the maintenance of good health. Their nutritive constituents serve as building material for the construction and renewal of cells, produce energy to put these cells into motion and give warmth to the body and supply the raw materials to the specialised cells needed for their productive activities. Natural nutrition, as provided by nature, thus ensures the normal functioning of all body organs. Cooked foods force human organs to work at about three to four times their normal capacity, bring about premature changes in them, cause various ailments and shorten the life span.

As against this, those who eat raw foods make use of the digestive organs at about one-fourth of their potential capacity. As a result, their organs are never overloaded or fatigued. The over-loading of the digestive organs results in over working of several accessory organs like the heart, liver, and the kidneys. The additional work performed by these organs soon has the effect of tiring them out and putting them out of action prematurely. This eventually causes ill health and reduces the life span of a person by several years.

Balancing Body Chemistry

Raw foods helps balance body chemistry. The tissues and cells of the body are composed of 16 chemical elements. The balance of equilibrium of these chemical elements in the body is an essential factor in the maintenance of health and healing of disease. The acid-alkaline balance plays a vital role in the balanced body chemistry. All foods, after digestion and absorption, leave either an acid or alkaline ash in the body, depending on their mineral composition.

The normal body chemistry is approximately 20 per cent acid and 80 per cent alkaline. To maintain this acid-alkaline balance, it is essential that one should eat 80 per cent of alkaline forming foods and 20 per cent of acid forming foods. Fresh,

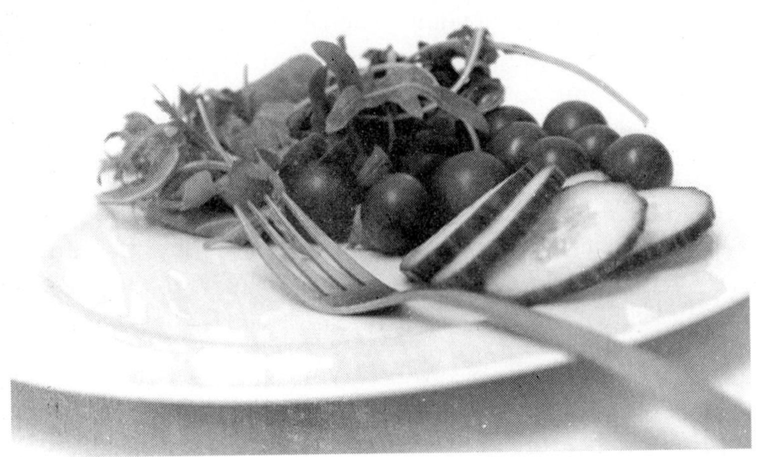

Raw foods like raw vegetables in the form of salad can help maintain good health and prevent diseases.

raw, uncooked fruits and raw vegetables are rich in mineral salts which are necessary for neutralizing acid waste products. In cooking foods, these mineral salts are lost to a large extent. Because of the large quantities of mineral salts they contain, in a form most suitable to the needs of the system, fresh fruits and raw vegetables are known as purifying foods. They possess eliminating, cleansing and healing properties.

Antioxidant Effects

The most important effect of raw foods on health is in its healing and preventive powers as disease-fighting dietary antioxidants. Many of the health problems are due to the perversity of oxygen. So far, scientists have linked destructive oxygen reactions to at least 60 different chronic diseases, as well as to ageing itself.

Raw foods like fresh fruits and raw vegetables, especially the deep coloured ones, contain strong antioxidants. When these foods are consumed in liberal quantities, the antioxidants contained in them are infused into the tissues and fluids where they can help resist the oxidant invasions. The dietary anti-oxidants can thus prevent all the damaging effects of oxidants on health.

Curative Power of Raw Foods

Hippocrates (460-357 B.C.), the father of medicine, said "let food be thy medicine and let medicine be thy food." The former part of the sentence is for the sick, the latter is for the healthy. For the sick, positive natural foods are the true medicine and not drugs, which are not conducive to health as all of them have adverse side-effects. For the healthy, natural foods are the means of freedom from disease. Hippocrats fully believed that natural foods have unlimited power to sustain health and restore it when lost.

There has been an increase in the variety of frequency of diseases in proportion to the process of the degeneration of food-stuffs through refining and cooking. Experiments conducted at various research laboratories throughout the world have clearly established the merit and value of raw foods in the treatment of several diseases. At the Royal Free Hospital in England, Dr. D.C. Hare put a group of arthritic patients on a totally raw food diet for two weeks and then a predominantly raw food diet for several more weeks. Practically all of the patients began to feel better within one to four weeks and marked improvement continued thereafter. Dr. W. Heupe, while working at the University Medical Polyclinic in Frankfurt, reported that a raw food diet aided in the treatment of diarrhoea of children, in heart and kidney diseases, and in obesity and diabetes.

The work of Dr. Kristine Nolfi of Denmark is most valuable in the field of healing through raw eating. She recovered from cancer after treating herself with an exclusive raw food diet and then opened an institution called Humlegaarden. Here, with great success she treated patients suffering from cancer and other diseases with exclusive diet of raw foods.

There is another important work of Dr. Joseph Evers of Germany in the field of healing through raw foods. He has treated successfully nearly 1,000 cases of multiple sclerosis with diets composed chiefly of raw vegetables, raw fruits, raw nuts, raw honey, raw grain sprouts, uncooked coarse rolled oats and whole meal bread.

The adoption of raw eating can thus free mankind from all diseases. Raw foods contain all the essential vitamins, minerals, trace elements and other constituents, whereas it is present in small amounts in refined and cooked foods.

CHAPTER 24

Wheat Grass: A Miracle Medicine

The wheat grass is a wonder plant. Dr. Ann Wigmore, the founder director of the Hippocrates Health Institute, Boston, U.S.A., is one of the proponents of the wheat grass therapy. According to her, "guided by spiritual mentality and nourished only by live uncooked food, the body will run indefinitely, unhampered by sickness." Dr. G.H. Earp-Thomas, a scientist and soil expert, isolated over one hundred elements from fresh wheat grass and concluded that it is a complete food.

Chlorophyll

The chief constituent of wheat grass is chlorophyll which nature utilises as a body cleanser, rebuilder and neutraliser of toxins. Dr. Fisher, a Noble Prize winner, used chlorophyll to treat, anaemia. As early as July, 1940, the American Journal of Surgery, reported 12,000 cases of peritonitis, brain ulcer, pyorrhoea and skin disorders cured by chlorophyll.

The chlorophyll molecule bears close resemblance to haemoglobin, the red pigmentation in human blood, and differs only in the central element which in blood is iron and in chlorophyll, magnesium. Owing to their close molecular resemblance, Frans Miller, another scientist, believed that chlorophyll is the natural blood building element for all plant eaters and humans.

Dr. Birscher, a research scientist, calls chlorophyll "concentrated sun power." According to him, "Chlorophyll increases the function of the heart, affects the vascular system,

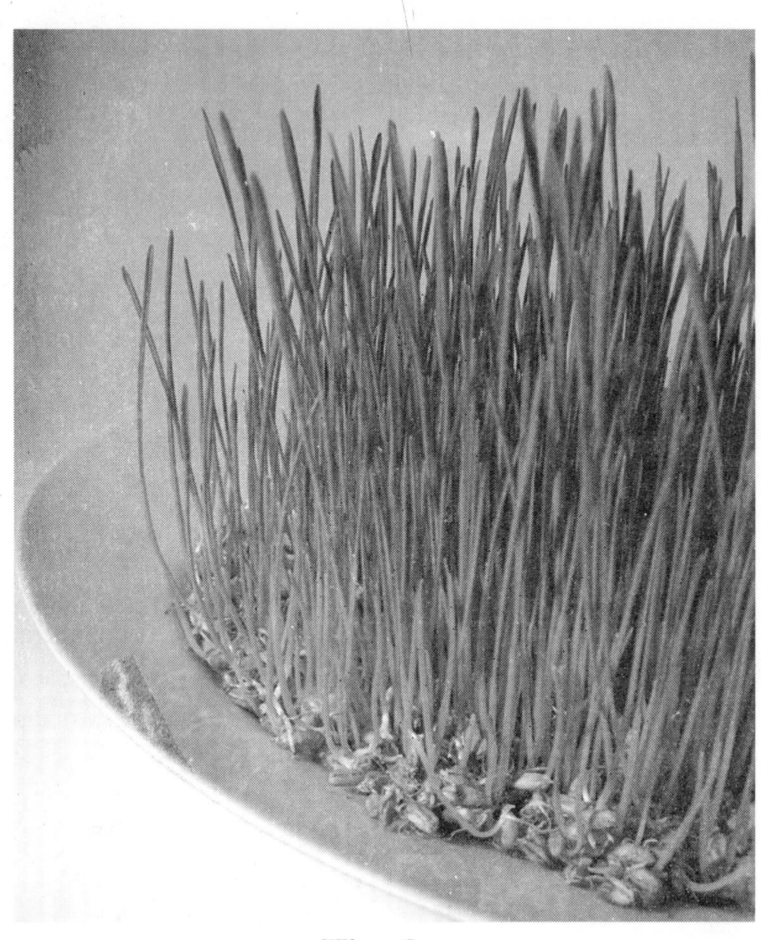

Wheat Grass

the intestines, the uterus and the lungs. It raises the basic nitrogen exchange and is therefore a tonic which, considering its stimulating properties, cannot be compared with any other."

Doctors Gurskin, Redpath and Davis at temple university used chlorophyll to successfully treat over one thousand patients for all forms of ear, nose and throat problems. Dr. Carroll Wright found chlorophyll effective in chronic ulcer.

Wheat Grass Juice Therapy

Wheat grass juice furnishes the body with vital nourishment, providing extra energy to the body. This juice contains nearly 70 per cent of chlorophyll. It is a rich source of vitamins A, B, C and contains minerals like calcium, iron, magnesium, phosphorus, potassium, sodium, sulphur, cobalt, and zinc. The chlorophyll contained in wheat grass juice is very beneficial for the body. It purifies the blood due to its high vitamin and mineral contents. This property is used by the body to cleanse and rebuild itself. By drinking this juice regularly, toxins can be neutralised. It thus helps to maintain good health.

Tooth Disorders

Wheat grass juice acts as an excellent mouth wash for sore throat and pyorrhoea. It also prevents tooth decay and toothache. It is therefore beneficial to chew wheat grass. By drawing out toxins from the gums, it checks bacterial growth.

Skin Diseases

It has been scientifically proved that chlorophyll arrests growth and development of harmful bacteria. Wheat grass therapy can thus be effectively used for skin diseases and ulcerated wounds. By retarding bacterial action, it promotes cell activity and normal regrowth. Regular drinking of wheat grass juice creates an unfavourable environment for bacterial growth. Poultice of wheat grass juice can be applied on the infected area, as it is an able sterilizer.

Digestive System Disorders

Wheat grass juice used as an enema helps detoxify the walls of the colon. The general procedure is to give an enema with lukewarm water. After waiting for 20 minutes, 100 to 125 ml.

of wheat grass juice enema is given. This should be retained for 15 minutes. This enema is very helpful in disorders of the colon, mucus, and ulcerative colitis, chronic constipation and bleeding piles.

Circulatory Disorders

The chlorophyll content present in wheat grass enhances heart and lung functions. Capillary activity also increases, while toxemia is reduced. By increasing iron content in the blood and thereby haemoglobin, lungs function better. Oxygeneration improves and the effect of carbon-dioxide is minimised. Wheat grass juice is thus highly beneficial in the treatment of circulatory disorders.

Other Diseases

Several other diseases can be treated successfully by regular drinking of wheat grass juice. These include: arthritis, psoriasis, premature greying and falling of hair, general weakness and debility, kidney stones, weak eyesight, abdominal pain, asthma, constipation and insomnia.

Many physicians at Hippocrates Health institute at Boston have tested the miraculous effectiveness of the wheat grass therapy. They have proved satisfactorily that wheat grass chlorophyll is a New Age food—medicine capable of alleviating the problems of sick humanity.

An exclusive diet of wheat grass can be used beneficially in treating diseases. In adopting this mode of treatment, the patient should undertake fast on wheat grass for seven days. This fast provides the body with all the nutrients of the richest living food in a form so concentrated and easy to digest that it provides virtually all the benefits of a complete fast with none of the dangers of total abstinence. Such a fast can pleasantly cleanse and nourish at the same time. One can be confident of complete safety and real health-building results.

To prepare for the wheat grass fast, it is essential for the patient to undertake repeated warm water enema so as to cleanse the body of accumulated waste products. It is necessary to eliminate this purification. The wheat grass fast consists of three or four wheat grass juice drinks each day plus two chlorophyll implants. If the patient does not like the taste or odour of the juice, he can take four implants instead of two, with same beneficial results.

Upon awakening, the patient should drink two glasses of warm water, mixed with the juice of one lemon and sweetened with molasses or honey. Then, the colon should be thoroughly evacuated with an enema to eliminate any debris clogging the inner walls of the colon. The patient should sip 120 ml of pure wheat grass chlorophyll three times a day at five-hourly intervals. Each drink may be diluted with water on 50 : 50 basis. While on wheat grass therapy, the patient should drink at least one litre of not-too-cold water each day, placing a small bunch of wheat-grass in each drink to purify it.

The patient may experience weakness during the wheat grass fast for one day or more. The quickest and most effective way to meet this crisis is to drink sesame milk. This drink is high in protein and calcium and should alleviate the sense of weakness.

While continuing the wheat grass juice fast, the patient would experience changes in the body. He may lose weight to the extent of 750 grams every day. To those overweight individuals who frequently experience digestive disorders, the wheatgrass fast provides their digestive systems a much needed rest.

During wheat grass fast, the chlorophyll will bring toxins stored away in cells or in fatty tissue into the bloodstream and then eliminate. This cleansing action may be accompanied by nausea, headache, fever and cramps. The patient should not get alarmed, but simply lie down and rest until he feels better. Relief may be obtained by chewing a little celery. Plenty of rest is essential during the cleansing period to enable the body to divest itself of the toxic accumulations resulting from wrong eating, medications and other abuses.

The wheat grass chlorophyll is very rapidly assimilated by the body. It can actually save human life when oral feeding is impossible. The colon is cleansed simultaneously, and, as is well known, most health problems begin in the colon. Constipation can be relieved by warm water enema or colonic massage. During wheat grass therapy, the patient should take sponge baths of warm water daily, followed by body rubs with a rough cloth to help circulation.

Immersing the feet in warm water for 15 to 20 minutes each day helps to eliminate the poisons from the system which the gravity has pulled down to the feet and ankles. It also aids in relaxation. Massage is also helpful.

How to Grow and Use Wheat grass

Wheatgrass can be grown in any sheltered place where the direct rays of the sun do not reach from about 11 a.m. to 3 p.m. and where the temperature is mild. The direct rays of the sun have a tendency to sap the strength from the grass. The round stalks flatten out and become limp. The chlorophyll seems to lack vigour compared to the chlorophyll extracted from grass protected from the direct rays of the sun.

For growing wheat grass a good variety of wheat should be soaked for eight to 10 hours. The water should then be

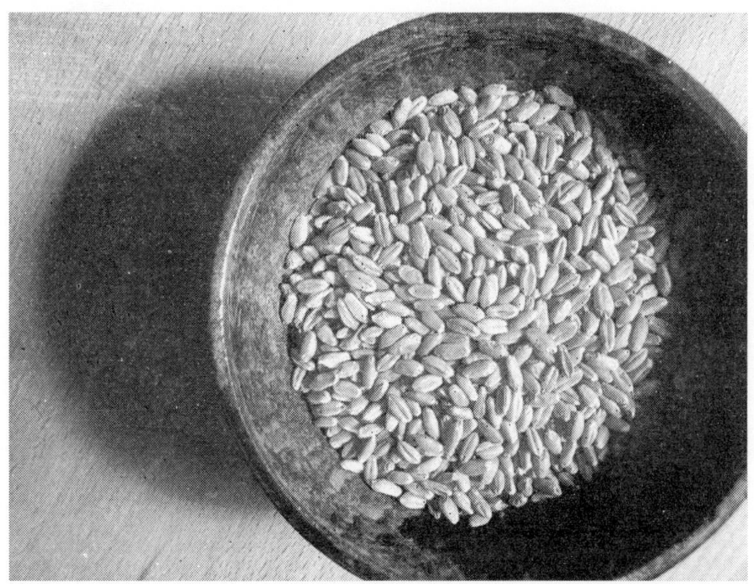

Ideally wheat should be soaked for atleast eight to ten hours for a good variety of wheat grass.

drained and those grains allowed to sprout for 15 hours. Earthen pots or wooden trays can be used to grow the wheat grass. They should be filled with compost manure and the wheat sprouts should be spared. They should be covered with a dark cloth or kept away from the sunlight in a room. They should be sprinkled with water once or twice a day and allowed to stay as such for six to seven days the grass grows five to seven inches high.

The grass can be cut with a scissor. It should be immediately washed and ground. Thereafter, the juice of the ground pulp should be extracted through a fine piece of cloth. To derive maximum advantage, the pulp should be ground and the juice extracted for two or three times. The juice so extracted should be taken immediately, as its efficacy reduces every minute and the medicinal value is completely lost after three hours.

CHAPTER 25

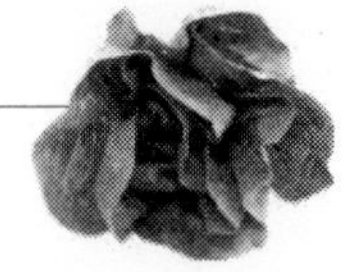

Health Hazards of Three White Products

There is a growing tendency in modern times to make the articles of diet as artificial and pleasing to the eye and tasty to the tongue, without any regard to their ultimate effect on health. This had led to the refining and demineralising of cereals and sugar and addition of salt to various foodstuffs to make them tasty and delicious. Fortunately, there is realisation now among the enlightened people that the artificial and concentrated dietary, to a large extent, is responsible for the vast array of present day diseases.

Foods such as bread, cereals and sugar are very acid-forming, if eaten in the refined state as white bread, white sugar and polished rice. But these foods are far less acid-forming in character if eaten in the natural state as natural brown sugar, whole meal bread and natural brown rice. Similarly, the excessive use of salt also leads to the formation of acids in the body.

Of the various artificial foodstuffs being used today for their delicious taste, white flour, sugar and salt, known as three Ws (white products) have been found especially harmful. They constitute serious health hazards and their excessive consumption can lead to several degenerative diseases. Their harmful effects are discussed in this chapter.

White Flour

Wheat is the most common cereal used throughout the world for making bread. It is a good source of energy. With its essential coating of bran, vitamins and minerals, it is an excellent health-building food.

The wheat grain is a seed which consists of three main parts, namely, the various outer coverings, endosperm and the germ or embryo. The outer coverings contain much indigestible fibre. Beneath them is the aleurone layer which is rich in protein. Inside is the endosperm which consists of an inner and outer portion. The germ or embryo which consists of the shoot and root. It is attached to the grain by a special structure, the scutellum.

The germ of the wheat is relatively rich in protein, fat and several of the B vitamins. So is the scutellum which contains 50 times more thiamine then the whole grain. The outer layers of the endosperm and the aleurone layer contain a higher concentration of protein, vitamins and phytic acid than the inner endosperm. The inner endosperm contains most of the starch and protein in the grain.

Wheat is usually ground into flour before use as food. In ancient times, wheat grains were crushed between two large stones. This method preserved all parts of the kernel and the product was called "whole wheat". If it is finely ground, it becomes whole wheat flour. The value of stone grinding is that the grain is ground slowly and it remains unheated, and a whole food. In modern times, steel roller mills have superseded stone grinding. These mills ground wheat hundred times faster, but they impoverish the flour by removing the precious wheat germ resulting in colossal loss in vitamins and minerals in the refining process. The following tables show the food value of various types of wheat (per cent per 100 grams).

Type of Wheat	Moisture gm	Protein gm	Fat gm	Minerals gm	Fibre gm	Carbohydrates gm	Energy gm
Wheat (whole)	12.8	11.8	1.5	1.5	1.2	71.2	346
Wheat Flour (whole)	12.2	12.1	1.7	2.7	1.9	69.4	341
Wheat Flour (refined)	13.3	11.0	0.9	0.6	0.3	73.9	348
Wheat Germ	5.2	29.2	7.4	3.5	1.4	53.5	397

Type of Wheat	Carotene Mcg.	Thiamine Mg.	Riboflavin Mg.	Niacin Mg.	Calcium Mg.	Phosphorus Mg.	Iron Mg.
Wheat (whole)	64	0.45	0.17	5.5	41	306	4.9
Wheat Flour (whole)	29	0.49	0.29	4.3	48	355	11 5
Wheat Flour (refined)	25	0.12	0.07	2.4	23	121	2.5

In the refining process of whole wheat, the precious wheat germ is destroyed. By doing so we remove the very life of the grain of wheat, because locked in the wheat germ is an oil which is man's greatest food. The wheat germ also contains all-important vitamin E, known as the anti-sterility factor of sex vitamin. The lack of this vitamin can also lead to heart diseases. The colossal loss of vitamins and minerals in the refined wheat flour has led to widespread prevalence of constipation and other digestive disturbances and nutritional disorders.

White Sugar

Sugar is the most common sweet carbohydrate used all over the world. There are many varieties of sugar, but only a few are included, to a considerable extent, in our diet. These are sucrose or cane sugar, dextrose or grape sugar, levulose or fruit sugar and lactose or milk sugar. Natural sugar contained in fruits is called fructose.

Cane sugar, also called the white sugar, is produced in enormous quantities. It is derived commercially from the sugar cane and beet root. When it is eaten, it is slowly converted into levulose and dextrose, for it cannot be utilised by the body in its native form. It must first undergo a digestive process as does starch. But, unlike starch, the digestion of cane sugar does not begin in the mouth, but is delayed until the sugar reaches the intestine.

There has been enormous increase in the consumption of sugar all over the world. Commensurate with the sharp rise of sugar consumption, there has been an alarming increase in the incidence of several diseases. There is mounting evidence from many medical sources that white sugar is extremely injurious to health. The heat and chemical process employed in the sugar refinery kills the vitamins and separates the mineral elements, protein and other substances from the sap, leaving nothing but pure sugar crystals, robbed of mineral elements and the life-sustaining vitamins.

White sugar has many great disadvantages. It is irritating and it is difficult to digest. It is called the vitamin-thief. Its high intake can rob the body of its vitamins made available to it by consumption of other foods. Excessive use of white sugar leads to gastric catarrh and hyperacidity. It is also associated with obesity, dental caries, diabetes and coronary heart diseases.

The white sugar supplies only calories without any nutritive value. It contains as many as 300 calories per 100 grams. It has been estimated that 90 per cent of overweight persons consume much more sugar than required. Eating sugar adds to calories. These are stored in the form of fat.

Another problem with sweet foods is that they can easily be overeaten because of their delicious taste. Cakes, pastries, biscuits and chocolates are some of the items that have a high sugar content and therefore have many calories. For instance, half a small bar of chocolate provides same amount of calories as five apples, but it does not contain the nutrients and fibre that the fruit provides. Thus, if two apples are eaten, it gives a sense of satisfaction due to its fibre content and less calories are ingested. On the other hand, while eating chocolates or sweets, more and more can be eaten without a sense of fullness and therefore more calories are ingested, leading to obesity.

The most harmful effects of sugar is on the teeth. It dissolves quickly in saliva and finds its way into the bacterial layer on the teeth, known as plaque. It feeds on sugar and converts it to acid. This acid eats away the enamel and causes cavities. This acid is produced within seconds of the sugar entering the mouth and attacks the tooth enamel as long as the sugar remains in contact with the teeth. For this reason, both the amount of sugar eaten and its frequency during the day, are important. Sugary foods like biscuits, cakes, fruits and drinks, taken often between the meals, therefore, play an important part in development of tooth decay. Sticky foods such as toffee, dry fruits that cling to the teeth are particularly harmful.

Dr. D.T. Quigley, M.D., an eminent medical authority, says, "Sugar is a concentrated carbohydrate, containing no vitamin or mineral of any kind. Every ounce of sugar that is taken reduces the ability to resist infection, as it furnishes only calories and none of the elements which protect against infection."

Natural sugars such as brown sugar, jaggery, unsulphured dark molasses and honey are preferable to refined white sugar, because they possess some vitamins and minerals. Raw honey also contains enzymes.

White Salt

Man's need for sodium chloride, the chemical name for the common salt, has been a subject of dispute since the beginning of medical practice. The first known salt mines have been found in the Austrian Tyrol and date from the late Bronze Age, about 1,000 B.C. It is not known accurately when man first began to use salt. However, salt was available in the early civilisations and Homer called it 'divine'.

Sodium Chloride is a chemical compound found in the sea, soil and it also occurs naturally in food. It is made up of two chemicals, namely, sodium, an element which never occurs in free form in nature, 40 per cent and chloride 60 per cent.

Sodium chloride is a major factor in maintaining acid-base equilibrium of the body. It is also needed for the working of various nerve impulses. It can help prevent catarrh. It promotes a clear brain, resulting in a better disposition and less mental fag. Because of its influence on calcium, sodium can also help dissolve any stones forming within the body—in the kidneys, urinary bladder and gall bladder. It is also essential for the production of hydrochloric acid in the stomach.

Thus, a certain amount of salt in the system is essential for life, but it is required in very small amounts, ranging from 10 to 15 grams daily, depending on the climate and occupation of the person. Many people, however, use too much salt. This puts an extra burden on the kidneys and may cause high blood pressure.

Too much salt in the body can result in oedema or swelling of the legs and ankles. This is due to incomplete elimination of salt through the kidneys. The blood pressure may rise and may not go down again until the excess sodium has been removed from the body.

Intake of too much salt can attract water, creating an artificial thirst. So a person drinks enormous quantities of water and this leads to obesity in due course. Excessive intake of salt can also lead to stomach ulcer, stomach cancer, hardening of arteries and heart diseases.

The adverse effects of excessive use of sodium chloride can be rectified by avoiding the use of common salt. Even foods rich in salt such as salted nuts, biscuits, meat, fish, chicken, egg, cheese, dried fruits, spinach, carrot and radish should be avoided. However, low-sodium foods like cereals, sugar, honey, fresh fruits, brinjals, cabbage, cauliflower, tomatoes, potatoes, onions, peas and pumpkin can be used.

It will also be advisable to omit salt altogether in case of all chronic diseases like high blood pressure, arthritis and allergies. In case total avoidance is not possible, it may be added in a very small quantity after cooking. This will prevent it from getting into every particle of the food, which will happen if salt is added before cooking. Salt added after cooking will be just superficial only to satisfy the taste.

CHAPTER 26

Health Hazards of Excessive Tea

Tea is one of the most widely consumed drinks. It is taken mainly as a hot drink for its stimulating effect. It helps to get over a tired feeling and one feels refreshed after drinking it. This reputation leads to tea drinking habit which in course of time becomes so deep rooted that it is difficult to give it up after some time.

The most active alkaloid principle in tea is caffeine. This is an addictive drug similar to cocaine in as much as it stimulates the central nervous system. These effects are short-lived but it has been observed that they lead to withdrawal symptoms of irritability, lethargy, headaches, anxiety and insomnia. This shows that it is quite a strong drug to constitute a potential health hazard.

The wide-spread consumption of tea is a striking example of the manner in which commercial forces cultivate poisonous habits in man for a profit. It is believed that almost a billion cups of tea per day are consumed all over the world. In India, even slogans like Roz Chai Piyo, Bauhat Din Jiyo (drink tea daily and live longer) were invented by the vested interests to mislead common people to believe that tea gives strength and vitality.

Tea is prepared from the leaves of an evergreen shrub belonging to Camellia family. The plant is native of South East Asia. In ancient times, the leaves were probably eaten or boiled into a beverage. The earliest record of its cultivation comes from China in the fourth century A.D. By the eighth century, it was quite popular in China and established in Japan. Over

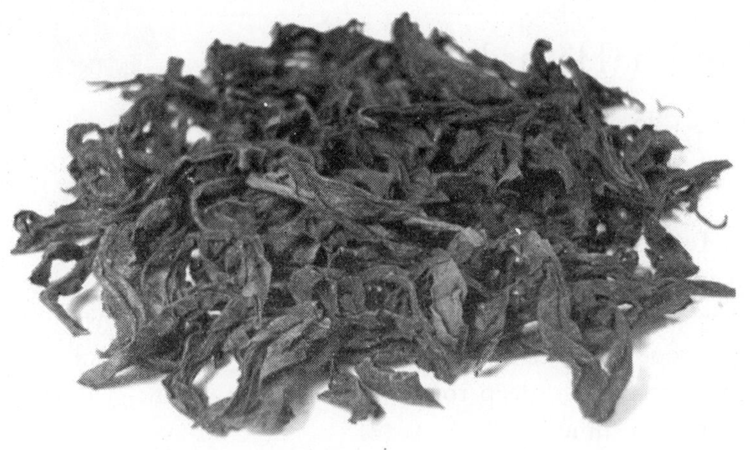

The use of tea is detrimental to health.

the next 600 years or so, the method of infusing tea in water slowly evolved.

Tea was not a popular drink in India even as late as 1940. The second world war brought about a sharp rise in the prices of commodities all over the world, including India, owing to the scarcity of food. As a result, the common man could not afford milk, due to six-fold increase in its price. Deprived of this nutritious food, they turned to tea as a substitute.

Composition

To ascertain the effect of tea on health, it is essential to know the chemical composition of tea leaves. On an average they contain moisture 5.0 to 8.0 per cent, aromatic oils 0.5 per cent, caffeine 2.5 to 5.0 per cent, nitrogen 4.75 to 5.5 per cent, soluble matter 38.0 to 45.0 per cent, tannin 7.0 to 14.0 per cent and minerals 5.0 to 5.75 per cent.

Of these ingredients, the most important are the alkaloids caffeine tannin and a small proportion of aromatic oil. The chief effects of tea are due to these ingredients. It is well-known that Indian tea is richer in all these chief ingredients than the Chinese tea.

It is not the composition of leaves alone that affects the health, but also the composition of infusion which is prepared by boiling tea with water. It is noted that caffeine comes out more rapidly than tannin and hence greater the period of infusion, the more is the amount of tannin, while the amount of caffeine will remain almost the same.

Harmful Effects

The use of tea is detrimental to health. Dr. P.C. Roy, the father of modern chemistry in India, equated tea drinking with the drinking of poison. The stimulating and restorative effects of tea are due to the action of caffeine on the nervous system. It affects the higher cerebral or psychic centres more than centres located in modulla and spinal cord. This results in heightening of intellectual faculties, relieving a feeling of fatigue and increasing the capacity for physical and mental work.

The harmful effects of tea in case of certain specific diseases are discussed herein in brief.

Indigestion

Tea is said to slow down digestion. Its daily intake causes indigestion as it impedes the action of 'ptyalin', a digestive ferment of saliva which acts on cooked starch. The inhibition of saliva seems to be due to tannin. This effect disappears if milk is added to it, as the protein of milk precipates the tannin. Tea is also said to delay stomach digestion. It can lead to gas formation, diarrhoea and constipation.

Kidney Disorders

A definite effect of caffeine in dieursis. Experiments show

that caffeine in five cups of tea increases the urine by 400 to 500 per cent. This continued stimulation of kidneys by caffeine may damage them. Tea may also promote kidney stones because of high content of oxalate.

Premenstrual Syndrome

Drinking tea can aggravate the symptoms of PMS. This was discovered by Dr. Annette Rossignol, an associate professor of public health at Oregon State University. He noted that women in China who drank one-half to four cups of tea a day were twice as likely to have PMS as non-tea drinkers. Drinking eight cups a day increased their PMS incidence about tenfold.

Incontinence

Drinking excess tea lead to incontinence or frequent and urgent impulse to urinate. In a study conducted at St. George's Hospital in London, it was discovered that caffeine can exert pressure on the bladder by causing the muscles surrounding it to contract, increasing the need to urinate in some incontinent individuals.

The respiratory and cardiac centres are also stimulated by caffeine as coronary arteries get dilated, resulting in an increase in the rate of blood flow. It is also said to increase the blood sugar level. The quickening of respiration lowers the level of carbonoxide and increases the heat production of the body by 10 to 20 per cent.

It is thus clear that tea, if taken in excess, causes indigestion, over excitability of the nervous system, irritability, palpitation and sometimes prostration. To minimize the harmful effects of tea, it should be infused by pouring boiling water over the leaves and the tea be allowed to draw for about four to five minutes, then the liquid should be poured into another pot. Mint and lemon grass should be added. This will help in relieving stomach disorders like flatulence and supply vitamins.

CHAPTER 27

Health Hazards of Coffee

Like tea, coffee is also one of the most widely consumed drinks all over the world. It is stimulant and helps get over a feeling of tiredness and fatigue. This leads to coffee drinking habit which is difficult to leave in course of time.

Most of the coffee's pharmacological impact comes from its high concentration of caffeine a psychoactive drug of great power, and the most active alkaloid principle in it. This is an addictive drug similar to cocaine in as much as it stimulates the central nervous system. These effects are short-lived, but it has been observed that they lead to withdrawal symptoms of irritability, lethargy, headaches and anxiety. This shows that it is quite a strong drug to constitute a potential health hazard. If taken in excess, it may cause psychiatric disturbances.

Coffee beans are the seeds of coffee trees that are widely cultivated in the tropics. There are a variety of coffee trees. Most of them are 10 to 15 ft. high, with evergreen leaves. Shade trees are necessary to protect them from excessive sun. They bear clusters of white flowers which develop into the beans. There are large plantations in India, Indonesia, Africa and Brazil.

Coffee is a native of Africa, where it has been cultivated for ages on the slopes of Abyssinia facing the Red Sea. The coffee tree crossed the sea and found its way into Arabia in the 15th century. The world derives its famous Mocha coffee from there.

Coffee drinking spread very rapidly in the East but entered

Europe more slowly. It was imported into England about 1652. But it was not until the 18th century that coffee drinking was generally adopted. It is, however, about two centuries, since it became an article of general consumption by the people of Europe. In the United States, about 96 per cent of the families drink coffee daily.

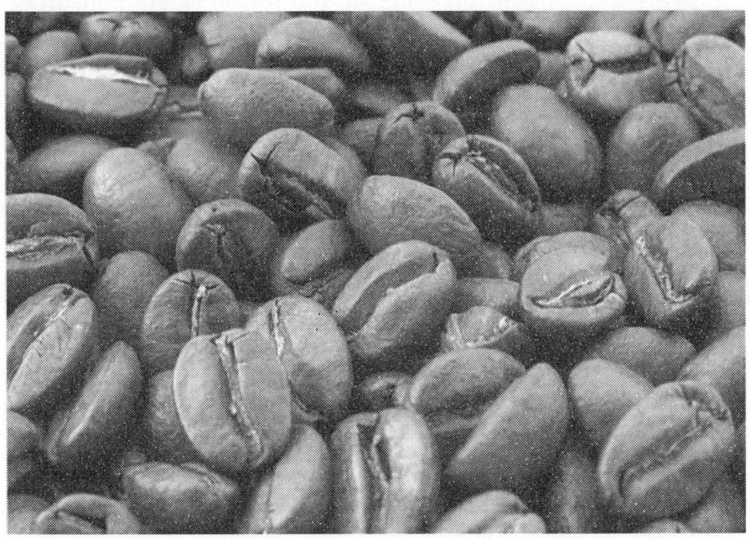

The most common side-effects of coffee are nervousness, irritability, heart palipitation and insomnia

Harmful Effects

Coffee is injurious to health. It is a more stimulating beverage than tea, as it contains greater amount of the active alkaloid principle, caffeine. Sir Robert Hutchison, an eminent nutrionist, found about 100 mg. of caffeine and 200 mg. of tannin in a cupful of coffee, made by infusing 69 g. in 450 ml of water.

Research studies have shown that coffee drinking has potential health hazards. They have linked it to heart disease, cancer, and even birth defects. The most common side-effects of coffee are nervousness, irritability, heart palpitation and insomnia. Some people experience a post-stimulation letdown that can make them as tired and lethargic as they were alert and energetic immediately after drinking. Herein are discussed in brief certain specific diseases which are caused or aggravated by excessive use of coffee.

Heart Disease

The most recent study on coffee's role in heart disease, done at Stanford University, found that sedentary men between 30 and 55, who drink three cups of coffee or more a day, may be at higher risk of developing heart disease than those who drink less coffee. A ten-year follow-up study of more than 1,00,000 individuals by Kaiser Permanent's Dr Klatsky suggested that four or more cups of coffee a day boosted chances of heart disease about 30 per cent in man and up to 60 per cent in women.

Dyspepsia

Coffee can bring an dyspepsia. The researchers at University of Michigan studied 55 people with this problem and found that half of them suffered digestive distress after drinking two cups of coffee a day. Even drinking decafeinated coffee caused indigestion. The researchers concluded that it may be due to acid in the coffee.

Constipation

Caffeine in coffee can contribute to constipation in some persons. One survey of 15,000 men and women by University of North Carolina researchers noted that those who were often constipated drank more coffee. This is attributable to the fact that the nerves of the colon may come to tolerate the constant stimulant effect of coffee and caffeine, and thus become sluggish, just as they often do when people become over dependent on stimulant-type laxatives. Another possible reason is that caffeine acts as a diuretic, disturbing the body fluid balance by drawing fluids out of the gut where they are needed to soften the stool. Thus the stools stay hard and become difficult to expel.

Diarrhoea

The use of coffee can also cause diarrhoea in some persons with sensitive colon. According to a British test, even a single cup of coffee, either caffeinated or decaffeinated, can stimulate muscle contractions in the bowel in at least one-third of the population. Further, caffeine is a diuretic that tends to rob the body of fluids that are most needed in diarrhoea. Thus, drinking coffee may induce or aggravate diarrhoea.

Gall Stones

Coffee can stimulate the gall bladder to bring about gall bladder attacks. This has been discovered by Bruce R. Douglas and his colleagues at the University Hospital in Leiden, Netherland. The Dutch investigators found in a test of healthy normal men and women that drinking as little as 115 ml. of decaffeinated coffee stimulated gall bladder contractions. The researchers advise people prone to gallstones to avoid all types of coffee.

Osteoporosis

Caffeine in coffee can cause osteoporosis by promoting excretion of calcium, thereby robbing bones of the minerals. A look at 3,170 older men and women, who participated in the famous Framingham Heart Study, indicated that two or more cups of coffee a day boosted the chances of breaking a hip by about 50 per cent. A recent Harvard study of 84,000 middle-aged women found that, those who drank more than four cups of coffee a day were about three times more likely to suffer hip fractures than women who drank little or no coffee.

Premenstrual Syndrome

Coffee drinking can lead to premenstrual syndrome which can become quite disabling to cause upset in life. Dr. Annette Rossignol, an associate professor of public health and Oregon State University, conducted a study of 841 female American students and found that those consuming caffeine in a cup of coffee per day were more prone to PMS. The more caffeine they consumed, the more severe their PMS symptoms.

Women's Other Problems

There are a number of studies that indicate a link between coffee and tea drinking and fibrocrystic breast disease, a condition characterised by benign breast lumps. Women with these conditions should therefore refrain from drinking these beverages. In 1994, The Journal of the American Medical Association reported that miscarriage and low-birthweight were linked to women's reported caffeine intake during pregnancy. This new study found that even the caffeine in a cup and a half of coffee could double the risk of miscarriage in the first trimester.

Research studies conducted by the University of California, San Diego, also indicate that women who drank a cup or more of coffee a day, were found to have significantly lower bone-density after they reached menopause.

Coffee should be completely given up by those suffering from peptic ulcer, heartburn and other gastro-intestinal disorders such as esophageal reflux, as it promotes gastric-acid secretion. People with hypertension, heart disease and anemia should also avoid coffee-drinking. It inhibits the absorption of iron. Researchers at Yale University recently found that caffeine produces a more pronounced reaction in people who have panic episodes than in normal healthy people.

To reduce the adverse effects of coffee on health, it should be prepared by drip method in which the brewed coffee goes through a filter or by percolator. Methods have been devised to remove most of the caffeine from coffee, making it caffeineless coffee. Coffee substitutes are made from roasted cereals. They resemble coffee in the bitter taste and aroma. Cereal coffee are wholesome and are used extensively by healthy-minded people and by those desirous of breaking the coffee habit.

Part III

Diseases and Their Natural Treatment

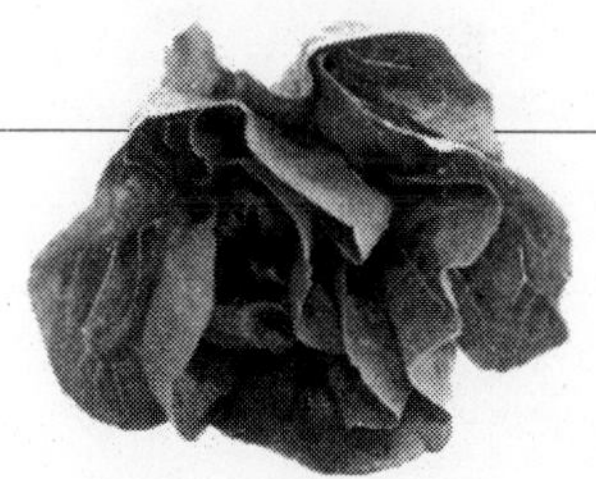

CHAPTER 28

Acne

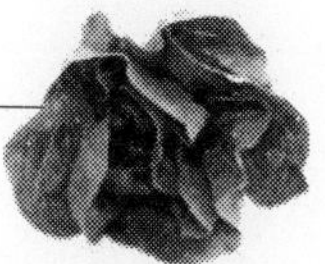

Acne is perhaps the most common chronic skin disease. It is an inflammatory condition of the sebaceous (that is fat or grease) glands and hair follicles usually found on the face, the neck, chest and shoulders. Nearly eight out of ten young people between the ages of 12 and 24 suffer from some degree of acne. It is closely related to the disturbance in the hormones experienced at puberty.

The majority of patients recover between the ages 20 and 30 years. But it is still common in men over 30 years. In women, it rarely lasts beyond the early thirties and is normally worse before each menstrual period. The disease causes a great deal of embarrassment at an age when people tend to be sensitive about personal appearance.

The skin, covering the entire body, is a marvellous and intricate mechanism. It serves three main purposes; namely, protection of the inner organism, regulation of body temperature and elimination of cell waste and systemic refuse. The skin is directly connected with and intimately bound up with the working of the whole system. All skin diseases, including acne, are the outcome of malfunctioning of the body as a whole.

Symptoms

Acne is characterized by the presence of comedones or blackheads, pimples, small superficial sebaceous cysts and scars. There are over half a dozen forms of acne. All of them

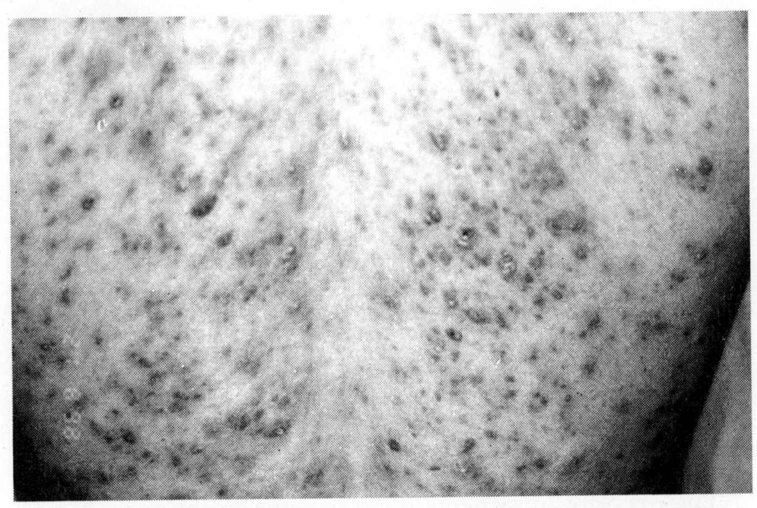

Acne vulgaris showing severe scarring on back.

are concerned with sebaceous glands or the glands connected with hair follicles. The most common form of acne is blackheads. The areas chiefly affected are the forehead, temples, cheeks, and chin, the chest and back. In rare cases, almost the entire body may be covered with blackheads with extensive scarring.

Causes

All forms of acne have their origin in wrong feeding habits, such as irregular hours of eating, improper food, excesses of starches and sugar, excess of fatty foods. Chronic constipation is another major cause of acne. If the bowels do not move properly, waste matter is not eliminated as quickly as it should be and the bloodstream becomes surcharged with toxic matter. The extra efforts of the skin to eliminate excess waste result in acne and other forms of skin disease. Yet another important cause of acne is a devitalised condition of the skin resulting from unhygienic living habits. Other causes of the disorder are excessive use of tea, coffee, alcohol or tobacco, strenuous studies, masturbation and sedentary habits which lead to indigestion and general debility.

Treatment

The treatment of acne by the administration of salve or ointment does not serve any purpose. They only suppress the action of the sebaceous glands temporarily. In nature cure, the main emphasis is on diet and certain water applications. To begin with the patient should resort to an all-fruit diet for about a week. In this regimen, there should be three meals a day, consisting of fresh juicy fruits, such as apples, pears, grapes, grape-fruit, pineapple and peaches. Citrus fruits, bananas, dried, stewed or tinned fruits should not be taken. Unsweetened lemon or plain water, either hot or cold, should be drunk and nothing else. During this period, warm-water enema should be taken daily to cleanse the bowels and ail other measures adopted to eradicate constipation.

After a week of all fruit diet, the patient can gradually adopt a well-balanced diet. Emphasis should be on raw foods, especially fresh fruits and vegetables, sprouted seeds, raw nuts and whole grain cereals, especially millet and brown rice. Further shorter periods on the all-fruits for three days or so may be necessary at a monthly interval till the condition of the skin improves.

Strict attention to diet is essential for recovery. Starchy, protein and fatty foods should be restricted. Meats, sugar, strong tea or coffee, condiments, pickles, refined and processed foods should all be avoided, as also soft drinks, candies, ice cream and products made with sugar and white flour.

Two vitamins, namely, niacin and vitamin A have been used successfully to treat acne. The vitamin therapy which may comprise niacin, 100 mg. three times daily and vitamin A in large doses upto 1,50,000 units per day should not exceed one month. Vitamin E is also vitally important to prevent scarring from acne and in removing old scars.

Another effective remedy in the realm of nutrition that seems to offer new promise of help for acne is zinc. It has shown dramatic results in some cases. Zinc should be taken in therapeutic doses of 50 mg. three times a day. After noticeable improvement it can be gradually reduced.

Local Treatment

As regards local treatment, hot fomentation should be applied to open up the pores and squeeze out the waste matter. Then rinse with cold water. Sun and air baths by exposing the whole body to sun and air are highly beneficial. The healing packs made of grated cucumber, oatmeal cooked in milk, and cooked, creamed carrots used externally, have been found to be effective.

The orange peel is valuable in the treatment of acne. The peel, pounded well with water on a piece of stone, should be applied to the affected areas. The lemon has also proved beneficial in removing pimples and acne. It should be applied regularly.

A teaspoonful of coriander juice, mixed with a pinch of turmeric powder, is another effective home remedy for pimples and blackheads. The mixture should be applied to the face after thoroughly washing it, every night before retiring.

The juice of raw potatoes, has also proved very valuable in clearing skin blemishes. This cleansing results from high content of potassium, sulphur, phosphorus and chlorine in the potato. These elements are, however, of value only when the potato is raw as in this state they are composed of live organic atoms.

A hot Epsom-salt bath twice a week will be highly beneficial in all cases of acne. This bath is prepared by adding one and a half kg. of Epsom-salt to 50 litres of water having a temperature of about 100°F. The patient should remain in the bath from 25 to 35 minutes till he perspires freely. After the bath the patient should cool off gradually.

CHAPTER 29

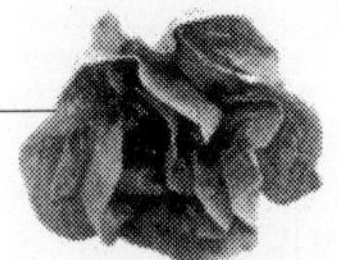

Alcoholism

Alcoholism refers to addiction to alcohol. It is a chronic disorder, in which a person is unable to refrain from frequent and excessive consumption of alcohol for physical or psychological reasons. The World Health Organisation (WHO) has listed alcoholism as one of the three most deadly killer diseases of the 20th century.

Alcoholism is also one of the most serious social problems. It often brings poverty and certain amount of crime and results in marital unhappiness and broken homes. It also leads to numerous traffic accidents.

Alcohol is not a product found in nature. It results from decomposition and as such belongs to a family of poisons. Ethyl alcohol, the main intoxicating ingredient in wine, beer and distilled liquor is a toxic drug which depresses the brain and nervous system. Alcohol cannot be called a food for it enters the alimentary canal and is not changed or digested in any way. It is quickly absorbed in the bloodstream and then travels to every part of the body, adversely affecting vital organs like brain and liver.

Symptoms

According to the WHO, "Alcoholics are those excessive drinkers whose dependence on alcohol has attained such a degree that it shows a noticeable mental disturbance or interference with their bodily or mental health, their interpersonal relations and their smooth social and economic functions, or who show the prodromal signs of such development."

Alcoholics have a puffy face with bloodshot eyes, a hoarse voice and a rapid pulse. They are suspicious, irritable and over-emotional. Vomiting, delirium, impaired judgement and disturbed sleep are some of the other symptoms.

The chronic alcoholic, who would rather drink than eat; fails to get enough vitamins. The few vitamins acquired by him are drained out of his system in the process of burning the alcohol in his body. Vitamin deficiency can lead to delirium tremors, convulsions, neuritis, disorders of the eyes and impaired memory. Excessive drinking often causes premature greying of hair due to vitamin deficiency. Chronic alcoholism results in a depletion of minerals in the body, particularly magnesium. Its lack produces symptoms like tremor of the hands, feet and tongue, convulsions, mental clouding and perspiration.

Excessive drinking imposes a strain on the liver. It gradually destroys its functions and often causes cirrhosis of the liver. It leads to disorders of the stomach and bowels. It can cause brain damage as brain cells are often affected by it. Alcohol also affects the heart which becomes weak and flabby.

Causes

Alcoholism results from intemperate drinking. Sometimes it sneaks upon a person comparatively rapidly; other times, years may pass before a person becomes a full-fledged alcoholic. A weak-minded person consoles himself by taking to drugs or alcohol. In doing so he simply tries to escape the situation rather than face it boldly.

A person generally takes to drinking as a means to enliven social life, to overcome anxiety or to induce sleep. He becomes an alcoholic if he gets dependent on alcohol physically and psychologically. He resorts to heavy drinking because of his maladaptive way of dealing with life's stresses.

Treatment

The chronic alcoholic first of all must make a firm resolve to stop drinking. He should abstain from alcohol all at once for the habit cannot be got rid of in gradual stages.

The most effective way to treat alcoholism is to build the body's nutritional integrity so as to prevent craving for stimulants like drinks. The patients should be put on a cleansing juice fast for at least 10 days in the beginning. During this period, he should have juice of an orange every two hours from 8 a.m. to 8 p.m. The juice may be diluted with warm water, if desired. If orange juice does not agree, vegetable juices may be taken. Each day while fasting, bowels should be cleansed of effete and poisonous matter thrown off by the self-cleansing process set up by the body. This can be achieved by warm water enema.

During the juice fast, the patient will usually feel no craving for alcohol. This will give a good 10-day start towards breaking the drinking habit and would help remove not only the physical dependence but also the psychological factors. After the initial fast on juices, the optimum diet of vital nutrients is essential. Such a diet should consist of whole grains, cereals, nuts, seeds and sprouts, fresh fruits and vegetables.

It is advisable that in the beginning of the treatment, the patient is given a suitable substitute to relieve the craving if and when such a craving occurs. The best substitute drink for alcohol is a glass of fresh fruit juice, sweetened with honey, if desired. In the alternative, wholesome candy may be taken. The patient should always have easily available juices, candy or other snacks to be taken between meals if he feels a craving for a stimulant.

All refined foods such as sugar, white rice, macaroni products and white flour and meat should be avoided. The patient should eat several small meals a day in preference to two or three large ones and avoid strong condiments such as pepper, mustard and chilli. He should not smoke as this will only increase his desire for alcohol.

Apples are considered valuable in the treatment of alcoholism as their, use removes intoxication and reduces the craving for wines and other intoxicating liquors. The raw celery juice is also considered useful. It has a sobering effect and is an antidote to alcohol.

In addition to proper nutrition, plenty of rest and outdoor exercise are necessary. The healthy condition of the appetite centre, which controls the craving for alcohol is improved by exercise. Yogic asans for general health such as padmasan, vajrasan, vakrasan, paschimotanasan, yogamudra, bhujangasan, halasan and shalabhasana and yogic kriyas like jalneti, kunjal and simple Pranayamas like kapalbhati, anuloma-viloma, shitali and sitkari will be beneficial.

Copious drinking of water, hot fomentations on the stomach and abdomen with a wet girdle pack between applications are also effective water treatments for alcoholism.

And finally, it will be advisable to follow the ten commandments to prevent alcoholism, offered by psychiatrist Dr. William B. Terhune. These are:

never drink when you "need one";

sip slowly;

space your drinks, taking a second drink 30 minutes after the first and a third an hour after the second;

dilute your alcohol;

keep an accurate and truthful record of the amount and number of drinks you take;

never conceal the amount of alcohol you drink;

do not drink on an empty stomach;

stop drinking on "signal" (signals are lunch, dinner, fatigue, sex stimulation, boredom, frustration and bedtime);

make it a rule never to take a drink to escape discomfort—either physical or mental; and

never, never take a drink in the morning thinking it will cure a hangover.

CHAPTER 30

Allergies

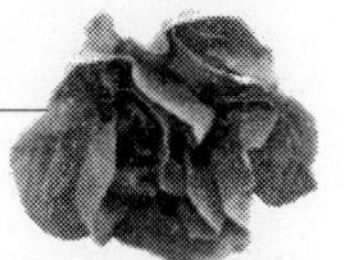

An 'allergy' can be described as sensitiveness of the body to a substance which does not normally affect other persons. There are innumerable substances in the environment which can cause mild to violent reactions in many people. These reactions range from true allergies due to intolerance of certain foods and substances, to those resulting from pollution.

Allergic reactions may occur within a few minutes of the patient coming in contact with the allergen, or they may be delayed for several hours or even several days. Almost any part of the body can be affected by allergies. The portion of the body which is affected is called a shock organ. Common sites are the nose and eyes, the skin, chest, intestines and ears.

Allergic reactions are caused by a wide range of substances and conditions. These include pollen, dust, cosmetics and animal hair; poisonous plants, serums, vaccines and drugs; physical agents such as heat, cold and sunlight; as well as a variety of foods. Among the numerous allergens in the food department, the more common ones are oranges, milk, eggs, wheat, fish, chocolates, cabbage, potatoes, tomatoes and strawberries.

Symptoms

The symptoms of allergy are as varied as the substances causing the reaction. These include recurring headache, migraine, dizziness, irritability, nervousness, depression, neuralgia, sneezing, conjunctivitis, diabetes, eczema, heart-burn, hay fever, indigestion, constipation, diarrhoea, gastric ulcer, asthma, overweight, high blood pressure, chest pain, heart attacks, a stuffy or runny nose, shortness of breath, swelling of the face and eyes, etc. The same food can cause different symptoms in different people. Many allergies are multiple and may be caused by multiple allergens.

Causes

Allergy is an indication of lowered resistance and internal disharmony caused by dietetic errors and faulty style of living. It is believed that the major cause of allergy is feeding babies such foods as cereals, meat, corns, whole milk, etc. before they reach the age of 10 to 12 months. These foods cause allergic reactions as babies lack the proper enzymes needed for their digestion before that age. Babies should be breast-fed for at least eight months as this is nature's way of providing all the required nutrients during this period.

Another important cause of allergy is today's processed foods loaded with numerous chemical additives, many of which cause powerful reactions. An allergic condition can result from diet imbalances. There can be a breakdown in the body's ability to handle sugar due to excessive intake of refined sugar and consequent blood sugar irregularities, or mineral and vitamin imbalances due to defective dietary patterns.

Emotional and psychological stress can also lead to allergies. According to Dr. Hans Salye, the world's premier researcher on stress, allergic symptoms are often nothing more than body's reaction to stress. A person can through chronic stress, become sensitive to common foods or commonplace substances like petrol fumes.

Treatment

There are various ways to tackle many of the allergic disturbances. First, the sources must be identified. This is a difficult one but not impossible task. Second, once the sources are discovered, they should be avoided. Third, and most important, general health and resistance should be built up to establish immunity to them.

There are two methods to detect disturbing foods. The first method is the trial-and-error elimination diet. This automatically eliminates many hazards and foods. Keep to organic, untreated, unprocessed foods as far as possible, and you will eliminate another set of hazards such as pesticides, various sprays and other poisons.

After having eliminated as many disturbing factors as possible, a self-search should be carried out to ascertain any suspicious symptoms from foods. It is advisable to try an eliminatory diet, excluding suspected foods for two weeks until the cause is detected. Occasionally, by changing the brand or the type, you can find a food substitute that does not upset you.

Another way to detect the cause of allergy is by Dr. Coca's "pulse test". The method is as follows: Check your pulse before a meal. Then limiting that meal to one food only, wait for half an hour after eating and take your pulse again. A slight increase is considered normal, even up to 16 extra beats. If your pulse does not rise above 84, you may be allergy-free. But if your pulse rises beyond that point, and remains high an hour after the meal, you have found your food allergy.

The best way, however, to prevent or overcome allergies is to strengthen the overall physical resistance so as not to fall an easy prey to every allergen that comes along. To start with, the patient should fast on fresh fruit juices for four or five days. Repeated short juice fasts are likely to result in better tolerance to previous allergies. After the fruit juice fast, the patient can take a mono diet of vegetables or fruits such as carrots, grapes or apples, for one week. After that one more food is added to the mono diet. A week later the third food is added and so on. After four weeks, the protein foods can be introduced, one at a time. In case an allergic reaction to a newly introduced food is noticed, it should be discontinued and a new food tried. In this way all real allergens can be eventually eliminated from the diet.

The body requires a large alkaline reserve for its daily activity. The many emergencies of acid formation through the day from wrong foods, fatigue, mental stress and lack of sleep can be met by the competency of the alkaline reserves. Boosting the normal body reserve of alkalines by liberal use of alkaline-forming foods is essential for those suffering from allergies.

The foods which should be excluded from the diet are tea, coffee, chocolate, cola drinks, alcohol, sugar, sweets and foods containing sugar, refined cereals, meats, fish, chicken, tobacco, milk, cheese, butter, smoked, salted, pickled foods and foods containing any chemical additives, preservatives and flavouring. These foods cause either toxic accumulations or over-stimulation of adrenal glands or strain on pancreatic enzyme production or may disturb the blood sugar balance.

For preventive purposes, the entire C complex vitamins—known as the bioflavonoids, are recommended. They gradually strengthen cell permeability to help immunise the body from various allergies, especially hay fever. Often the addition B_5 or pantothenic acid brings great relief to allergy sufferers. Multiple allergies may result from poor adrenal gland functioning.

In such cases liberal amounts of pantothenic acids help cure them, although the recovery will take several weeks. An adequate intake of vitamin E is also beneficial as this vitamin possesses effective anti-allergic properties, as some studies have shown.

An exciting remedy for allergy has been discovered by an Indian physician, Dr. Hemant Pathak. He found that the use of five drops of castor oil in a little juice or water taken on an empty stomach in the morning, is highly beneficial for allergies in the intestinal tract, skin and nasal passages. Dr. Pathak, who is an expert in Chinese medicine, has reported numerous cases of allergic protection by this method.

For allergic conditions in which an element of stress is present, it is essential to employ such methods as relaxation, exercise, meditation and mind control. These methods will reduce or remove stress and thereby contribute towards the treatment of allergies. Yogic asanas like yogamudra ardhmatsyendrasana, sarvangasana, shavasana and anuloma-viloma, pranayama are also beneficial.

CHAPTER 31

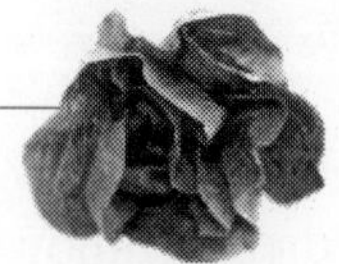

Amnesia

Amnesia refers to partial or complete loss of memory. The latter, however, is almost inconceivable as no intellectual functions are possible without memory. Different types and degrees of amnesia are found in old age and other organic conditions.

Symptoms

The most common form of this disease is verbal amnesia. In this condition, the patient forgets words or names. A very uncommon form of amnesia is temporary loss of memory, in which a person even forgets his own identity, including his name, age, family background and any recollection of the past. In case of poor memory caused by brain weakness, the patient may suffer from mild headache, intolerance to noise and inability to concentrate.

Causes

The main cause of amnesia is the impairment of brain cells by diseases directly or indirectly affecting them through a poor blood supply due to circulatory diseases. Poor memory also results from dullness of intellect and weakness of brain. Many cases are, however, largely psychological in origin, caused by anxiety neurosis, resulting from lack of attention in persons obsessed with their own problems. Temporary loss of memory may result from an injury.

Treatment

Diet has a profound effect on the mental health of a person. Even a single nutritional deficiency can cause anxiety neurosis in susceptible people. Persons suffering from amnesia should avoid tea, coffee, alcohol, chocolate and cola, all white flour products, sugar, food colourings, chemical additives, white rice and strong condiments.

The diet should be restricted to three meals. Fruits can be taken in the morning for breakfast with milk and a handful of nuts and seeds. Lunch may consist of steamed vegetables, whole wheat chappatis and a glass of buttermilk. For dinner, green vegetable salad and all available sprouts such as alfalfa seeds and mung beans, cottage cheese or a glass of buttermilk would be ideal. The patient should take liberally phosphorus-rich foods like cereals, pulses, nuts, fruit juices and milk. Cow's milk is especially beneficial and the patient should take as much of this milk as he can safely digest.

Certain home remedies have been found beneficial in the treatment of amnesia. The most remarkable of these is the use of brahmi booti, botanically known as (Bacopa scruphulariaceae). About seven grams of this herb should be dried in the shade and ground in water, along with seven kernels of almond and four and a half decigrams of pepper, strained and sweetened with 25 grams of sugar. This should be drunk every mornings for a fortnight on an empty stomach.

Almond (badam) is very valuable in poor memory caused by brain weakness. It contains unique properties to remove brain debility and to strengthen it. This dry fruit preserves the vitality of the brain and cures ailments originating from nervous disorders. Almonds should be immersed in water for an hour or so and their upper red coating removed. They should then be made into a fine paste by rubbing them on a stone slab with sandalwood and taken mixed with butter or alone, inhaling 10 to 15 drops of almond oil through the nose is also beneficial in the treatment of brain weakness.

Walnut (akhrot) is another unique dry fruit valuable in brain weakness. Its value will be enhanced if it is taken with figs or raisins. If it is intended to be consumed alone, about 20 grams of walnuts should be taken every day.

Apples (seb) are useful in amnesia. The various chemical substances contained in this fruit such as vitamin B_1, phosphorus and potassium help the synthesis of glutamic acid. This acid controls the wear and tear of nerve cells. Eating an apple with honey and milk is beneficial in the treatment of lack of memory and mental irritability. It acts as a very effective nerve tonic and recharge the nerves with new energy and life.

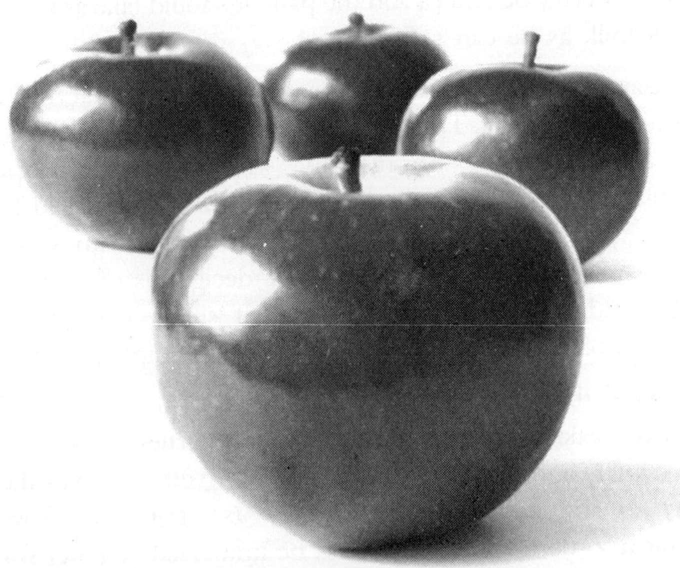

Apples are ueful in amnesia

The patient must gain control over his nervous system and channelise his mental and emotional activities into restful harmonious vibrations. This can be achieved by ensuring sufficient rest and sleep under right conditions. He must also learn the art of scientific relaxation and meditation which will go a long way in curing amnesia.

Relaxation enables the muscles to work more efficiently and eliminates fatigue by promoting venous blood circulation throughout the body. The best method of relaxation is to practice shavasana or the 'dead pose'.

Meditation will help create an amount of balance in the nervous system. This will enable the glands to be in a correct state of hormonal balance and thereby help in curing amnesia. Regularity of time, place and practice are very important in meditation. Regularity conditions the mind to slow down its activities with minimum delay. The most effective times are early dawn and dusk, when the atmosphere is serene and peaceful.

CHAPTER 32

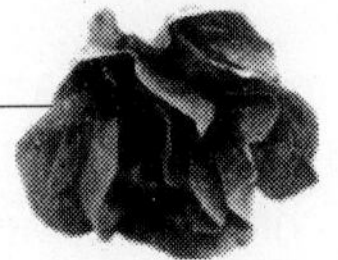

Anaemia

Anaemia, which means "lacking in blood", is among the most common diseases affecting human beings. It denotes a shortage of rich red blood cells and colouring matter and usually results from consumption of refined foods.

The blood flowing in our veins and arteries is really living tissue. Nearly half of it consists of red blood cells which carry oxygen to the tissues. Approximately one trillion (10,000 million) new blood cells are formed in the bone marrow daily. The raw materials required in the production of these cells are iron, proteins and vitamins, especially folic acid and B_{12}.

The red colouring matter, called haemoglobin, is a protein which is composed of an organic iron compound called 'heme". The globin is a sulphur-bearing protein which makes up 96 per cent of the molecule. The formation of haemoglobin thus depends on adequate dietary supplies of iron and protein. Red cells have a lifespan of approximately 120 days and are destroyed and replaced daily. Each person should have 100 per cent haemoglobin or about 15 grams to 100 cc of blood, and a blood count of five million red cells per millimeter. A drop in the haemoglobin content, results in anaemia and a consequent decreased ability of the blood to carry oxygen to the tissues.

Symptoms

A haggard look, with lines of strain, premature wrinkles, grayish skin, and dull and tired looking eyes are the main symptoms of anaemia. Other symptoms include poor memory, weakness, dizziness, fatigue, lack of energy, shortness of breath on exertion, slow healing of wounds, headaches, mental depression, pale fingernails, lips and ear lobes. The patient usually complains of weakness, easy fatigue, lack of energy and dizziness.

Causes

There are two principal causes of anaemia. It can result from reduced or low formation of red blood cells either due to defects in the bone marrow or an inadequate intake of iron, vitamins and protein. Heavy loss of blood due to injury, bleeding piles and heavy menstruation may also cause anaemia. A lack of digestive acid or hydrochloric acid needed for digestion of iron and proteins may also result in anaemia. Emotional strain, anxiety and worry usually interfere with the manufacture of hydrochloric acid in the body. Anaemia can also be caused by a variety of drugs which destroy vitamin E or by others which inactivate the nutrients needed in building blood cells. Chronic diseases such as tuberculosis, when accompanied by hemorrhage, may also result in anaemia.

Other little-known causes of anaemia are intestinal parasites or worms. Hookworm, pinworms, round worms and tapeworms feed on the blood supply as well as on the vitamins. Twenty-five hookworms can consume fifteen grams of blood every 24 hours; a tapeworm can cause acute shortage of vitamin B_{12}. Symptoms of intestinal worms are itching at the rectum, restlessness at night with bad dreams, diarrhoea, foul breath, dark circles under the eyes and a constant desire for food. Garlic can help get rid of some types of intestinal parasites. Fresh papaya and grated raw carrot are also effective. After successful treatment for intestinal worms, perfect cleanliness should be observed to prevent recurrence.

The Cure

Anaemia is much more easily prevented than corrected. A liberal intake of iron in the formative years can go a long way in preventing iron-deficiency anaemia.

Diet is of the utmost importance in the treatment of anaemia. Almost every nutrient is needed for the production of red blood cells, haemoglobin, and the enzymes, required for their synthesis. Refined food like white bread, polished rice, sugar, and desserts rob the body of the much-needed iron. Iron should always be taken in its natural organic form as the use of inorganic iron can prove hazardous, destroying the protective vitamins and unsaturated fatty acids, causing serious liver damage and even miscarriage and delayed or premature births. The common foods rich in natural organic iron are wheat and wheat grain cereals, brown rice and rice polishings; green leafy vegetables, cabbage, carrot, celery, beets, tomatoes, spinach; fruits like apples, berries, cherries, grapes, raisins, figs, dates, peaches and eggs. It has been proved that a generous intake of iron alone will not help in the regeneration of haemoglobin. The supplies of protein, too, should be adequate. The diet should, therefore, be adequate in proteins of high biological value such as those found in milk, cheese and egg. Copper is also essential for the utilisation of iron in the building of haemoglobin.

Vitamin B_{12} is a must for preventing or curing anaemia. This vitamin is usually found in animal protein and especially in organic meats like kidney and liver. A heavy meat diet is often associated with a high haemoglobin and high red cell count, but it has its disadvantages. One cause of anaemia is intestinal putrefaction, which is primarily brought on by a high meat diet. Moreover, all meats are becoming increasingly dangerous due to widespread diseases in the animal kingdom. There are, however, other equally good alternative sources of vitamin B_{12} such as dairy products, like milk, eggs and cheese, peanuts. Wheat germ and soyabeans also contain some B_{12}. Vegetarians should include sizeable amounts of milk, milk products and eggs in their diet.

For prevention of anaemia, it is essential to take the entire B-complex range which includes B_{12}, as well as the natural foods mentioned above. Eating lacto-avo products, which are complete proteins, and which also contain vitamin B_{12}, is good insurance against the disease. Brewer's yeast is a good source of complete protein.

A liberal intake of ascorbic acid is necessary to facilitate absorption of iron. At least two helpings of citrus fruits and other ascorbic acid rich foods should be taken daily.

Mention must be made of beets which are extremely important in curing anaemia. Beet juice contains potassium, phosphorus, calcium, sulphur, iodine, iron, copper, carbohydrates, protein, fat, vitamins B_1, B_2 niacin B_6, C and vitamin P. With its high iron content, beet juice regenerates and reactivates the red blood cells, supplies the body with fresh oxygen and helps the normal function of vesicular breathing.

Water Treatment

A cold water bath is among the most valuable curative measures in anaemia. The patient should be given carefully graduated cold baths twice daily. Cold friction, hot epsom salt bath for five to 10 minutes once a week and an occasional cabinet steam bath are also recommended. Full sun baths are especially beneficial as sunlight stimulates the production of red cells.

There are other important factors which are helpful in curing anaemia. Deep breathing and light exercise like walking and simple yoga asanas should be undertaken to tone up the system. Sarvangasana paschomittanasana, uttanpadasana and shavasana are recommended. Massage also helps to keep the blood level high.

CHAPTER 33

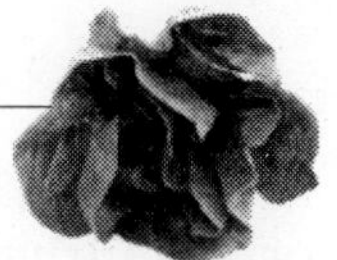

Anal Fissure

An anal fissure is a crack in the skin surrounding the anus, the excretory opening from the bowel. The irritation usually extends down to the muscle fibres. It is generally associated with other bowel disorders.

Symptoms

Anal fissure is very painful. The patient feels a sharp pain on passing motions. There may be bleeding and very often itching round the anus. Any stretching of this area cause intense distress.

Causes

The most common cause of anal fissure is chronic constipation and the resultant hard motions, which damage the tissue and the mucous membrane. Once this had been done, the fissure is reopened at the passage of subsequent motions and further infected by the faeces. However, the root cause of this disorder is, wrong feeding.

Treatment

The treatment for anal fissure should aim at softening the stools, keep them regular and avoid constipation, to begin with, the patient should fast on raw juices for about five days. Juices of orange, mosambi, pineapple and carrot may be taken during this period. The patient should drink a glass of juice every two hours from 8 a.m. to 8 p.m. mixed with water on 50 : 50 basis. A warm-water enema should be administered daily to cleanse the bowels.

After the juice fast, the patient may adopt an exclusive diet of fresh fruits for further five days. In this regimen, he should take fresh juicy fruits such as orange, apple, pineapple, pear, peach, papaya and grapes at five-hourly intervals. Thereafter, he may gradually embark upon a well-balanced diet.

The most important factor in curing anal fissure is a natural and simple diet. This should consist of unrefined foods such as whole grain cereals, honey, molasses and lentils, green leafy vegetables, especially spinach, french beans, tomatoes, lettuce, onion, cabbage, turnip, pumpkin, beets and carrot; fresh fruits, especially pears, grapes, figs, papaya, mangoes, grapefruit, gooseberries, guava and oranges; dry fruits such as figs, raisins, apricots and dates, milk products in the form of butter, ghee and cream.

Gentle instillation of about 60 grams of olive oil into the rectum will be beneficial in the treatment of anal fissure. It will soften the hardened stool. This should be repeated daily as needed.

Sugar and sugary foods should be strictly avoided because sugar steals the B Vitamins from the body, without which the intestines cannot function normally. Foods which result in constipation and anal fissure, are products made of white flour, rice, cakes, pastries, biscuits, cheese, fleshy foods, preserves and white sugar.

Drinking adequate quantities of water is beneficial not only for constipation but also for cleansing the system, diluting the blood and washing out poisons. Water, should, however, not be taken with meals as it dilutes the gastric juices essential for proper digestion. It should be taken either half an hour before or an hour after meals.

Generally, all fruits, except banana and jackfruit, are

beneficial in the treatment of constipation and anal fissure. Certain fruits like pears and grapes are, however, more effective and should be taken liberally by the patient. Drinking hot water with sour lime juice and a little salt is also an effective remedy for treating this condition.

The daily dry friction should form a regular feature of the treatment for anal fissure. The affected part should be bathed several times daily with hot and cold fomentations. A piece of linen material should be wrung out in hot water and applied for two or three minutes. The hot application should be repeated three times for the same length of time. This should be followed by a cold application. This order should always be adopted, namely three hot applications followed by one cold application.

Fresh air and regular physical exercises are also essential. Yogic asanas beneficial in the treatment of this diseases are uttanpadanasana, pavanmuktasana, vajrasana, yogamudra, bhujangasana, shalabhasana and shavasana.

CHAPTER 34

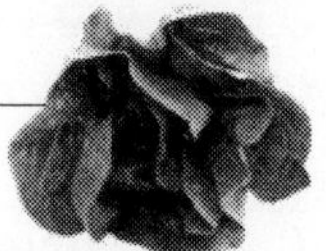

Anorexia Nervosa

Anorexia nervosa refers to loss of appetite resulting from nervous anxiety. This worrying condition is self-induced and seen mainly in young women. It is considered to be a psychological disorder which begins in efforts to slim. The women reduces the intake of food more and more until, she is virtually eating nothing and becomes very thin. She develops a distorted image of her own body and is not able to realize that it is very harmful and that it spoils the appearance rather than enhance it.

Symptoms

A women suffering from anorexia nervosa refuses to eat, sleeps very little, although she remains very active. She may lose weight upto 25 per cent of the normal weight. There may be a stoppage of menstruation and lack of sexual desire. She is often impatient, irritable and depressed. In course of time, emaciation become severe and may even result in death, if not treated properly.

Causes

Women suffering from this condition tend to have a somewhat neurotic personality. They set very high standards for themselves, and any failure to reach their idea of perfection results in much heart-searching. This attitude extends their search for an 'ideal' slim body. Fear of failure in any undertaking also plays a part in the onset of the disease. Specific criticism may be the final precipitating factor in the food refusal, as for instance, a chance joking remark from a school fellow about fatness.

Failure to eat an adequate nutritious diet can lead to metabolic upset and serious illness. Inspite of appearing to have a super-abundance of energy, the patient is living off bodily reserves and in the very advanced stages, the body chemistry is irreversibly upset.

Treatment

At the outset, patients suffering from anorexia nervosa must be helped to understand their problems so that they can begin to help themselves on to the road to normality again. Much loving understanding and support from family and friends will be needed.

To begin with, the patient should fast on orange juice and water for three to five days. The procedure is to take the juice of an orange in a glass of warm water every two or three hours during the day. If orange juice does not agrees, carrot juice mixed with water may be taken. Each day while fasting, the bowels should be cleansed of the poisonous matter thrown off by the self-cleansing process now set up by the body. This can be achieved through warm-water enema. After the juice fast, the patient may adopt an all-fruit diet for further two or three days. In this regimen, she should take three meals a day of fresh juicy fruits, such as apple, pear, orange, pineapple, grapes and papaya at five-hourly interval. Thereafter she may adopt a restricted diet of easily digestible foods, consisting of lightly-cooked vegetables, juicy fruits and buttermilk for about 10 days.

After the restricted diet, the patient may, depending on the progress, gradually embark upon a well-balanced diet consisting of seeds, nuts and grains, vegetable and fruits. The emphasis should be on fresh fruits and raw vegetables. The patient should avoid white sugar, and white flour as well as products made from them, tea, coffee and fried foods.

The application of ice-bag over the stomach for half an hour before meals will be beneficial in the treatment of this condition. Another usual application is wet girdle pack for an hour daily. The procedure is as follows: A thin cotton underwear should be wrung in cold water and worn by the patient. Above this, wet underwear, a thick dry cotton underwear should be worn. A cold hip bath taken once daily will also go a long way in curing anorexia. The procedure for this bath has been explained in chapter 3 on Therapeutic Baths'.

Certain home remedies have been found beneficial in the treatment of anorexia nervosa. The most important of this is the use of orange (santra). It gives rest to the digestive organs and supplies nutrition in a most easily assimilable form. It also stimulates the flow of digestive juices thereby improving digestion and increasing appetite. It creates suitable conditions for the development of friendly bacteria in the intestine.

The use of sour grapes (khata angoor) is another effective remedy for anorexia nervosa. The juice of these grapes should be used in kneading the flour before preparing the bread. This bread should be used continuously for two to three weeks. It will tone up the stomach and create good appetite.

Lime (niboo) is also a valuable remedy for loss of appetite. A preparation made from this fruit and ginger has been found very effective in overcoming this condition. About five ml. of the juice of lime should be mixed with an equal quantity of the juice of ginger and a gram of rock salt should be added to this mixture. It should then be placed in sunlight for three days and a teaspoon should be taken after each meal. This will tone up the digestive system and improve appetite.

The apple (seb) is another fruit useful in anorexia nervosa. It helps digestion by stimulating the flow of pepsin in the stomach.

Garlic (Lahsoon) possess special property to stimulate the digestive tone of the system and improve appetite. A soup prepared from this vegetable can be of immense help to a patient suffering from anorexia nervosa. This soup can be reinforced with lemon juice for better results.

The use of ginger (adrak) has also proved valuable in the loss of appetite. About five grams of this vegetable should be ground and licked with a little salt for the treatment of this condition.

Other measures beneficial in the treatment of anorexia nervosa are daily sun and cool air baths, out-of-door life and general and abdominal massage.

CHAPTER 35

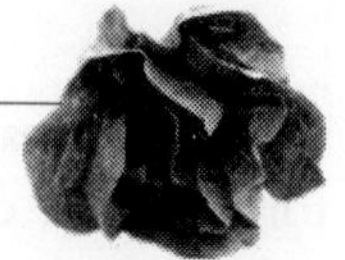

Appendicitis

Appendicitis is the most common of all serious intestinal disorders. It refers to an inflammation of the vermiform appendix. It presents itself in acute and chronic forms and affects both the sexes equally. This disease now accounts for about half the acute abdominal emergencies occurring between the ages of 10 to 30. It is more frequent in developed countries than underdeveloped countries.

The appendix is a small tube located at the end of the caecum, the first part of the large intestine. It is called vermiform appendix as it resembles a worm. It is usually eight to ten cm long. Its structure is made of the same tough fibrous outer covering that protects the entire alimentary canal. There is a layer of muscular tissue under the outer covering and further a layer of lymphoid tissue. The function of the appendix, which is performed by this lymphoid tissue, is to neutralise the irritating waste material generated in the body or the organic poisons introduced through the skin or membranes.

Symptoms

Appendicitis usually begins with a sudden pain in the centre of the abdomen, which gradually shifts to the lower right side. The pain may be preceded by general discomfort in the abdomen, indigestion, diarrhoea or constipation. The patient usually has a mild fever varying from 100° to 102°F. Nausea is common, and the patient may vomit once or twice. The muscles of the right side of the abdomen become tense and

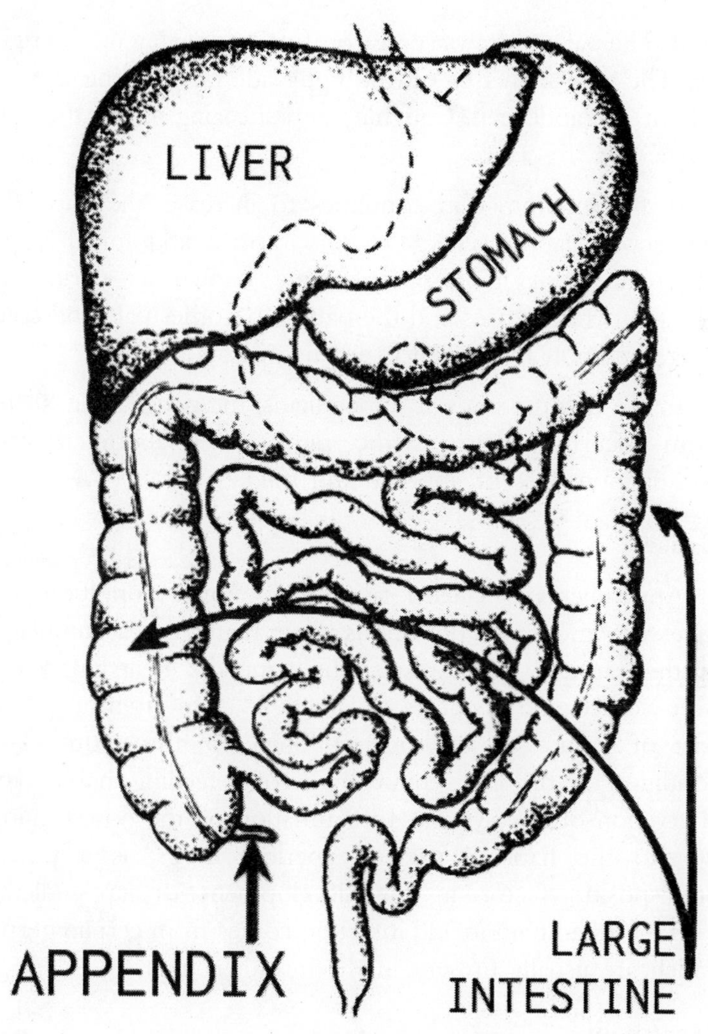

Diagram showing poisition of appendix

rigid. The patient draws some comfort by drawing up the right leg. The pain increases on the right side on pressing the left side of the abdomen. Coughing and sneezing makes the pain worse.

If the inflammation continues to increase, the appendix may rupture and discharge its pus into the abdominal cavity. This may result in a serious state known as peritonitis. The temperature rises and the patient becomes pale and cold. This condition may call for urgent operation.

In the chronic state of appendicitis, the patient may suffer from recurrent pain in the right lower abdomen with constipation, loss of appetite and mild nausea.

Causes

Appendicitis is caused by a toxic bowel condition. An excessive amount of poisonous waste material is accumulated in the caecum. As a result, the appendix is irritated and over-worked and becomes inflamed. It is an attempt on the part of nature to localise and 'burn up' the toxins. This condition is brought about by wrong feeding habits and enervation of the system. Inflammation of the bowel lining, due to the habitual use of aperient drugs, is a potent predisposing factor in the development of appendicitis. Further inflammation and infection comes from certain germs which are usually present in the intestinal tract.

Treatment

The patient should be put to bed immediately at the first symptoms of severe pain, vomiting and fever. Rest is of utmost importance in the treatment of this disease. The patient should resort to fasting which is the only real cure for appendicitis. Absolutely no food should be given. Nothing except water should enter the system. Low enemas, containing about one pint (½ litre) of warm water should be administered every day for the first three days to cleanse the lower bowel. Hot compresses may be placed over the painful area several times daily. Abdominal packs, made of a strip of wet sheet covered by a dry flannel cloth bound tightly around the abdomen, should be applied continuously until all acute symptoms subside.

When the acute symptoms subside by about the third day, the patient should be given a full enema, containing about 1½ litre of warm water and this should be repeated daily until all inflammation and pain have subsided. The patient can be given fruit juices from the third day onwards. This simple treatment sensibly applied will overcome an appendicitis attack.

After spending three days on fruit juices, the patient may adopt an all-fruit diet for a further four or five days. During this period, he should have three meals a day each meal of fresh juicy fruits. Thereafter, he should adopt a well-balanced diet based on three food groups namely, (i) seed, nuts and grains, (ii) vegetables and (iii) fruits.

In case of chronic appendicitis, a short fast should be followed by a full milk diet for two to three weeks. In this regimen, a glass of milk should be taken every two hours from 8 a.m. to 8 p.m. on the first day, a glass every hour and a half the next day and a glass every hour the third day. Then the quantity of milk should be gradually increased so as to take a glass every half an hour, if such a quantity can be tolerated comfortably. After the full milk diet, the patient should gradually embark upon a well-balanced diet, with emphasis on fresh fruits and green leafy vegetables.

Certain vegetable juices, especially carrot juice, in

combination with the juices of beets and cucumbers, have been found valuable in the treatment of appendicitis. Regular use of tea made from fenugreek seeds has also proved helpful in preventing the appendix from becoming a dumping ground for excess mucous and intestinal waste.

The patient of appendicitis should adopt all measures to eradicate constipation, if it is habitual. Much relief can be obtained by the application of hot fomentation and abdominal packs every morning and night. An abdominal massage is also beneficial. Once the waste matter in the caecum has moved into the colon and thence eliminated, the irritation and inflammation in the appendix will subside and surgical removal of the appendix will not be necessary. The surgical operation should be resorted to only in rare cases, when the appendix has become abscessed.

CHAPTER 36

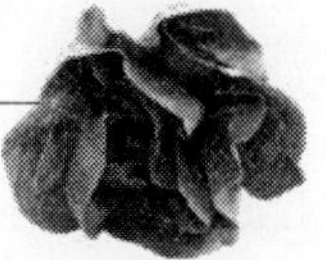

Arteriosclerosis

Arteriosclerosis is one of the most common diseases of the blood vessels. It refers to a thickening of the walls of the arteries due to the presence of calcium or lime. It has become a common ailment in modern times, accounting for much of the disability and high death rate among older people.

Arteriosclerosis is usually preceded by atherosclerosis, a kind of degeneration or softening of the inner lining of the blood vessel walls. The most risky places for such degeneration are the coronary vessels of the heart and the arteries leading to the brain. Arteriosclerosis results in the loss of elasticity of the blood vessels, with a narrowing of the smaller arteries, which interferes with the free circulation of the blood. These changes may gradually extend to capillaries and veins.

Arteriosclerosis is more frequent in men than women, especially in the younger age-group. It has been estimated that 40 per cent of all men over 40 years have a significant degree of obstruction of their coronary arteries and this can lead to heart attacks at any time.

Symptoms

The symptoms of arteriosclerosis vary with arteries involved. Signs of inadequate blood supply generally appear first in the legs. There may be numbness and coldness in the feet and cramps and pains in the legs even after light exercise. If the coronary arteries are involved, the patient may have sharp pains, characteristic of angina pectoris. When arteries leading to the brain are involved, the vessel may burst, causing haemorrhage in the brain tissues. A cerebral vascular stroke, with partial or complete paralysis of one side of the body may result, if there is blockage with a blood clot. It may also lead to loss of memory and a confused state of mind in elderly people. If arteries leading to the kidneys are involved, the patient may suffer from high blood pressure and kidney disorders.

Causes

The most important cause of arteriosclerosis is excessive intake of white sugar, refined foods and high fat diet, rich in cholesterol. A sedentary life and excesses of all kinds are the major contributing causes. Hardening of the arteries may also be caused by other diseases such as high blood pressure, obesity, diabetes, rheumatism, Bright's disease, malaria, syphilis. Emotional stress also plays an important part, and heart attacks are more common during the periods of mental and emotional disturbances, particularly in those engaged in sedentary occupations. Heredity also plays its role and this disease runs in families.

Treatment

If the causes of arteriosclerosis are known, remedial action should be taken promptly to remove them. To begin with the patient should resort to a short juice fast for five to seven days. All available fresh, raw vegetables and fruit juices in season may be taken. Grape-fruit juice, pineapple juice, lemon juice and juices of green vegetables are especially beneficial. A warm water enema should be used daily to cleanse the bowels during the period of fasting.

After the juice fast, the patient should take optimum diet made up from three basic food groups, namely (i) seeds, nuts and grains, (ii) vegetables and, (iii) fruits, with emphasis on raw foods. Plenty of raw and sprouted seeds and nuts should be used. Cold pressed vegetables oils, particularly safflower oil, flax seed oil and olive oil should be used regularly.

Further, short fasts on juices may be undertaken at intervals of three months or so, depending on the progress being made.

The patient should take several small meals instead of a few large ones. He should avoid all hydrogenated fats and an excess of saturated fats, such as butter, cream, ghee and animal fat. He should also avoid meat, salt and all refined and processed foods, condiments, sauces, pickles, strong tea, coffee, white sugar, white flour and all products made from them. Foods cooked in aluminium and copper utensils should not be taken as toxic metals entering the body are known to be deposited on the walls of the aorta and the arteries. Smoking, if habitual, should be given up as smoking constricts the arteries and aggravates the condition.

Recent investigations have shown that garlic and onions have a preventive effect on the development of arteriosclerosis. Vitamin C has also proved beneficial as it helps in the conversion of cholesterol into bile acids.

One of the most effective home remedies for arteriosclerosis is the lemon peel. It is believed to be one of the richest known sources of vitamin P. It strengthens the entire arterial system. Shredded lemon peel may be added to soups and stews, or sprinkled over salads. To make a medicine, the peel of one or two lemons may be cut up finely, covered with warm water and allowed to stand for about 12 hours. A teaspoonful may be taken every three hours, or immediately before or after a meal.

Parsley is another effective home remedy for arteriosclerosis. It contains elements which help to maintain the blood vessels, particularly the capillaries and arterial system in a healthy condition. It may be taken as a beverage by simmering it gently in the water for a few minutes and partaking several times daily.

The beet juice has also proved valuable in arteriosclerosis. It is an excellent solvent for inorganic calcium deposits. Juices of carrot and spinach are also beneficial. These juices can be taken individually or in combination. Formula proportions found helpful when used in combination are carrot 300 ml and spinach 200 ml to prepare 500 ml of juice.

The patient should undertake plenty of outdoor exercise and eliminate all mental stress and worries. Prolonged neutral immersion baths at bed time on alternate days is beneficial. This bath is administered in a bath tub which should be properly fitted with hot and cold water connection. The bath-tub should be fitted with water at a temperature ranging from 92° to 98° F and the patient should lie in it for an hour or so. The head should be kept cold with a cold compress.

CHAPTER 37

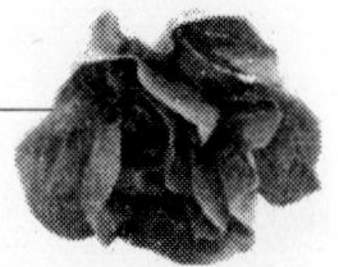

Arthritis

The word 'arthritis' means 'inflammation of joints'. It comes from two Greek words, *athron* meaning joints and *itis* meaning inflammation. It is a chronic disease process. In the early stages, the whole body is usually involved and one or two joints may become completely deformed, leaving the patient handicapped and somewhat weakened.

Arthritis assumes various forms, the most frequent being osteoarthritis and rheumatoid arthritis. Inflammation is the main feature of arthritis, which is a reaction of the joint tissues to some form of damage or injury.

Osteoarthritis

Osteoarthritis is a degenerative joint disease which usually occurs in the older age-group. It results from structural changes in the articular cartilage in the joints, usually those which are weight-bearing such as the spine and knees.

The chief symptoms of osteoarthritis are pain and stiffness in the joints. The pain usually increases after exercise. Other symptoms include watery eyes, dry neck, leg cramps, allergies, arteriosclerosis, impairment in the functioning of the gall-bladder and liver disturbances. The possible causes include malnutrition, continuous physical stress, obesity, glandular insufficiency, calcium deficiency and shortage of hydrochloric acid.

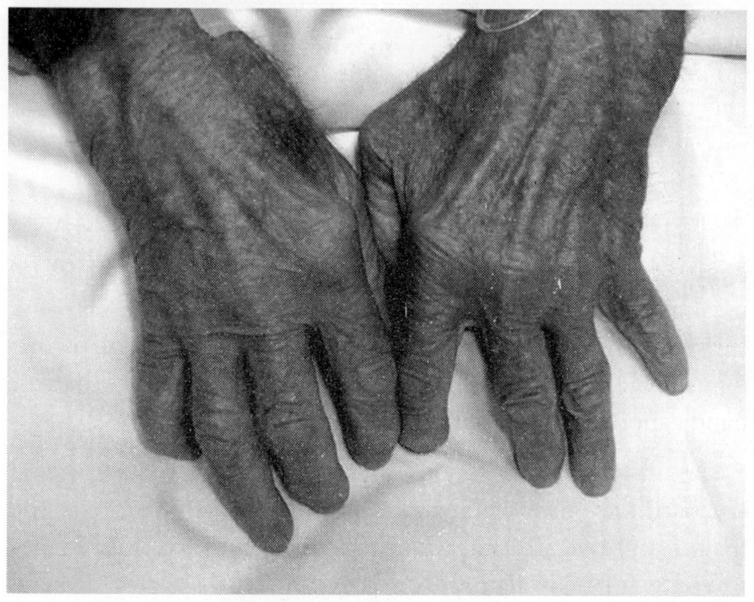

Advanced rheumatoid arthritis showing twisted hands and puffiness of the metacarpel points.

Rheumatoid Arthritis

Rheumatoid arthritis is a serious disease which affects not only the joints of the fingers, wrists, hips, knees and feet but also the muscles, tendons and other tissues of the body. The disease is due to an inflammatory process of the synovium or lining of the joints accompanied by swelling and eventual deformity.

Rheumatoid arthritis is often called the "cooked food disease". It usually develops gradually over several months with persistent pain and stiffness in one or more joints. Ultimately the whole body is affected. Symptoms include anaemia, colitis, constipation, gall-bladder disturbances, low blood pressure, deformed hands and feet. The condition may be caused by hormonal imbalance, physical and emotional stress, infection, severe fright, shock and injury. Hereditary factors may also be responsible for the onset of this disease.

Treatment

The diet of the arthritis patient should be planned along alkaline lines and should include fruits and vegetables for protection and proteins and carbohydrates for energy. It may consist of a couple of fresh raw vegetables in the form of a salad and at least two cooked vegetables. Cabbage, carrot, celery, cucumber, endive, lettuce, onion, radishes, tomatoes and watercress may be used for raw salad. The cooked vegetables may include asparagus, beets, cauliflower, cabbage, carrots, celery, brinjal, mushroom, onions, peas, beans, spinach, tomatoes, squash and turnips.

In severe cases, it will be advisable to put the patient on raw vegetables juice therapy for about a week. Green juice, extracted from any green leafy vegetable, mixed with carrot, celery and red beet juice, is specific for arthritis. The alkaline action of raw juices dissolves the accumulation of deposits around the joints and in other tissues. Fresh pineapple is also valuable as the enzyme in fresh pineapple juice, bromelain reduces swelling and inflammation in osteoarthritis and rheumatoid arthritis. Repeated juice fasts are recommended at intervals of every two months.

The raw potato juice therapy is considered one of the most successful biological treatment for rheumatic and arthritic conditions. It has been used in folk medicine for centuries. The old method of preparing potato juice was to cut the potato into thin slices, without peeling the skin, and place them overnight in a large glass filled with cold water. The water should be drunk in the morning on an empty stomach. Fresh juice can also be extracted from potatoes and drunk diluted with water on 50 : 50 basis, first thing in the morning.

Black gingelly seeds, soaked overnight in water, have been found to be effective in preventing frequent joint pains. The water in which the seeds are soaked should also be taken along with the seeds the first thing in the morning. Drinking water kept overnight in a copper container also serves the same purpose. This water has traces of copper which helps strengthen the muscular system. For the same reason wearing a copper ring or bracelet will also help.

Warm coconut oil or mustard oil, mixed with camphor, should be massaged in case of stiff and aching joints. It will increase blood supply and reduce inflammation and stiffness on account of gentle warmth produced while massaging. Camphorated oil is an ancient rubefacient used for the purpose.

The lime has also been used as a home remedy for arthritis since long. The citric acid found in lime is solvent of the uric acid which is the primary cause of arthritis. Other remedies found useful in relieving pains in the joints include green-gram soup mixed with crushed garlic cloves and a teaspoonful of powdered fenugreek seeds in warm water taken everyday.

Sea bathing is considered beneficial in the treatment of arthritis. The natural iodine in the sea water is said to relieve arthritis pain. As is well-known, iodine regulates the acid-alkaline balance in the blood and tissues, helps to repair and regenerate worn out tissues and nourishes the skeletal structure. It enters into the thyroid gland's secretion. The hormone uses this iodine to nullify germs in the bloodstream and to create a self-cleansing of internal toxemia.

If sea bathing is not possible, the patient should relax for

30 minutes every night in a tub of warm water in which a cupful of sea salt has been mixed. The minerals in the sea salt, especially iodine, can be absorbed through the skin pores. This will help correct an internal imbalance.

The body should be kept warm at all times. Joints should not be bandaged tightly as this limits movement and interferes with the free circulation of blood. There should be plenty of indirect ventilation in the bedroom. Rest is of greatest importance to arthritics, who should not overdo their work, exercise or recreational activities.

Constipation should be avoided as it poisons the system and adds to the irritation and inflammation of the joints. Light exercises such as walking, hiking and swimming are beneficial. Maintaining a normal body weight is also an important factor in preventing arthritis. Obesity places excess stress on weight-bearing joints and interferes with the smooth functioning of tendons, ligaments and muscles.

The yogic asanas helpful in curing arthritis are trikonasana, bhujangasana, shalabhasana, naukasana, vakrasana and shavasana. Arthritis patients should practice these asanas regularly. Yogic kriyas like jalneti and kapalbhati and pranayamas such as anuloma viloma, ujjai and bhramari are also beneficial.

The patient should be given a lukewarm enema for a few days to cleanse the bowels. Neutral immersion baths, hot foot baths, ultrasonic diathermy and exposure of the affected parts to infra-red rays, a knee pack applied for an hour every night, steam baths and a massage once a week are beneficial in the treatment of arthritis. All general cold water treatments, such as cold baths and cold sprays, should be avoided.

CHAPTER 38

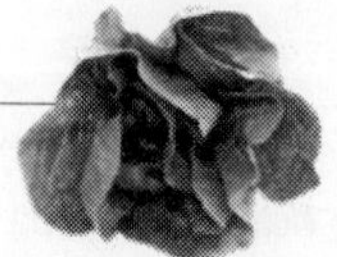

Asthma

Asthma is an ancient Greek word meaning 'panting or shortdrawn breath'. It is the most troublesome of the respiratory diseases, causing chest tightness, recurring periods of wheezing, shortness of breath and coughing.

Symptoms

Patients suffering from asthma appear to be gasping for breath. Actually, they have more trouble exhaling than inhaling because the air passages of the small bronchi become clogged and constricted with mucus, thus making it difficult for the patient to breathe out. All asthmatics have more difficulty at night, especially during sleep.

The onset of asthma is either gradual or abrupt. Sudden onsets are often preceded by a spell of coughing which may be associated with itching of the chin, the back of the neck or chest. When the onset is gradual, the attack is usually brought on by respiratory infection. A severe attack causes an increase in heartbeat and respiratory rates and the patient feels restless and fatigued. There may be coughing, tightness in the chest, profuse sweating and vomiting. There may also be abdominal pain, especially if coughing is severe. Foggy weather aggravates the symptoms.

An asthmatic attack begins when the bronchial tubes in the lungs become constricted. The tubes having become narrow, the inhaled air becomes trapped in the tiny air sacs at the end of the tubes, making the release of breath difficult. The wheezing sound identified with asthma is produced by the air being pushed through the narrowed bronchi.

Causes

Mainly bronchial in its symptoms, asthma is caused by a variety of factors. For many it is an allergic condition resulting from the reaction of the system to the weather, food, drugs, perfumes and other irritants which vary with different individuals. Allergies to dust are the most common. Some persons are sensitive to the various forms of dust like cotton dust, wheat dust and paper dust, some pollens, animal hair, fungi and insects, especially cockroaches. Foods which generally cause allergic reactions are wheat, eggs, milk, chocolates, beans, potato, pork and beef.

For others, asthma may result from the abnormal body chemistry involving the system's enzymes or a defect in muscular action within the lungs. Quite often, however, asthma is precipitated by a combination of allergic and non-allergic factors including emotional tension, air pollution, infections and hereditary factors. It has been estimated that when both parents have asthma or hay fever, in 75 to 100 per cent cases, the offspring also has allergic reactions.

Treatment

Modern medical system has not been able to find a cure for this crippling disease. Drugs and vaccines have only limited value in alleviating symptoms. Most of these are habit forming and the dose has to be increased from time to time to give the same amount of relief. The frequent introduction of drugs in the system, while giving only temporary relief, tends to make asthma chronic and incurable. Allergy—which is the immediate cause of asthma—itself is an indication of lowered resistance and internal disharmony caused by faulty eating and bad habits. This is the root cause and the real cure lies in return to nature.

The natural way to treat asthma consists of stimulating the functioning of slack excretory organs, adopting appropriate diet patterns to eliminate morbid matter and reconstruct the body, and practising yogasanas, yogic kriyas and pranayamas to permit proper assimilation of food and to strengthen the lungs, digestive system and circulatory organs.

The patient should be given an enema to clean the colon and prevent auto-intoxication. Mud-packs applied to the abdomen will relieve the fermentation caused by undigested food and will promote intestinal peristalsis. Wet packs should be applied to the chest to relieve the congestion of the lungs and strengthen them. The patient should be made to perspire through steam bath, hot foot bath, hot hip bath and sun bath. This will stimulate the skin and relieve congested lungs.

The patient should fast for a few days on lemon juice with honey and thereafter resort to a fruit juice diet to nourish the system and eliminate the toxins. Gradually, solid foods can be included. The patient should, however, avoid the common dietic errors. Ideally, his diet should contain a limited quantity of carbohydrates, fats and proteins which are acid-forming foods, and a liberal quantity of alkaline foods consisting of fresh fruits, green vegetables and germinated gram. Foods which tend to produce phlegm such as rice, sugar, lentils and curds as also fried and other difficult-to-digest foods should be avoided. Breakfast may consist of prunes, orange or berries or a few black raisins with honey. Lunch and dinner should consist of a salad of raw vegetables such as cucumber, lettuce, tomato, carrot and beets, one or two lightly cooked green vegetables and wheat bread. The last meal should preferably be taken before sunset or at least two hours before going to bed.

Asthmatics should always eat less than their capacity. They should eat slowly, chewing their food properly. They should drink eight to 10 glasses of water a day, but should avoid taking water or any liquid with meals. Spices, chillies and pickles, too much tea and coffee should also be avoided.

Asthma, particularly when the attack is severe, tends to destroy the appetite. In such cases, do not force the patient to eat. He should be kept on fast till the attack is over. He should, however, take a cup of warm water every two hours. An enema taken at that time will be very beneficial.

Honey is considered highly beneficial in the treatment of asthma. It is said that if a jug of honey is held under the nose of an asthma patient and he inhales the air that comes into contact with the honey, he starts breathing easier and deeper. The effect lasts for about an hour or so. This is because honey contains a mixture of 'higher' alcohols and ethereal oils and the vapours given off by them are soothing and beneficial to the asthma patient. Honey usually brings relief whether the air flowing over it is inhaled or whether it is eaten or taken either in milk or water. It thins out accumulated mucous and helps its elimination from the respiratory passages. It also tones up the pulmonary parenchyma and thereby prevents the production of mucous in future. Some authorities recommend one year old honey for respiratory disease.

Another effective remedy for asthma is garlic. The patient should be given daily garlic cloves boiled in thirty gms of milk as a cure for early stage of asthma. Steaming ginger tea with minced garlic cloves in it, can also help to keep the problem under control and should be taken both in the morning and evening. Turmeric is also regarded as an effective remedy for bronchial asthma. The patient should be given a teaspoonful of turmeric powder with a glass of milk two or three times daily. It acts best when taken on an empty stomach.

During the attack, mustard oil mixed with little camphor should be massaged over the back of the chest. This will loosen up phlegm and ease breathing. The patient should also inhale steam from the boiling water mixed with caraway seeds, known as *ajwain* in the vernacular. It will dilate the bronchial passage.

The patient should also follow the other laws of nature. Air, sun and water are great healing agents. Regular fasting once a week, an occasional enema, breathing exercises, fresh air, dry climate, light exercises and a correct posture go a long way in treating the disease.

The patient should perform yogic kriyas such as jalneti, vamanadhouti and yogic asanas such as ekpaduttanasana, yogamudra, sarvangasana, padmasana, bhujangasana, dhanurasan, vakrasana, ardh-matsyendrasan, shalabhasan, paschimottanasana and shavasana. Pranayamas like kapalbhati, anuloma-viloma, ujjayi, suryabhedana and bhramari are also highly beneficial.

The patient should avoid dusty places, exposure to cold foods to which he is sensitive, mental worries and tensions. Asthmatic should be made to feel that they are not sick, and with slight adjustments, can live a full life.

CHAPTER 39

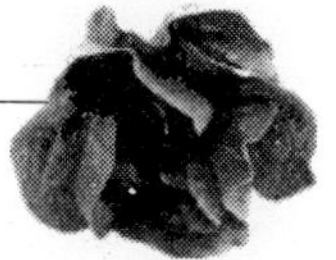

Backache

Backache, one of the most common ailments, is widely prevalent these days due to sedentary living habits and hazardous work patterns. The psychological conditions associated with emotional stress, which bring about spasm of the muscles, may also cause backache. As the back bears the weight of the entire body it gives way when it has to carry an extra load in the case of persons who are overweight.

The back, a complex structure of muscles, bone and elastic tissue, is known as the life-bone of the body. The spine is made of 24 blocks of bone piled one on top of the other. Sandwiched between these bony blocks are cushions of cartilage and elastic tissues called intervertebral discs. The vertebral discs act as shock absorbers for the back. Mobility would be impossible without discs.

Sometimes these cushions rupture and the pulp protrudes a little. The process is erroneously called a 'slipped' disc. If the cushion disappears entirely, the result is known as a degenerated disc. In slipped-disc trouble, the nerve is affected in such a way that the pain radiates down the thigh and leg. If the disc 'slips' in the neck area, it causes numbness and pain radiates to the arms.

Disc trouble does not occur suddenly but builds up over a long time. The backbone forms a protective arch over the vertebrae and spinal cord and protects the spinal nerves that are interwoven through the spinal column. There is a close relationship between the bones, discs, joint muscles and nerves

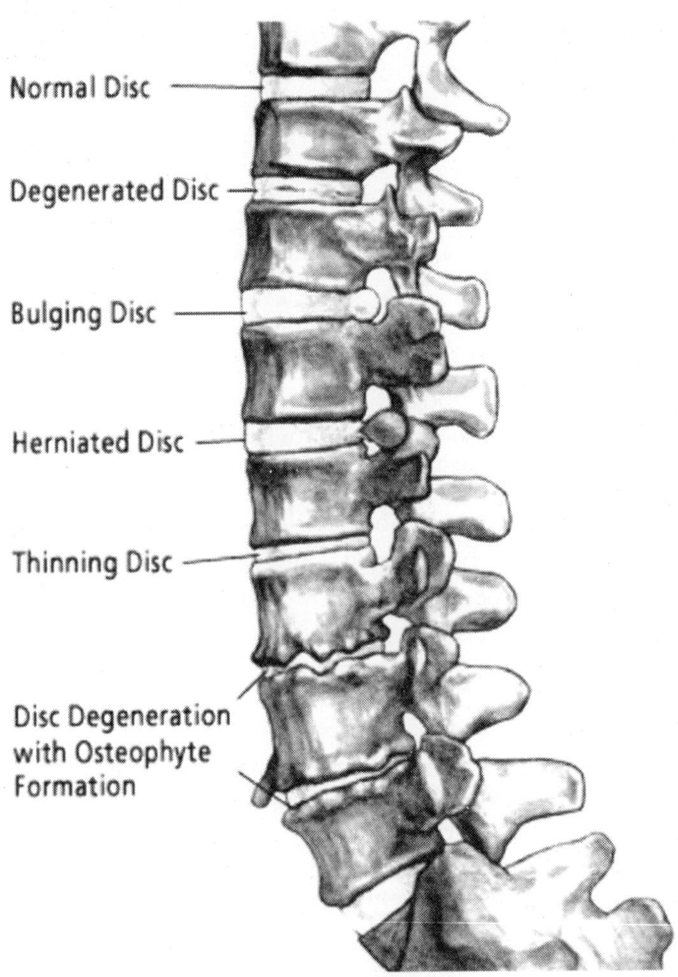

Disc Problems

in the back and the slightest problem or injury to the back or neck area can have disastrous effects.

Symptoms

In most cases of backache, the pain is usually felt either in the middle of the back or lower down. It may spread to both sides of the waist and the hips. With acute pain, the patient is unable to move and is bedridden.

About 90 per cent of backache patients suffer from what is called cervical or lumber spondylosis. It is a degenerative disorder in which the vertebral bone or the intervertebral disc becomes soft and loses shape. As a result of this, the spine loses its flexibility.

Causes

The main causes of backache and spondylosis are muscular tension, joint strain, poor posture and incorrect nutrition resulting from dietetic errors and lack of exercise. Acute or chronic illnesses like kidney or prostate problems, female disorders, influenza and arthritis, may also lead to backache. Other causes include stress and strain resulting from sitting for a long time, improper lifting of weights, high heels and emotional problems which may cause painful muscle cramping.

Poor posture results from soft chairs and coaches, which facilitate slouching and sitting incorrectly. Shoes with high heels place a tremendous strain on the back and other muscles of the body. Sleeping on too soft a mattress which results in an improper back and neck posture, can cause tension, headaches and pain in the upper and lower back.

Another major cause of back problems and tense muscles is lack of exercise. Modern conveniences have made office work easier. The easy life can lead to obesity which puts a great strain on the back. When muscles are not exercised and remain weak, the chances of injury to them is increased manifold.

Treatment

Drugs prescribed to relieve pain or relax muscles in backache disorders do not cure common back problems. These can become habit forming and may actually perpetuate the disease in case of excessive intake.

Certain safety measures, especially for people in sedentary occupation, are necessary to relieve and prevent backache. The most important of these is exercise which improves the supply of nutrients to spinal discs, thereby delaying the process of deterioration that comes with age and eventually affects everybody. Safe exercises include walking, swimming and bicycling. The latter should be done keeping the back upright. Controlling one's weight is another important step towards relieving backache as excess weight greatly increases the stress on soft back tissues.

Those with sedentary occupations should take a break to stand up every hour. Soft cushioned seats should be avoided and position should be changed as often as possible. Persons with back problems should sleep on a firm mattress on their sides with knees bent at right angles to the torso. They should take care never to bend from the waist down to lift any object but instead should squat close to the object, bending the knees but keeping the back straight, and then stand up slowly.

Neck tension arising from long hours at the desk or behind the wheel of the car can be relieved by certain neck exercises. These include rotating the head clockwise and anti-clockwise, allowing the head to drop forward and backwards as far as possible and turning the head to the right and left as far as possible several times. These exercises help to loosen up contracted neck muscles which may restrict blood supply to the head.

The diet of those suffering from backache should consist of a salad of raw vegetables such as tomato, carrot, cabbage, cucumber, radish, lettuce and at least two steamed or lightly cooked vegetables such as cauliflower, cabbage, carrot, spinach and plenty of fruits, all except bananas. The patients should have four meals daily. They may take fruits and milk during breakfast, steamed vegetables and whole wheat chappatis during lunch, fresh fruit or fruit juice in the evening and a bowl of raw salad and sprouts during dinner.

The patients should avoid fatty, spicy and fried foods, curd, sweetmeats, sugar, condiments as well as tea and coffee. Those who smoke and take tobacco in any form should give them up completely.

Proteins and vitamin C are necessary for the development of a healthy bone metrix. Vitamin D, calcium, phosphorus and the essential trace minerals are essential for healthy bones. Foods that have been processed for storage to avoid spoiling have few nutrients and should be eliminated from the diet. Vitamin C has proved helpful in relieving low-back pain and averting spinal disc operations.

Hot fomentations, alternate sponging or application of *radiant* heat to the back will also give immediate relief. Yogic asanas which are beneficial in the treatment of backache are bhujangasana, shalabhasana, halasana, uttanpadasana and shavasana.

The back can be strengthened through proper nutrition, exercise and relaxation and in the process general health will also improve.

CHAPTER 40

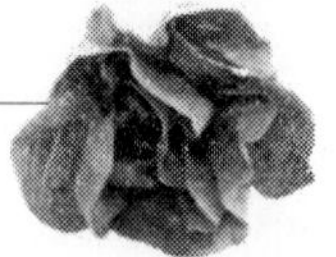

Boils

The boils, known as furuncle in medical parlance, are tender swellings in the skin surrounded by large red areas. They are infections of the sweat glands or hair follicles of the skin. They commonly occur during summer.

Symptoms

Boils can occur anywhere on the body, but they appear most often on the face, eyelids, back of the neck, upper back and buttocks. They specially favour places where clothing rubs such as the area on the collar line. Boils occurring round the eyes and nose are especially serious because their poisons can spread to the brain.

At first, a painful red nodule appears on the skin. This grows bigger and then breaks down in the middle for the pus to collect and looks yellow under the skin. It creates a great deal of irritation and itching. There may be a single boil, or several may develop in the same area or different areas at or about the same time, or they may come in successive crops. The swellings may not be limited to one hair follicle but may extend to many follicles. There may therefore be many openings when the boils ripen and discharge. Fever may sometimes accompany the boils.

Causes

Boils are mainly caused by stapphylococcus germs which enter the sweat glands or hair follicles. They can be transmitted from one person to another and in fact, some live harmlessly on the skin all the time and in infected areas like cuts or pimples. The essential cause of this disorder is thus bacterial. However, several factors predispose to the growth of bacteria in hair follicle. Of these, the chief factor is a toxic condition of the blood stream due to faulty diet and wrong style of living. Boils generally appear when a person is in a run-down and devitalised condition.

Treatment

A thorough cleansing of the system is essential to the treatment of boils. To begin with, the patient should be placed on an exclusive diet of fresh juicy fruits for two or three days. A warm-water enema should be administered daily, if possible, during this period to cleanse the bowels.

After the all-fruit diet, the patient may be allowed to adopt a well-balanced diet. The emphasis should be on whole grain cereals, raw vegetables and fresh fruits. Further periods on an all-fruit diet may be necessary, depending on the general health-level and bodily condition of the patient. In case constipation is habitual, all possible measures should be adopted to overcome it.

The patient should avoid tea, coffee, starchy and sugary foods especially, cakes, pastries, sweets, chocolates, white sugar and white bread. He should also avoid all condiments, pickles and sauces.

The use of garlic and onion has proved most effective among the several home remedies found beneficial in the treatment of boils. The juice of garlic or onion may be applied externally on the boils to help ripen them and also to break them and evacuate the pus. Equal quantity of the juices of these two vegetables can also be applied with beneficial results.

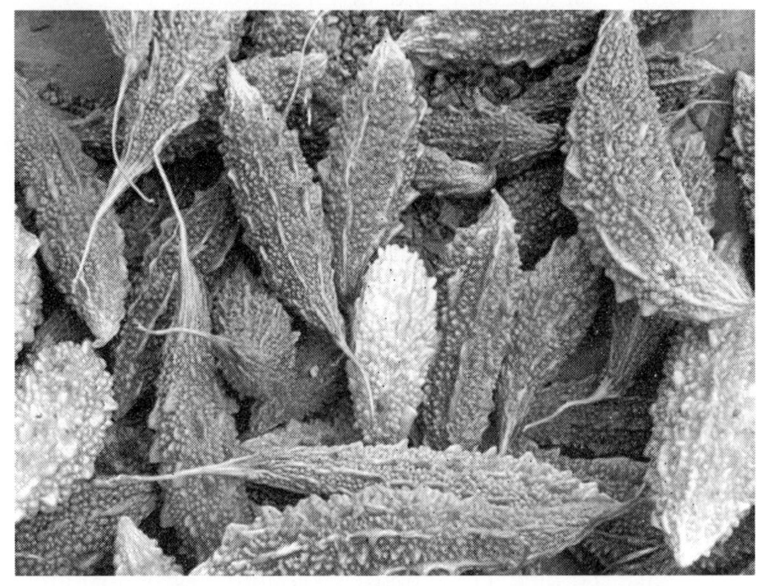

Bitter Gourd (Karela) is an efficient home remedy for boils.

Bitter Gourd (karela) is another effective home remedy for boils. A cupful of fresh juice of this vegetable, mixed with a teaspoon of lime juice, should be taken, sip by sip, on an empty stomach daily for few days in treating this condition.

Betel leaves (pan-ka-patta) are a valuable remedy for boils. A leaf is gently warmed till it gets softened. It is then coated with a layer of castor oil. The oiled leaf should be spread over the inflammed part. It should be replaced every few hours. After a few application, the boil will rupture, draining all the purulent matter. The application can be made at night and removed in the morning.

Cumin seeds (jeera) are beneficial in the treatment of boils. The seeds of black cumin should be ground in water and made into a paste. This paste can be applied to boils with beneficial results.

An application of turmeric (haldi) powder to boils speeds up the healing process. In case of fresh boils, a few dry roots of turmeric are roasted and the ash is dissolved in a cupful of water and applied over the affected portion. This solution enables the boils to ripen and burst.

Warm moist compresses should be applied three or four times a day over the tender area. This will help to bring the boil to a head and encourage easy drainage. Other helpful measures in the treatment of boils are daily dry friction in the morning, cold sponge, physical and breathing exercises. Fresh air and outdoor exercises are also essential for toning up the system.

CHAPTER 41

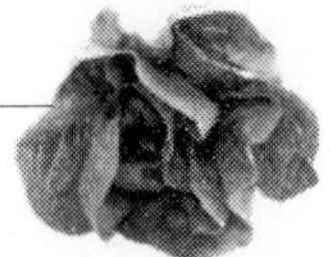

Bronchitis

Bronchitis refers to an inflammation of the mucous membrane lining the bronchi and bronchial tube within the chest. It is a breathing disorder affecting the expiratory function. In most cases, some infection also occurs in the nose and throat. It is a disease endemic to cold, damp climates, but may occur anywhere.

Bronchitis may be acute or chronic. In chronic cases, the disease is of long duration. It is more serious than the acute type as permanent changes may have occurred in the lungs, thereby interfering with their normal movements. Chronic bronchitis is more frequent in males than in females and mortality rate is also higher in males.

Symptoms

In most cases of bronchitis, the larynx, trachea and bronchial tubes are acutely inflamed. The tissues are swollen due to irritation. Large quantities of mucus are secreted and poured into the windpipe to protect the inflamed mucous membranes. The phlegm, when expelled is found to be viscid and purulent. There is usually a higher fever, some difficulty in breathing and a deep chest cough. Other symptoms are hoarseness and pain in the chest and loss of appetite. Breathing trouble continues till the inflammation subsides and mucus is removed.

Causes

The chief cause of bronchitis is wrong feeding habits. The

habitual use of refined foods such as white sugar, refined cereals and white-flour products results in the accumulation of morbid matter in the system and collection of toxic waste in the bronchial tube. Another important cause of this disease is smoking. Excessive smoking irritates the bronchial tubes and lowers their resistance so that they become vulnerable to germs breathed in from the atmosphere. Other causes of bronchitis are living or working in stuffy atmospheres, use of drugs to suppress earlier diseases and hereditary factors. Changes in weather and environment are common factors for the onset of the disease.

Treatment

In acute cases of bronchitis, the patient should fast on orange juice and water till the acute symptoms subside. The procedure is to take the juice of an orange in a glass of warm water every two hours from 8 a.m. to 8 p.m. Thereafter, the patient should adopt an all-fruit diet for two or three days. In case of chronic bronchitis, the patient can begin with an all-fruit diet for five to seven days, taking each day three meals of fresh juicy fruits. After the all-fruit diet, the patient should follow a well-balanced diet of seeds, nuts and grains, vegetables and fruits. For drinks, unsweetened lemon water or cold or hot plain water may be taken. The patient should avoid meats, sugar, tea, coffee, condiments, pickles, refined and processed foods, soft drinks, candies, ice-cream and products made from sugar and white flour.

One of the most effective remedies for bronchitis is the use of turmeric powder. A teaspoonful of this powder should be administered with a glass of milk two or three times daily. It acts best when taken on an empty stomach.

Another effective remedy for bronchitis is a mixture of

dried ginger powder, pepper and cloves taken in equal quantities three times a day. It may be licked with honey or infused with one's daily tea. The powder of these three ingredients have antipyretic qualities and are effective in dealing with fever accompanied by bronchitis. They also tone up the metabolism of the patient.

Onions possess expectorant properties that liquefies phlegm and prevents its further formation. One teaspoon of raw onion juice, the first thing in the morning will be highly beneficial in such cases.

A simple hot poultice of linseed should be applied over the front and back of the chest. It will greatly relieve pain. Poultices act by diluting the vessels of the surface and thereby reducing the blood pressure. The heat of the poultice acts as a cardiac stimulant. A poultice should be applied neatly and carefully and should be often renewed, so that it does not hamper respiration. Turpentine may be rubbed over the chest with fomentation for the same object.

Hot Epsom-salts bath every night or every other night will be highly beneficial during the acute stages of the attack. This bath is prepared by dissolving three lbs. of Epsom-salts to 60 litres of water having a temperature of 100° F. The patient should remain immersed in the bath for about 20 minutes. In case of chronic bronchitis, this bath may be taken twice a week. Hot towels wrung out and applied over the upper chest are also helpful. After applying three hot towels in turn for two or three minutes each, one should always finish off with a cold towel. A cold pack should also be applied to the upper chest several times daily in acute conditions. The procedure is to wring out some linen material in cold water, wrap two or three times round the affected part and cover it with some flannel, The pack can remain for about an hour at a time.

Fresh air and outdoor exercises are also essential for the treatment of bronchitis and the patient should take a good walk every day. He should also perform yogic kriyas such as jalneti and vamandhouti and yogic asanas such as ekpaduttanasana, yogamudra, bhujangasana, shalabhasana, padmasana and shavasana. Simple pranayamas like kapalbhati, anuloma-viloma, ujjai and bhramari are also highly beneficial.

CHAPTER 42

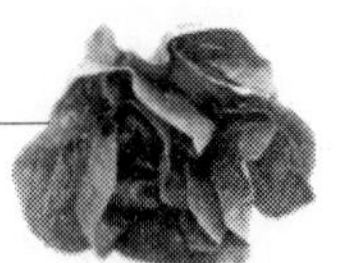

Cancer

The word 'cancer' comes from the latin 'carcinoma' meaning crab. It is the most dreaded disease and refers to all malignant tumours caused by the abnormal growth of a body cell or a group of cells. It is today the second largest killer in the world, next only to heart ailments. The term covers more than 200 diseases.

The majority of cancers occur in the age group 50-60. Sex does not affect the incidence of the disease. It however, affects the site of growth. In men, cancer is usually found in the

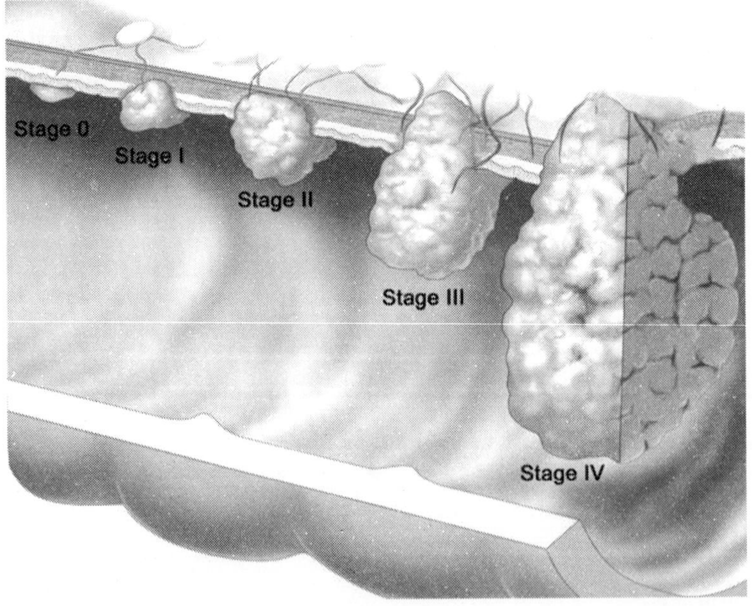

Colon Cancer

intestines, the prostate and the lungs. In women, it occurs mostly in the breast tissues, uterus, gall-bladder and thyroid.

Symptoms

The symptoms of cancer vary according to the site of the growth. The American Cancer Society has prescribed seven signs or danger signals in general which may indicate the presence of cancer. These are; a sore that does not heal; change in bowel or bladder habits; unusual bleeding or discharge; thickening or lump in breast or elsewhere; indigestion or difficulty in swallowing; obvious change in a wart or a mole, and a persistent and nagging cough or hoarseness. Other symptoms may include unexplained loss of weight, particularly in older people, a change in skin colour and changes in the menstrual periods, especially bleeding between periods.

Causes

The prime cause of cancer is not known. Certain cancer-causing substances, known as carcinogens, however, increase the chances of getting the disease. About 80 per cent of cancers are caused by environmental factors. Forty per cent of male cancers in India are linked with tobacco, a known cancer-causing agent. The consumption of *pan,* betelnut, tobacco and slaked lime has been linked with cancer of the tongue, lips, mouth and throat. Cigarette and *bidi* smoking and *hukka* puffing are linked with lung and throat cancers. Heavy consumption of alcoholic drinks can cause oesophagal, stomach and liver cancers. Occupational exposure to industrial pollutants such as asbestos, nickel, tar, soot and high doses of X-rays can lead to skin and lung cancers and leukaemia. Other factors contributing to cancer are viral infections, trauma, hormone imbalance and malnutrition. Many well-known biologists and naturopaths, however, believe that a faulty diet is the root cause of cancer. Investigations indicate that the cancer incidence is in direct proportion to the amount of animal protein, particularly meat, in the diet. Dr. Willard J. Visek, a renowned research scientist explained recently a link between excessive meat-eating and cancer. According to him, the villain is ammonia, the carcinogenic by-product of meat digestion.

Treatment

The effective treatment of cancer consists of a complete change in diet, besides total elimination of all environmental sources of carcinogens, such as smoking and carcinogenic chemicals in air, water and food. There has recently been a surge of popular interest in the concept that diet is not just a minor, but rather a major, factor in both the development and the prevention of cancer. The disease can be prevented and even treated by dietary programmes that include 'natural foods' and the use of megavitamin supplements.

As a first step, the patient should cleanse the system by thoroughly relieving constipation and making all the organs of elimination—the skin, lungs, liver, kidneys and bowels—active. Enemas should be used to cleanse the colon. For the first four or five days, the patient should take only juicy fruits like oranges, grapefruits, lemons, apples, peaches, pears, pineapples and tomatoes. Vegetable juices are also useful, especially carrot juice.

After a few days of an exclusive fruit diet, the patient may be given a nourishing alkaline-based diet. It should consist of 100 per cent natural foods, with emphasis on raw fruits and vegetables, particularly carrots, green leafy vegetables, cabbage, onion, garlic, cucumber, asparagus, beets and tomatoes. A minimum requirement of high quality protein, mostly from vegetable sources such as almonds, millet, sesame seeds, sprouted seeds and grains, may be added to the diet.

Dr. Ann Wigmore of Boston, U.S.A., the well-known naturopath and a pioneer in the field of living food nutrition, has been testing the effect of a drink made of fresh wheatgrass in the treatment of leukaemia. She claims to have cured several cases of this disease by this method. Dr. Wigmore points out that by furnishing the body with live minerals, vitamins, trace elements and chlorophyll through wheatgrass juice, it may be able to repair itself.

Johanna Brandt, the author of the book *The Grape Cure* has advocated an exclusive grape diet for the treatment of cancer. She discovered this mode of cure in 1925, while experimenting on herself by fasting and dieting alternately in the course of her nine-year battle with cancer. She claimed to have cured herself by this mode of treatment. She recommends a fast for two or three days so as to prepare the system for the change of diet.

After the short fast, the patient should have a grape meal every two hours from 8 a.m. to 8 p.m. This should be followed for a week or two, even a month or two, in chronic cases of long standing. The patient should begin the grape cure with a small quantity of 30, 60 to 90 grams per meal, gradually increasing this to double the quantity. In course of time, about 250 grams may safely be taken at a meal.

Recent researches have shown that certain vitamins can be successfully employed in the fight against cancer and that they can increase the life expectancy of some terminal cancer patients. According to recent Swedish studies vitamin C in large doses can be an effective prophylactic agent against cancer. Noted Japanese scientist, Dr. Fukunir Morishige, and his colleagues who have been examining the healing potential of vitamin C for the last 30 years, have recently found that a mixture of vitamin C and copper compound has lethal effects on cancer.

According to several studies, vitamin A exerts an inhibiting effect on carcinogenesis. It is one of the most important aids to the body's defence system to fight and prevent cancer. Dr. Leonida Santamaria and his colleagues at the University of Pavia in Italy have uncovered preliminary evidence suggesting that beta-carotene, a precursor of vitamin A may actually inhibit skin cancer by helping the body thwart the cancer-causing process known as oxidation.

Recent studies from all over the world suggest that a liberal use of green and yellow vegetables and fruits can prevent cancer. The 20-year old, ongoing Japanese study found that people who ate green and yellow vegetables every day had a decreased risk of developing lung, stomach and other cancers. A Harvard University study of more than 1,200 elderly Massachusetts residents found that those who reported the highest consumption of carrots, squash, tomatoes, salads or leafy green vegetables, dried fruits, fresh strawberries or melon had a decreased risk of cancer.

The other useful measures are plenty of rest, complete freedom from worries and mental stress and plenty of fresh, pure air.

CHAPTER 43

Cataract

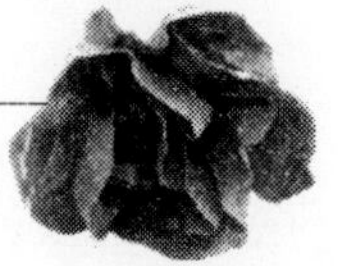

Cataract is among the most common eye diseases. The term actually means a waterfall, and refers to the opacity of the crystalline lens of the eye on the assumption that the condition is caused by the humour of the brain falling over the pupil.

The crystalline lens, through which light travels into the interior of the eye, is situated just behind the iris, or coloured portion of the eye. In cataract, this lens becomes opaque, hence seriously hampering the entrance of light into the eye. Blindness ensues when no light rays can permeate the opacity of the lens. According to the modern medical system, a surgical operation to remove the lens or a major portion of it is the only way to get rid of the disease. The patient is provided with suitable glasses after the operation to enable him to see well enough to carry on his normal duties.

Symptoms

The first sign of cataract is blurred vision. The patient finds it difficult to see things in focus. As the cataract progresses, the patient may get double vision or spots or both. There is a gradual increase in blindness. At first, vision in twilight may be better than in full daylight since light is admitted round the more widely-dilated pupil in the dark. In advance stage, objects and persons may appear merely blobs of light. In the final stage, there is a grayish-white discoloration in the pupil.

Causes

Cataract is often found in association with other defects of the eye. There are four factors which contribute to the loss of transparency of the lens. These are stagnation of the fluid current in the lens resulting from blood condition; deterioration in the nutrition of the lens which diminishes the vitality and resistance of the delicate lens fibres; deposits between the lens fibres of acids and salts which have an irritating effect on the lens tissues and exert an increasing pressure on its delicate fibres, clouding whole lens in the absence of appropriate measures.

As in the case of most diseases, poisons in the blood stream due to dietetic errors and a faulty style of living is the real cause of cataract. The toxic matter in the blood stream spreads throughout the body to find shelter in any available weak spot. It strikes the lens if that part has become weak through strain, excessive use of the eyes and local irritation. The condition becomes worse with the passage of time and then a cataract starts developing. Other causes of cataract are stress and strain, excessive intake of alcoholic drinks, sugar, salt, smoking, certain physical ailments such as gastro-intestinal or gall-bladder disturbance, diabetes, vitamin deficiencies, especially of vitamin C, fatty acid intolerances, ageing, radiation and side-effects of drugs prescribed for other diseases.

Some specialists believe that the most important cause of many cataracts is poor nutrition. This may be true even in case of the type of cataract commonly called senile or ageing cataract. The cause may be a lifetime of malnutrition. Dr. Morgan Raiford, an opthalmologist who has studied cataracts for many years, considers faulty nutrition to be a basic factor in cataract. He has found from experience that prevention of cataract is initiated by improving nutrition.

Treatment

Cataract is one of the most stubborn conditions to deal with. If it has become deep-seated, nothing short of a surgical operation will help in overcoming the trouble. If, however, the cataract is in the early stages, there are good chances of getting over the ailment by natural means. Even advanced cases can be prevented from becoming worse.

A thorough course of cleansing the system of the toxic matter is essential. To start with, it will be beneficial to undergo a fast for three to four days on orange juice and water. A warm water enema may be taken during this period. After this initial fast, a diet of very restricted nature should be followed for two weeks. In this regimen, breakfast may consist of oranges or grapes or any other juicy fruit in season. Raw vegetable salads in season, with olive oil and lemon juice dressing, and soaked raisins, figs or dates should be taken during lunch. Evening meals may consist of vegetables such as spinach, fenugreek, drum sticks, cabbage, cauliflower, carrot, turnips, steamed in their own juices, and a few nuts or some fruits, such as apples, pears and grapes. Potatoes should not be taken. No bread or any other food should be added to this list.

After two weeks on this diet, the cataract patient may start on a fuller diet on the following lines:

Breakfast: Any fresh fruits in season, except bananas.

Lunch: A large mixed raw vegetable salad with wholemeal bread or chappatis and butter.

Dinner: Two or three steamed vegetables, other than potatoes, with nuts and fresh fruit.

The short fast followed by a restricted diet should be repeated after three months of the commencement of the treatment and again three months later, if necessary. The bowels should be cleansed daily with a warm water enema during the fast, and afterwards as necessary.

The patient should avoid white bread, sugar, cream, refined cereals, rice, boiled potatoes, puddings and pies, strong tea or coffee, alcoholic beverages, condiments, pickles, sauces, or other so-called aids to digestion.

There is increasing evidence to show that in several cases cataracts have actually been reversed by proper nutritional treatment. However, the time needed for such treatment may extend from six months to three years. Adelle Davis, one of America's best-known nutritionists, has pointed out that animals develop cataracts if deprived of pantothenic acid and amino acid, tryptophane and vitamin B_6 needed for tryptophane assimilation. She states that the diet of the cataract patient should be high in B_2, B_6, as well as whole B-complex, pantothenic acid, vitamin C, D, E and other nutrients.

The aniseed is considered a useful remedy for cataract. The patient should take about six grams of aniseed daily in the morning and evening. Equal weights of aniseed and coriander powder mixed with brown sugar is also beneficial in the treatment of this disease and the mixture should be taken in doses of 12 grams in the morning and evening. Another valuable remedy for cataract is to grind seven kernels of almonds and half a gram of pepper together in water, and then drink the mixture after sifting and sweetening the mixture with sugar candy. It helps the eyes to regain their vigour.

Simultaneous with the dietary treatment, the patient should adopt various methods of relaxing and strengthening the eyes. These include moving the eyes gently up and down, from side to side and in a circle, clock-wise and anti-clockwise; rotating the neck in circles and semi-circles and briskly moving the shoulders clock-wise and anti-clockwise. The patient should also resort to palming which is highly beneficial in removing strain and relaxing the eyes and its surrounding tissues. The procedure has been outlined in chapter 40 on defective vision.

The epsom salt bath is highly beneficial and should be taken twice a week. The patient should remain in the bath from 25 to 35 minutes till he perspires freely. After the bath the patient should cool off gradually. Closed eyes should also be bathed at least twice daily with hot water containing epsom salt—a tablespoonful of salt to a large cupful of hot water.

In cases where the cataract has been caused by stress, an antistress diet rich in protein, vitamin B, C, E, pantothenic acid and nutrients is essential to overcome the trouble. If a cataract has already developed, the diet will help prevent its occurrence in the other eye.

Fresh air and gentle outdoor exercises, such as walking, are other essentials to the treatment. Exposure to heat and bright light should be avoided as far as possible.

CHAPTER 44

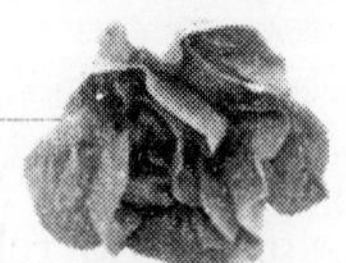

Cervical Spondylosis

Cervical spondylosis is a degenerative disease of cervical region of the spine. It results from degeneration of intervertebral disc and consequent pressure on the cervical nerve roots or cervical spinal cord. It is an arthritic process involving the vertebrae, and is often associated with osteoarthritis in the rest of the skeleton.

The spine is a vital part of the back which is known as life bone of the body. It is made of 24 blocks of bone piled one on top of the other. Sandwiched between these bony blocks are cushions of cartilage and elastic tissues, called intervertebral discs. The vertebral discs act as shock absorbers for the back. Mobility would be impossible without these discs. Cervical spondylosis occurs due to the narrowing of the space between the cervical vertebrae resulting in the compression of the nerves.

Symptoms

The main symptom in cervical spondylosis is nagging and severe pain, which may spread over to both sides of shoulders, back side of neck, the collar bone and head side. In some cases, pain may occur in both the arms and fingers. Another important symptom of this disease is stiffness, which may be acute or chronic. It may lead to the restricted movements, which may be partial or complete. Other symptoms of cervical spondylosis are numbness and tingling or complete loss of sensation on the affected side, headache and giddiness.

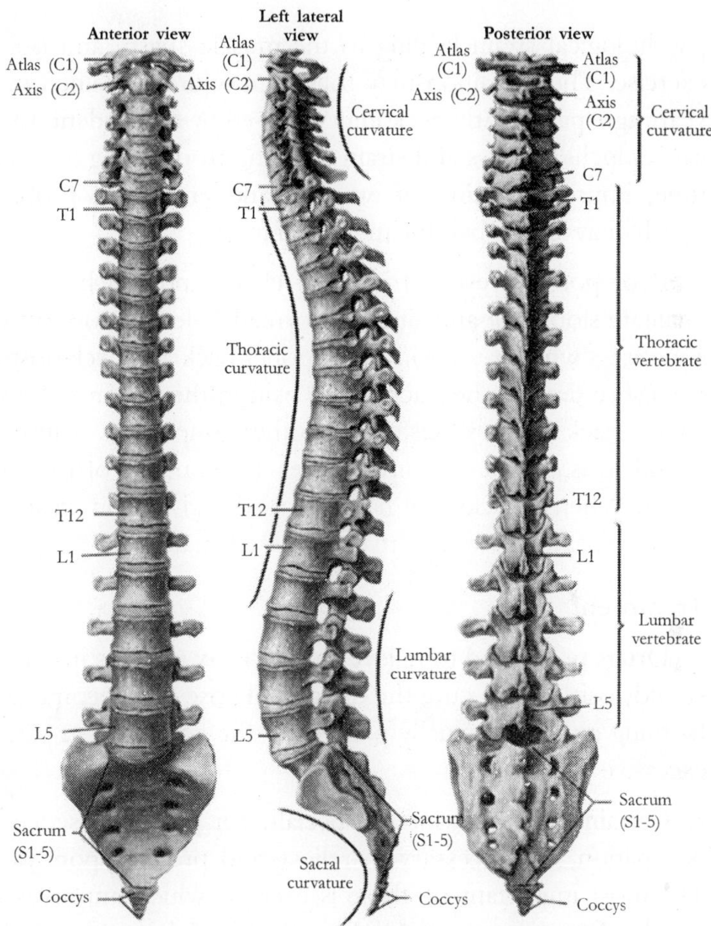

Cervial spondylosis results from degeneration of intervertebral disc and consequent pressure on the cervical nerve roots or cervical spinal cord.

Occasionally, there may be weakness of the muscles of the arm or hand. Diagnosis can be confirmed by an X-ray of the spine.

Causes

The main causes of cervical spondylosis are injury, faulty posture, incorrect nutrition resulting from dietic errors, psychological strain leading to the muscle spasm and lack of exercise. The condition may follow an injury, sustained many years ago, particularly neck injury, caused by an accident. Other causes include stress and strain resulting from sitting for a long time, improper lifting of weights and emotional problems which may cause painful muscle cramps.

Poor posture results from soft chairs and coaches, which facilitate slouching and sitting incorrectly. Sleeping on too soft a mattress which results in an improper back and neck posture, can cause tension, headaches and pain in the upper and lower back. Lack of exercise is another important cause of spondylosis. Modern conveniences have made office work easier. When muscles are not exercised and remain weak, the chances of injury to them is increased manifold.

Treatment

Drugs prescribed to relieve pain or relax muscles in cervical spondylosis do not cure the diseases. Those can become habit forming and may actually perpetuate the condition in case of excessive intake.

Certain safety measures, especially for people in sedentary occupation, are necessary to relieve and present spondylosis. The most important of these is exercise which improves the supply of nutrients to spinal discs, thereby delaying the process of deterioration that comes with age. Safe exercise include walking, swimming and bicycling. The latter should be done keeping the back upright.

Other exercises found beneficial in the treatment of cervical spondylosis are joint movements like folding and unfolding of fingers, moving the wrists up and down, rotating them in both clock-wise and anti-clock-wise direction, folding and unfolding of the forearms and rotating the shoulder clockwise and anti-clock-wise, head and neck exercises like moving the neck up and down, moving to the sides, rotating the neck clock-wise and anti-clock-wise and nodding the neck from one shoulder to another. All these exercises should be undertaken three times daily.

Those with sedentary occupations should take a break to stand up every hour. Soft cushioned seats should be avoided and position should be changed as often as possible. The patient should sleep on a firm mattress on their sides with knees bent at right angles to the torso. He should use thin pillow or avoid it altogether.

The diet of persons suffering from spondylosis should consist of salad of raw vegetables such as tomato, carrot, cabbage, raddish, lettuce and at least two steamed or lightly cooked vegetables such as cauliflower, cabbage, carrot, spinach and plenty of fruits. The patients should have four meals daily. They may take fruits and milk for breakfast, steamed vegetables and whole wheat chappatis during lunch, fresh fruit or fruit juice in the evening and a bowl of raw salad and sprouts during dinner.

The patient should avoid fatty, spicy and fried foods, sour curd, sweets, sugar, condiments as well as tea and coffee. Those who smoke and take tobacco in any form should give up completely.

The patient should take adequate amounts of Proteins and Vitamin C as they are essential for the development of a healthy bone metrix. Vitamin D, Calcium, Phosphorous and the essential trace minerals are also necessary for healthy bones.

Foods that have been processed for storage to avoid spoiling have few nutrients and should be eliminated from the diet. The use of garlic has been found beneficial in the treatment of spondylosis. Two or three capsules of this vegetable should be taken daily in the morning. It will give good results. An oil prepared from garlic and rubbed on the affected part will give great relief. This oil is prepared by frying 10 cloves of garlic in 60 grams of oil in a frying pan. They should be fried slowly till they are brown. After it is cooled, it should be applied vigorously on the affected part and allowed to remain there for three hours. The patient may thereafter have a warm bath. This treatment should be continued for atleast 15 days.

Relief from pain can be obtained by taking lemon juice mixed with common salt twice or thrice daily. A piece of the chebulic myrobalan (harad or haritaki) taken after principal meals also gives quick relief.

Other measures found valuable in cervical spondylosis are mild oil massage to the neck, shoulders and hands, hot fomentation for five to 10 minutes twice a day, five to 10 minutes of exposure to the Infra red rays. Yogic asanas which are beneficial in the treatment of spondylosis are bhujangasana, shalabhasana, vakrasana, uttanpadasana and shavasana.

CHAPTER 45

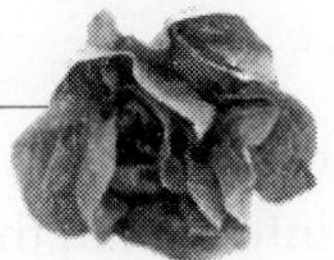

Chicken Pox

Chicken pox is a common infectious and highly contagious disease. It is common during childhood and children between the ages of five and nine are affected more than any other age group. Infants under six months seem to have some immunity against this disease. In most cases, the older the child, the more severe the attack. The disease occurs more frequently in cooler weather.

Symptoms

Chicken pox usually begins with a low grade fever, a mild headache, loss of appetite and a feeling of weakness. Then rashes appear on the skin, first as tiny red spots, mostly on the upper back or chest. In more severe cases, rashes may also appear on the face and lower extremities. The spots turn into blisters and many of them become pustules and form scabs, which fall off.

Lesions come in successive crops, so that some are drying whilst others are beginning to form. The extent of the rash varies from person to person. Some patients have only a few spots, while others have in the mouth, ears, and nose, as well as over most of the body limbs. The skin is cleared after a few days and the patient feels well again. The duration of this disease ranges from 10 to 21 days, but is usually between 14 and 17 days.

Causes

Chicken pox is caused by a virus, in children, it is a

comparatively mild illness, so it is good to succumb to the infection in the early years. An attack of this disease in an adult can be quite severe.

Chicken pox spreads by contact with persons suffering from this disease. It can also spread by inhalation of dust contaminated by dried scabs. The real cause of the disease, as in most cases of fevers, however, is persistent wrong feeding, leading to a natural healing crisis.

Treatment

The patient should be kept in bed in a well-ventilated room in isolation until all the scabs fall off. The nails should be cut short to prevent frequent scratching, as scratching can introduce infection and the spots thus infected will take longer to clear than usual and may leave permanent scars. Wearing cotton gloves at night will avoid the risk of scratching while the patient is a sleep. Itching can be reduced by the application of talcum powder.

The patient should be given plenty of fruit and vegetable juices in the beginning of the treatment. Lemon juice will be especially beneficial. If possible, warm water enema should be taken daily to cleanse the bowels.

Application of mud packs on the abdomen twice a day in the morning and evening and repeated application of chest pack will be beneficial. The procedure for these packs has been explained in Chapter 4 on 'Curative powers of Earth' and Chapter 3 on 'Therapeutic Baths'. Lukewarm water baths can be given every day to relieve itching. For better results, neem leaves can be added to this water.

As the condition improves, the patient can be placed on an all-fruit diet for further two or three days. Thereafter, he may be allowed to gradually adopt a well-balanced diet, with emphasis on fresh fruits and raw vegetables.

Certain home remedies have been found beneficial in the treatment of chicken pox. The use of cider vinegar is one such remedy. Half a cup of cider vinegar should be added to a bath of warm water. This will relieve irritating condition of the skin.

A bath of oatmeal is considered a natural remedy for relieving the itch due to chicken pox. This bath is prepared by cooking two cups of oatmeal in two litres of water for 15 minutes. This mixture is then put into a cloth bag, preferably cotton, and a string is tied tightly around the top. This bag is allowed to float in a tub of warm water, swishing it around, until the water becomes silky. It should, however, be ensured that the bag is not broken. The patient with chicken pox must splash in the water, with the pouch of oatmeal in the tub. The water should go over all the scalds. However the patient should, not be allowed to catch cold.

Green pea water is another effective remedy for relieving irritation of the skin, the water in which the fresh peas have been cooked can be used for this purpose.

Baking soda is also a popular remedy to control the itching in chicken pox. Some baking soda should be put in a glass of water. The patient should be sponged with this water, so the soda dries on. This will keep him away from scratching the eruptions.

A soup prepared from carrots and corriander has been found valuable in chicken pox. About 100 grams of carrot and 60 grams of fresh corriander leaves should be cut into small pieces and boiled for a while. The residue should be discarded and the soup should be taken once a day.

The use of Vitamin E oil is useful in chicken pox. It will

have healing effect. The marks of chicken pox will fade away by this application.

A mild sedative herbal tea can also prove beneficial in the treatment of this disease. This tea can be prepared from any of the herbs like camomile (babunah), basil (tulsi), marigold (zergul) and lemon balm (billilotan). A little cinnamon (dalchini), honey and lemon may be added to this tea. It should be sipped very slowly several times a day.

CHAPTER 46

Cholera

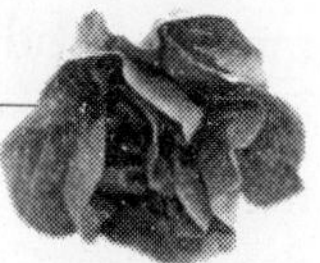

Cholera is one of the most severe diseases of the intestines. It is a serious affliction, involving the lower part of the small bowel. It is a waterborne disease and is common during the monsoons. The mortality rate for this disease has been quite high.

The disease strikes suddenly and fills the intestinal canal with bacilli which die rapidly and leave the person quickly, alive or dead. It comes as a fell epidemic and creates havoc but subsides quickly in the locality. Those who are susceptible to it are carried away and those who are left alive are immuned to it. Thus after an epidemic in a non-endemic area, there is no revisitation in the locality for two or three years.

The original home of cholera is Bengal in India. It spread from this country during the 19th century in a series of epidemics along the trade routes. It reached Japan and also Astrakhan, in Russia, in 1817. The disease spread to Moscow in 1826, Berlin in 1831 and London and Paris in 1832. Subsequently, it spread to Canada and several countries in Europe. However, by 1895, cholera had disappeared from Europe.

Symptoms

Cholera appears in three stages. In the first stage, the patient suffers from mild diarrhoea and vomiting, which worsens rapidly. The motions become watery, containing no faecal matter. The patient experiences severe cramps in the abdominal muscles and limbs, resulting due to lack of salts. The temperature rises but the skin is generally cold and blue and the pulse is weak. The intake of water to quench thirst dilutes the body salts still further, and makes the cramps worse.

In the second stage of collapse, the body becomes colder, the skin dry, wrinkled and purple. Voice becomes weak and husky while the urine looks dark and formation is less, or altogether absent. It is in this 'algid' stage that the patient may die, as early as 24 hours after the onset of the symptoms.

In the third stage, recovery follows in favourable cases. All the changes seem to reverse themselves, the fluid loss decreases and there is improvement in the general condition. Even at this stage, a relapse may occur or the patient may sink into a condition resembling typhoid fever. The condition may deteriorate over a period of two or three weeks. During this stage of reaction, the temperature may rise, and the patient may be in danger from pneumonia.

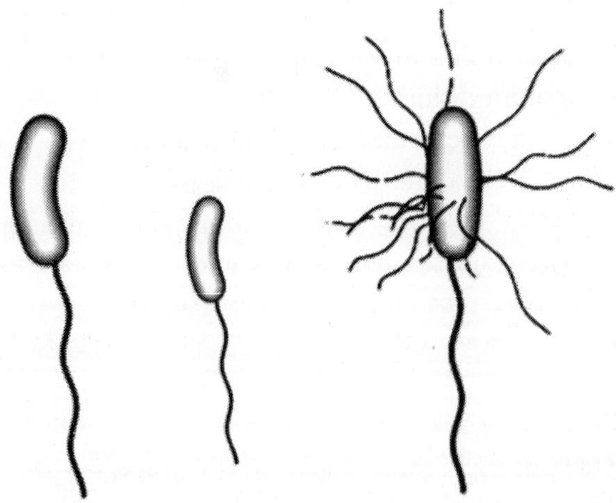

Cholera Bacteria

Causes

Cholera is caused by a short, curved, rod-shaped germ known as vibrio cholerae. This germ produces a powerful poison or endotoxin. It is spread by flies and water contaminated by the germs. The real cause of the disease, however, is the toxic and devitalized condition of the system brought about by incorrect feeding habits and faulty style of living. This condition facilitates invasion of cholera germs.

Treatment

The treatment should in the beginning aim at combating the loss of fluids and salts from the body. To allay thirst, water, soda water or tender coconut water should be given for sipping although these may be thrown out by vomiting. Therefore, only small quantities of water should be given repeatedly, as these may remain for sometime within the stomach and a stay of every one minute means some absorption. Ice may be given for sucking. This will reduce internal temperature and restrict the tendency to vomit. Intravenous infusions of saline solution should be given to compensate for the loss of fluids and salts from the body. The patient may require five litres or more a day. Care should, however, be taken to avoid waterlogging the patient. Potassium may be added to the infused fluid. Rectal saline may sometimes prove useful for adults. Normally, half a litre of saline, with 30 grams of glucose, should be given per rectum every four hours until urine is passed freely.

After the acute stage of cholera is over, the patient may be given tender coconut water and barley water in very thin form. When the stools begin to form, he should be given buttermilk. As he progresses towards recovery, rice softened to semi-solid form mixed with curd, may be given.

The patient should not be given solid food till he has fully recovered. Liquid and bland foods, which the patient can ingest without endangering a reoccurrence of the malady, are best. Lemon, onion, green chillies, vinegar and mint should be included in the daily diet during an epidemic of cholera.

Home Remedies

Certain home remedies have been found beneficial in the treatment of cholera. The foremost among these is the use of lemon (*bara nimbu*). The juice of this fruit can kill cholera bacilli within a very short time. It is also a very effective and reliable preventive food item against cholera during the epidemic. It can be taken in the form of sweetened or salted beverages for this purpose. Daily intake of lemon with food can also prevent cholera.

The root bark of guava (*amrud*) is another valuable remedy. It is rich in tannins and can be successfully employed in the form of concentrated decoction in cholera. It will arrest vomiting and symptoms of diarrhoea.

According to Culpeper, an eminent nutritionist for children and young people, nothing is better to purge cholera than the leaves and flowers of peach (*arhu*). They should be taken in the form of syrup or conserve. The leaves of drumstick (*sanjana*) tree are also useful in the treatment of this disease. A teaspoon of fresh leaf-juice, mixed with honey and a glass of tender coconut water, can be given two or three times as a herbal medicine in the treatment of cholera.

Onion is very useful in cholera. About 30 grams of this vegetable and seven black peppers should be finely pounded in a pestle and given to the patient. It allays thirst and restlessness and the patient feels better. The fresh juice of bitter gourd (*karela*) is another effective medicine in the early stages of cholera.

Two teaspoons of this juice, mixed with an equal quantity of white onion juice and a teaspoon of lime juice, should be given.

Cholera can be controlled only by rigid purification of water supply and proper disposal of human wastes. In case of slightest doubt about the contamination of water, it must be boiled before use, for drinking and cooking purposes. All foodstuffs must be kept covered and vegetables and fruits washed with a solution of potassium permanganate before consumption. Other precautions against this disease include avoiding all uncooked vegetables, thorough washing of hands by all those who handle food, and elimination of all contacts with the disease.

CHAPTER 47

Cirrhosis of the Liver

Cirrhosis of the liver refers to all forms of liver disease characterised by a significant loss of cells. It is one of the most serious hepatic diseases. The liver gradually contracts in size and becomes hard and leathery.

The liver is one of the most important glandular organs in the body. It is located high up on the right side of the abdomen just under the diaphragm. It is a vast chemical laboratory which performs many important functions. It produces bile, cholesterol, lecithin, blood albumin vital to the removal of tissue wastes, prothrombin essential to the clotting of blood and numerous enzymes. It inactivates hormones no longer needed, synthesises many amino acids used in building tissues and breaks proteins into sugar and fat when required for energy. It stores vitamins and minerals. It also destroys harmful substances and detoxifies drugs, poisons, chemicals and toxins from bacterial infections. Liver damage interferes with all of these functions.

In cirrhosis of the liver, although regenerative activity continues, the progressive loss of liver cells exceeds cell replacement. There is also progressive distortion of the vascular system which interferes with the portal blood flow through the liver. The progressive degeneration of liver structure and function may ultimately lead to hepatic failure and death.

Symptoms

In the early stages of the disease, there may be nothing

more than frequent attacks of gas and indigestion, with occasional nausea and vomiting. There may be some abdominal pain and loss of weight. In the advanced stage, the patient develops a low grade fever. He has a foul breath, jaundiced skin and distended veins in the abdomen. Reddish hairlike markings, resembling small spiders, may appear on the face, neck, arms and trunk. The abdomen becomes bloated and swollen, the mind gets clouded and there may be considerable bleeding from the stomach.

Causes

Excessive use of alcohol over a long period is the most potent cause of cirrhosis of the liver. It has been estimated that one out of 12 chronic alcoholics in the United States develops cirrhosis. The disease can progress to end-stage of hepatic failure if the person does not abstain from alcohol. Cirrhosis appears to be related to the duration of alcohol intake and the quantity consumed daily. Recent researches indicate that the average duration of alcohol intake to produce cirrhosis is 10 years and the dose is estimated to be in excess of 500 ml of alcohol daily.

Poor nutrition can be another causative factor in the development of cirrhosis and a chronic alcoholic usually suffers from severe malnutrition as he seldom eats. Other causes of cirrhosis are excessive intake of highly seasoned food, habitual taking of quinine for a prolonged period in tropical climate, and drug treatments for syphilis, fever and other diseases. It may also result from a highly toxic condition of the system in general. In fact, anything which continually overburdens the liver cells and leads to their final breakdown can be a contributing cause of cirrhosis.

Treatment

The patient should be kept in bed. He must abstain completely from alcohol in any form. He should undergo an initial liver cleaning programme with a juice fast for seven days. Freshly extracted juices from red beets, lemon, papaya and grapes may be taken during this period. This may be followed by the fruit and milk diet for two to three weeks.

In this regimen, the patient should have three meals a day, each of fresh juicy fruits and milk. The fruits may include apples, pears, grapes, grape fruit, oranges, pineapples and peaches. One litre of milk may be taken on the first day. It should be increased by 250 ml. daily upto two to two and a half litres a day. The milk should be fresh and unboiled, but may be slightly warmed if desired. It should be sipped very slowly.

After the fruit and milk diet, the patient may gradually embark upon a well-balanced diet of three basic food groups, namely (i) seeds, nuts and grains (ii) vegetables and (iii) fruits, with emphasis on raw organically grown foods. An adequate high quality protein diet is necessary in cirrhosis. The best complete proteins for liver patients are obtained from raw goat's milk, home-made raw cottage cheese, sprouted seeds and grains and raw nuts, especially almonds. Vegetables such as beets, squashes, bitter gourd, egg-plant, tomato, carrot, radishes and papaya are useful in this condition. All fats and oils should be excluded from the diet for several weeks.

The patient should avoid all refined, processed and canned foods, sugar in any form, spices and condiments, strong tea and coffee, fried foods, all preparations cooked in ghee, oil or butter and all meats rich in fat. The use of salt should be restricted. The patient should also avoid all chemical additives in food and poisons in air, water and environment.

Warm water enema should be used during the treatment to cleanse the bowels. If constipation is habitual, all steps should be taken for its eradication. Application of alternate compress to liver area followed by general wet sheet rub will be beneficial. The morning dry friction and breathing and other exercises should form a regular daily feature of the treatment.

CHAPTER 48

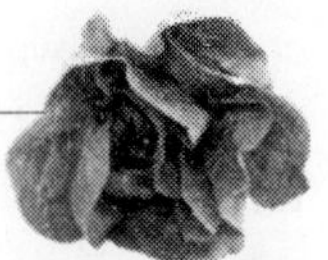

Colitis

Colitis is an inflammation of the colon or large intestine. There are two types of colitis: mucus and ulcerative. Mucus colitis is a common disorder of the large bowel, producing discomfort and irregular bowel habits. Chronic ulcerative colitis is a severe prolonged inflammation of the colon or large bowel in which ulcers form on the walls of the colon, resulting in the passing of bloody stools with pus and mucus. Both forms of colitis are the results of prolonged irritation of the delicate membrane which lines the walls of the colon.

Normally, it is the function of the colon to store waste material until most of the fluids have been removed to enable well-formed soft stools, consisting of non-absorbable food

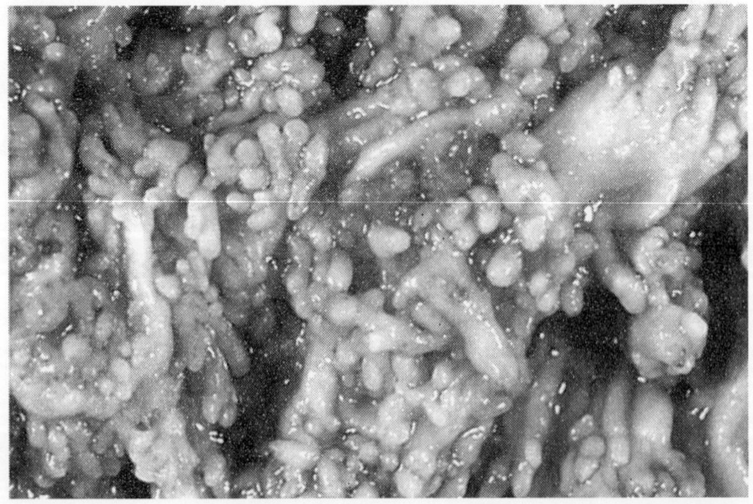

Chronic Ulcerative Colitis

materials to be passed. Persons who suffer from an irritable colon have irregular and erratic contractions which are specially noticeable on the left side.

Symptoms

Chronic ulcerative colitis usually begins in the lower part of the bowels and spreads upwards. The first symptom of the trouble is an increased urgency to move the bowel, followed by cramping pains in the abdomen and bloody mucus in the stools. As the disease spreads upwards, the stools become watery and more frequent and are characterised by rectal straining. All this loss of blood and fluid from the bowels results in weakness, fever, nausea, vomiting, loss of appetite and anaemia.

The patient may develop a bloated feeling because the gas is not absorbed or expelled normally. Some patients suffer from constipation alternating with periods of loose bowel movements. Still others may suffer from a persistent diarrhoea for years together. The patient is usually malnourished and may be severely underweight. He may suffer from frequent insomnia.

Ulcerative colitis in its severe form may also lead to nutritional problems. The improper assimilation of the ingested foods due to inflammatory conditions may cause deficiency diseases. This may gradually result in nervous irritability, exhaustion and depression. In very severe cases, the patient may even develop suicidal tendencies.

Causes

The main cause of colitis is chronic constipation and the use of purgatives. Constipation causes an accumulation of the hard faecal matter which is never properly evacuated.

Purgatives used as a 'cure' only increase irritation. Often, colitis is caused by a poorly digested roughage, especially of cereals and carbohydrates, which causes bowel irritation. The disease may also result from an allergic sensitivity to certain foods especially milk, wheat and eggs. Often, the intake of antibiotics may upset the bacterial flora in the intestines and interfere with proper digestion.

Severe stress may also produce ulcerative colitis. During any form of severe stress, outpouring of adrenal hormones causes such destruction of body protein that at times parts of the walls lining the intestines are literally eaten away. Such stress also depletes the body of pantothenic acid. Experiments on animals have shown that they can develop ulcerative colitis when they are kept on diets deficient in pantothenic acid.

Treatment

The usual treatment of colitis with suppressive drugs is based on the assumption that colitis is due to germ infection, which it is not. The suppressive drugs drive back into the system the toxic matter in the colon which nature is endeavouring to eliminate in the form of mucus. They suppress the symptoms temporarily, without removing the cause. In such cases, the symptoms recur and colitis becomes chronic. Plain warm water or warm water with a little olive oil used as a wash-out is the only method of softening and removing the accumulations of hardened matter sticking to the walls of the colon.

Diet plays an important part in the treatment of colitis. It is advisable to observe a juice fast for five days or so in most cases of ulcerative colitis. The juices may be diluted with a little boiled water. Papaya juice, raw cabbage and carrot juices will be especially beneficial. Citrus juices should be avoided. The bowel should be cleansed daily with a warm water enema.

After the juice fast, the patient should gradually adopt a diet of small, frequent meals of soft cooked or steamed vegetables, rice, *dalia* (coarsely broken wheat), well ripened fruits like banana and papaya, yogurt and home-made cottage cheese. Sprouted seeds and grains, whole meal bread and raw vegetables may be added gradually to this diet after about 10 days. All food must be eaten slowly and chewed thoroughly.

Foods which should be excluded from the diet are white sugar, white bread and white flour products, highly seasoned foods, highly salted foods, strong tea, coffee and alcoholic beverages and foods cooked in aluminium pans.

Ripe bananas are highly beneficial in the treatment of ulcerative colitis, being bland, smooth, easily digested and slightly laxative. They relieve acute symptoms and promote the healing process.

An effective remedy for ulcerative colitis is the use of butter-milk. (It is the residual milk left after the fat has been removed from yogurt by churning.) Buttermilk enema twice a week is also soothing and helps in re-installing a healthy flora in the colon.

Another valuable remedy for colitis is tender coconut water, it is soothing to the soft mucosa of the colon. Cooked apple also aids the healing of ulcerative conditions because of its ample concentration of iron and phosphorus.

The patient should have a bowel movement at the same time each day and spend 10 to 15 minutes in the endeavour. Straining at stools should be avoided. Drinking two glasses of water the first thing in the morning will stimulate a normal bowel movement. An enema may be used if no bowel movement occurs.

Complete bed rest and plenty of liquids are very important. The patient should eliminate all causes of tension, adjust to his disability and face his discomfort with patience.

CHAPTER 49

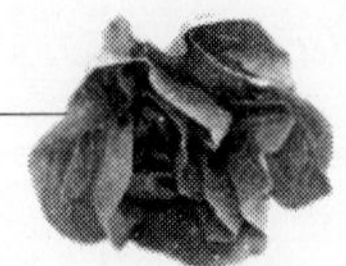

Common Cold

The common cold, also known as "acute coryza," is an inflammation of the upper respiratory tract and is caused by infection with virus. It occurs more often than all other diseases. A person suffers from this disease three times in a year on an average. A cold usually lasts from three to ten days. The patient feels miserable for the first three days or so.

Symptoms

The first signs of a cold are a feeling of soreness of the throat and congestion of the nasal passage. Although the disease normally begins in the nose and throat, it affects all parts of the body. Its usual symptoms are a running nose, sneezing, a rise in temperature, headache, sore throat, chill, aches and pains in the body and loss of appetite. The skin around the nostrils may become sore.

Causes

The common cold results from exposure to a virus. Its intensity however, depends upon the state of health of the person and environmental factors. Lowered vitality, allergic disorders of the nose and throat, chilling of the body, lack of sleep, depression, fatigue and factors such as sudden changes in temperature, dust and other irritating inhalations are important contributory causes for the development of a cold.

The real cause of a cold, however, is the toxic condition of the body brought about by wrong feeding habits such as an excessive intake of starch, carbohydrates, proteins and other acid-forming foods. A cold is, therefore, nature's simplest way of expelling toxic waste from the human system. The duration of the cold will depend on the amount of poisons accumulated in the body and the rapidity with which they are expelled.

Treatment

To treat a cold by means of customary suppressive drugs like aspirin and codeine only paves the way for future trouble of a more serious nature. For such a treatment puts a sudden stop to the eliminative process then taking place and forces the toxic matter back into the tissues again. Moreover, drugs have no effect on the duration of the cold. It has been aptly said that a cold can be cured in a week by taking medicines; otherwise it will subside in seven days.

The only real treatment for colds is a proper diet. The best way to begin the treatment is to put the patient on a fast for two days. Nothing should be taken during this period except warm water mixed with lemon juice and honey or fruit juice and hot water. A liquid diet of fruit juice in large amounts is necessary to neutralise the acid condition of the blood and hot drinks are needed to help clear the kidneys. Pineapple juice in particular is highly beneficial. A warm water enema should be used daily to cleanse the bowels during this period.

The short juice fast may be followed by an exclusive fresh fruit diet for three days. In this regimen, the patient should have three meals a day of fresh juicy fruits such as apples, pears, grapes, grapefruit, oranges, pineapple, peaches, melon or any other juicy fruit in season. Bananas, dried or stewed or tinned fruits, should not be taken. No other foodstuff should be added to the diet as otherwise the whole value of the treatment is lost.

After the exclusive fruit diet, the patient should gradually embark upon a well-balanced diet of three basic food groups, namely (i) seeds, nuts and grains (ii) vegetables and (iii) fruits. It is advisable to avoid meat, fish, eggs, cheese and starchy foods for a few days.

The patient should strengthen the system as a whole by taking a diet which supplies all the vitamins and minerals the body needs. Vitamin C, however, heads the list of these nutrients. It protects one against infection and acts as a harmless antibiotic. It is found in citrus fruits, green leafy vegetables, sprouted Bengal and green grams.

According to Dr. Linus Pauling, a noble prize-winning scientist, the regular use of this vitamin in the optimum daily amount will prevent the common cold and if a cold has already appeared, large doses of this vitamin will relieve the symptoms and shorten its duration. He estimates that one to two grams or 100 mg. to 200 mg. per day is approximately the optimum amount of this vitamin. His advice is to swallow one or two 500 mg. tablets of vitamin C at the appearance of first sign of the cold and continue the treatment by taking an additional tablet every hour.

Lime is the most important among the many home remedies for common cold. It is highly beneficial in all types of cold and fevers. It should be taken well diluted. Vitamin C-rich lime juice increases resistance, decreases toxicity and reduces the duration of the illness. Lime juice should be diluted in a glass of warm water, and a teaspoonful of honey should be added to it. It forms an ideal remedy for a cold and dry cough.

Garlic soup is an ancient remedy to reduce the severity of cold. Garlic contains antiseptic and antispasmodic properties besides several other medicinal virtues. The volatile oil in garlic flushes out the system of all toxins and thus helps bring down fever. Garlic oil combined with onion juice, diluted with water and drunk several times a day, has also been found in several studies to be extremely effective in the treatment of the common cold.

Ginger is also an excellent food remedy for colds and coughs. Ginger should be cut into small pieces and boiled in a cup of water; it should then be strained and half a teaspoon of sugar added to it. It should be drunk while it is still hot, in case of colds. Ginger tea, prepared by adding a few pieces of ginger into boiled water before adding tea leaves, is also an effective remedy for colds and for fevers resulting from cold.

Turmeric, with its antiseptic properties, is an effective remedy for colds and throat irritations. Half a teaspoonful of fresh turmeric powder mixed in 30 grams of warm milk is a useful prescription for these conditions. Turmeric powder should be put in a hot ladle. Milk should then be poured in it and boiled over a slow fire. In case of a running cold, smoke from the burning turmeric should be inhaled. It will increase the discharge from the nose and will bring quicker relief.

Water Treatment

A hot water bath, if it can be taken without undue exposure, is recommended as it helps relieve much of the congestion in the chest and nasal membranes. Hot packs or fomentations are excellent for treating chest and head colds. Steam bath, hot foot bath and hot hip bath are also beneficial as they stimulate perspiration. Steam inhalation will help relieve the congestion of the nasal tissues. Gargling with hot water mixed with salt is beneficial for a sore throat. Cold chest packs should be applied two or three times a day as they will relieve congestion of lungs and help in eliminating the accumulated mucus.

Other useful measures in the treatment of common cold are mild sunbath, fresh air and deep breathing, brisk walks, sound sleep, adjustment of one's clothes and habits to the requirements of the season, so as to nullify the effect of weather fluctuations.

Yogasanas like bhujangasana, shalabhasana, dhanurasana and yogamudra in vajrasana, yogic kriyas such as jalaneti and vamandhouti and pranayamas such as kapalbhati, anuloma-viloma and suryabhedana are beneficial in the treatment of the common cold.

CHAPTER 50

Common Fever

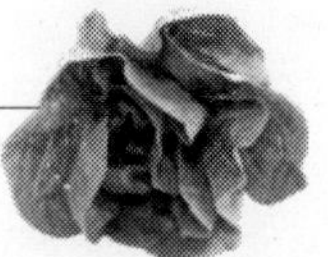

Fever refers to a condition of the body in which the temperature goes beyond the normal. It is also characterised by disturbance in normal functioning of the system. It is a common ailment which occurs both in children and adults.

The average temperature of the body in health ranges between 98.4°F and 99.5°F or 36.9°C and 37.5°C. It is liable to marginal variations, depending on the intake of food, the amount of exercise and the temperature surrounding the atmosphere. The lowest temperature of the body is between the hours 1.30 a.m. to 7 a.m. and the highest between 4 p.m. and 9 p.m.

The temperature can be taken by a clinical thermometer, which is basically a bulb of mercury connected to a narrow tube inside a glass case. There are marked degrees of temperature upon this thermometer. As the mercury is warmed, it rises up the tube and the body temperature is that at which the mercury stops. To get a true reading of the body temperature, it should not be measured after undue exertion, or after a hot drink—either of which activities cause the temperature to rise and so give a false reading.

Symptoms

Fever generally begins by a slight shivering, pain in various parts of the body, particularly the head, thirst and great lassitude. The urine is scanty. There may be constipation, nausea and vomiting. The pulse and respiration are speeded up. Then finally, there is profuse sweating, a copious flow of concentrated urine and general relief of symptoms.

A high temperature is often accompanied by delirium. If the temperature of the body during an attack of fever reaches 106°F, the condition is known as pyrexia. It is an indication of danger. If the temperature goes beyond 107°F for any length of time, death may be inevitable.

Causes

The term fever has a very wide application. It is the symptoms of a body's fight against infection. It is one of the most common features of several diseases. In many cases, it is a secondary symptom of the disordered state of the body with which it is associated.

The real cause of all fevers, including common fewer, however, is the accumulation of morbid matter in the system due to wrong feeding habits and unhygenic conditions of living. Fever is thus, a natural attempt on the part of the body to rid itself of toxic matter. It is not the result of germ infection, as is generally believed. If it was true, all persons exposed to an infection should get it.

Treatment

Fever being a natural healing crisis, it should be helped to run its normal course. Any interference with this natural process by administration of drugs will only enable the body to retain the morbid matter which caused this condition. If dealt with in natural way, the common fever, where there are no complications, will subside in two or three days.

The patient should be put on a fast on orange juice and water in the beginning of the treatment. The procedure is to take the juice of an orange in a glass of warm water every two hours from 8 a.m. to 8 p.m. It will provide energy, increase urinary output and promote body resistance against infection, thereby hastening recovery. Warm-water enema should be given daily to cleanse the bowels during this period.

Cold compresses may be applied to the head in case the temperature rises above 103°F. If this method does not succeed, cold pack may be applied to the whole body. The procedure is to wring out a sheet or large square piece of linen material in cold water, wrap it twice around the body and legs of the patient and then cover completely with a small blanket or similar warm material. This pack should be applied every three hours during the day while temperature is high and kept on for one hour or so each time. Hot water bottles may be applied to the feet and also against the sides of the body.

After the temperature has come down to normal and the tongue has cleared, the patient may adopt an all-fruit diet for further two days. In this regimen, he should take three meals a day of fresh juicy fruits such as apple, pear, grapes, orange, pineapple, peach, melon or any other juicy fruit in season. For drinks, unsweetened lemon water or plain water, either hot or cold may be taken. Thereafter, the patient may gradually embark upon a well-balanced diet, with emphasis on fresh fruits and raw or lightly-cooked vegetables.

Certain home remedies have been found beneficial in the treatment of common fever. The use of the leaves of holy basil (*Tulsi*) is the most effective of these remedies. A decoction made of about 12 grams of these leaves, boiled with half a litre of water, should be administered with milk, sugar and powdered cardamom (*chhoti elaichi*). This will bring down the temperature.

A tea made from fenugreek (*methi*) seed is equal in value to quinine in reducing fevers. It is particularly valuable as a cleansing and soothing drink. Fenugreek seeds, when moistened with water become slightly mucilaginous, and hence the tea made from them has the power to dissolve sticky substances like mucus.

CHAPTER 51

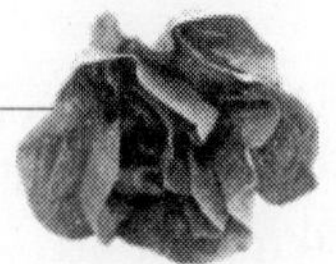

Conjunctivitis

Conjunctivitis refers to the inflammation of the conjunctiva, the thin transparent membrane covering the front of the eye. It is also known as "sore eyes" and is a very common form of eye trouble. It spreads from person to person through direct contact. Overcrowding, dirty surroundings and unhealthy living conditions can cause epidemics of this ailment.

Symptoms

The eyeball and under side of the eyelids become inflamed. At first, the eyes are red, dry and burning. Later, there may be a watery secretion. In more serious cases, there is pus formation. During sleep, this material dries, making the eye-lashes stick together.

Causes

Medical science believes that conjunctivitis results from bacterial infection, viruses or eye-strain. Prolonged work under artificial light and excessive use of the eyes in one way or the other no doubt contributes towards the disease. But its real cause can be traced to a catarrhal condition of the system resulting from general toxaemia due to dietetic errors and faulty style of living. The patient generally suffers from colds or other ailments indicative of a general catarrhal condition.

The Cure

The treatment of conjunctivitis through salves and ointments does not cure the disease. To be effective, treatment must be constitutional. A thorough cleansing of the system and adoption of natural laws in diet and general living alone can help eliminate conjunctivitis.

The best way to commence the treatment is to adopt an exclusive fresh fruit diet for about seven days. The diet may consist of fresh juicy fruits in season such as apple, orange, pears, grapes pineapple and grapefruit. Banana should, however, not be taken. No other foodstuff should be added to this diet.

Those who have a serious trouble should undertake a juice fast for three or four days. The procedure is to take the juice of an orange, in a glass of warm water, if desired, every two hours from 8 a.m. to 8 p.m. Nothing else should be taken as otherwise the value of the fast will be lost, if orange juice disagrees, carrot juice may be taken. A warm water enema should be taken daily during the period of fasting.

The short juice fast may be followed by an all-fruit diet for further seven days. Thereafter, the patient may adopt a general diet scheme on the following lines:—

Breakfast: Any fresh fruits in season, except bananas.

Lunch: Large mixed raw vegetable salad with whole meal bread or chappatis and butter.

Dinner: Two or three steamed vegetables, other than potatoes, with nuts and fresh fruit.

The patient should avoid an excessive intake of starchy and sugary foods in the form of white bread, refined cereals, potatoes, puddings, pies, pastry, sugar, jams and confectionery, which cause the general catarrhal condition as well as conjunctivitis. He should also avoid the intake of excessive quantities of meat and other protein and fatty foods, strong tea and coffee, too much salt, condiments and sauces.

Raw juices of certain vegetables, especially carrots, and spinach, have been found valuable in the treatment of conjunctivitis. The combined juices of these two vegetables have proved very effective. 200 ml. of spinach juice should be mixed with 300 ml. of carrot juice in this combination.

Vitamin A and B_2 have also been found valuable in the treatment of conjunctivitis. The patient should take liberal quantities of natural foods rich in these two vitamins. Valuable sources of vitamin A are: whole milk, curds, butter, carrots, pumpkin, green leafy vegetables, tomatoes, mangoes and papaya. Foods rich in vitamin B_2 are green leafy vegetables, milk, almonds, citrus fruits, bananas and tomatoes.

As regards local treatment to the eyes themselves, a cold foment renders almost immediate relief by chasing away an overactive local blood supply. The procedure is as follows:

Fold a small hand towel. Saturate it with cold water. Squeeze out excess water and mould towelling gently over both eyes. Cover it with a piece of warm cloth to retain the temperature. Repeat the process as soon as the foment gets warmed. Carry out the procedure for one hour. After terminating the wet pack, treatment cover the eyes with a dry towel. Lie back and relax. The damaged eye tissues will quickly return to normal. The treatment should be repeated every night for a week, even though the problem may clear up with the first treatment itself.

Eye Exercises

The eye muscle exercises outlined in chapter 43 on cataract and palming outlined in chapter 57 on defective vision are also beneficial in the treatment of conjunctivitis.

CHAPTER 52

Constipation

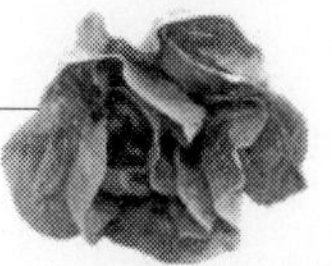

Constipation is a common disturbance of the digestive tract. In this condition, the bowels do not move regularly, or are not completely emptied when they move.

Constipation is the chief cause of many diseases as such a condition produces toxins which find their way into the blood stream and are carried to all parts of the body. This results in weakening of the vital organs and lowering of the resistance of the entire system. Appendicitis, rheumatism, arthritis, high blood pressure, cataract and cancer are only a few of the diseases in which chronic constipation is an important predisposing factor.

The number of motions required for normal health varies from person to person. Most people have one motion a day, some have two a day, while others have one every other day. However, for comfort and health, at least one clear bowel movement a day is essential and considered normal.

Symptoms

The most common symptoms of constipation are infrequency, irregularity or difficulty of elimination due to hard faecal matter. Among the other symptoms are a coated tongue, foul breath, loss of appetite, headache, dizziness, dark circles under the eyes, depression, nausea, pimples on the face, ulcer in the mouth, constant fullness in the abdomen, diarrhoea alternating with constipation, varicose veins, pain in the lumber region, acidity, heart burn and insomnia.

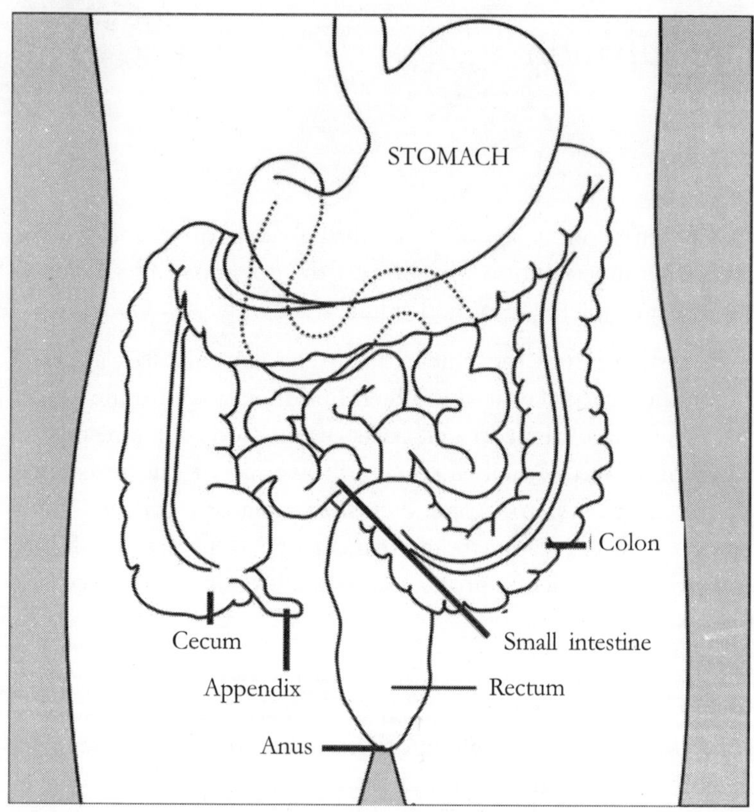

Digestive System

Causes

The most important causes for chronic constipation are wrong diet and a faulty style of living. All foods in their natural state contain a good percentage of 'roughage' which is most essential in preserving natural balance of foods and also in helping peristalsis—the natural rhythmic action by means of which the food is passed down the alimentary canal. Much of the food we eat today is very deficient in natural bulk or roughage and this results in chronic constipation.

Intake of refined and rich food lacking in vitamins and minerals, insufficient intake of water, consumption of meat in large quantities, excessive use of strong tea and coffee, insufficient chewing, overeating and wrong combination of foods, irregular habits of eating and drinking may all contribute to poor bowel function. Other causes include faulty and irregular habit of defecation, frequent use of purgatives, weakness of abdominal muscles due to sedentary habits, lack of physical activity and emotional stress and strain.

Diseases such as tumours or growths, a sluggish liver, colitis, spastic condition of the intestine, hyperacidity, diseases of the rectum and colon, bad teeth, uterine diseases, diabetes, use of certain drugs for treating other ailments, abnormal condition of the lower spine and enlargement of the prostate glands can also cause chronic constipation.

Treatment

The most important factor in curing constipation is a natural and simple diet. This should consist of unrefined food such as whole grain cereals, bran, honey, molasses and lentils; green and leafy vegetables, especially spinach, french beans, tomatoes, lettuce, onion, cabbage, cauliflower, Brussels sprouts, celery, turnip, pumpkin, peas, beets, asparagus, carrot; fresh fruits, especially pears, grapes, figs, papayas, mangoes, grapefruit, gooseberries, guava and oranges; dry fruits such as figs, raisins, apricots and dates; milk products in the form of butter, ghee and cream.

The diet alone is not enough. Food should be properly chewed-each morsel for at least 15 times. Hurried meals and meals at odd times should be avoided. Sugar and sugary foods should be strictly avoided because sugar steals B vitamins from the body, without which the intestines cannot function normally. Foods which constipate are all products made of white flour, rice, bread, pulses, cakes, pastries, biscuits, cheese, fleshy foods, preserves, white sugar and hard-boiled eggs.

Regular drinking of water is beneficial not only for constipation but also for cleaning the system, diluting the blood, and washing out poisons. Normally six to eight glasses of water should be taken daily as it is essential for digesting and dissolving food nutrients so that they can be absorbed and utilised by the body. Water should, however, not be taken with meals as it dilutes the gastric juices essential for proper digestion. Water should be taken either half an hour before or an hour after meals.

Generally all fruits, except banana and jack fruit, are beneficial in the treatment of constipation. Certain fruits are however, more effective. Bael fruit is regarded as best of all laxatives. It cleans and tones up the intestines. Its regular use for two or three months throws out even the old accumulated faecal matter. Though generally used to check diarrhoea, bael contains both laxative and constipative properties. It hardens the stools when they are loose and serves as a laxative when the bowels are constipated. It should be preferably used in its original form and before dinner. About 60 grams of the fruit will suffice for an adult.

Pears are regarded the next best fruit beneficial in the treatment of constipation. Patients suffering from chronic constipation should better adopt an exclusive diet of this fruit or its juice for few days, but in ordinary cases a medium-sized pear taken after dinner or with breakfast will have the desired effect. The same is true of guava which, when eaten with seeds, gives roughage to the diet and helps in the normal evacuation of the bowels.

Grapes have also proved highly beneficial in overcoming constipation. The combination of the properties of the cellulose, sugar and organic acid in grapes make them a laxative food. Their field of action is not limited to clearing the bowels only. They also tone up the stomach and intestines and relieve the most chronic constipation. One should take at least 350 grams of grapes daily to achieve the desired results. When fresh grapes are not available, raisins soaked in water can be used. Raisins should be soaked in a tumblerful of drinking water for 24 to 48 hours. This would swell them to the original size of the grapes. The raisins should be eaten early in the morning. The water in which raisins are soaked should be drunk along with the soaked raisins.

Drinking hot water with sour lime juice and half a teaspoon of salt is also an effective remedy for constipation. Drinking water which has been kept overnight in a copper vessel, the first thing in the morning will bring good results. Linseed is extremely useful in difficult cases of constipation. A teaspoon of linseed swallowed with water before each meal provides both bulk and lubrication.

In all ordinary cases of constipation, an exclusive fruit diet for about seven days would be the best way to begin the treatment. For long-standing and stubborn cases, it would be advisable to have a short fast for four or five days. This will drive out the packed contents of the bowels, eliminate toxins and purify the blood stream. Weak patients may take orange juice during the period of fasting. After the all-fruit diet or the short fast, as the case may be, the patient should gradually embark upon a balanced diet comprising adequate raw foods, ripe fruits and whole grain cereals. In some cases, further short periods on fruits or short fasts may be necessary at intervals of two months or so, depending on the progress being made.

The bowels should be cleansed daily through a warm water enema for a few days at the commencement of the treatment.

A cold friction bath taken daily in the morning can help cure constipation. An alternate hot and cold hip bath taken before retiring to bed is also beneficial. Abdominal exercise and manual or mechanical vibratory massage have a refreshing and stimulating effect in many cases.

Toning up the muscles also helps in the treatment of constipation. Fresh air, outdoor games, walking, swimming, gardening and exercise play an important role in strengthening and activating the muscles, thereby preventing constipation.

Certain yogic asanas also help to bring relief from constipation as they strengthen the abdominal and pelvic muscles and stimulate the peristaltic action of the bowels. These asanas are: bhujangasana, shalabhasana, yogamudra, dhanurasana, halasana, paschimotanasana. Pranayamas such as anuloma-viloma and bhastrika and jalaneti kriya are also helpful.

CHAPTER 53

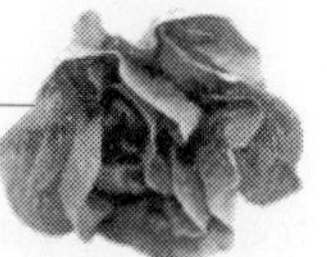

Corns

Corns refer to localized thickening of the skin. Thickening of the skin over a large area is called a callosity, and is usually protective, whereas corn is relatively small and painful.

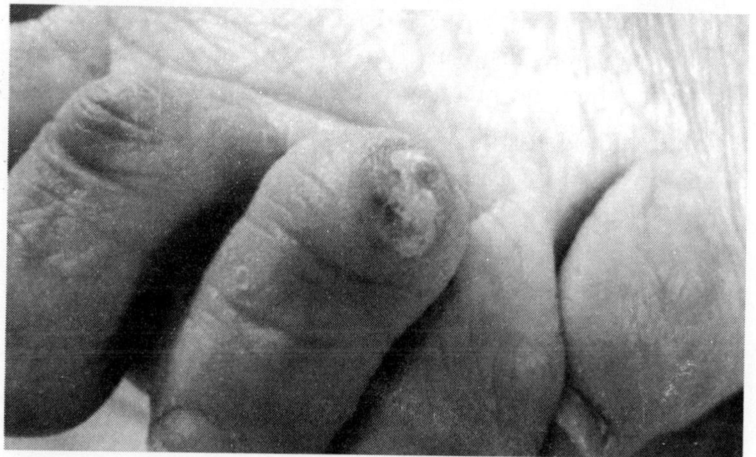

Corn over the toe

Symptoms

Corns are usually found over the joins of the toes and on the soles of the feet. They are shaped like a pyramid with the apex pointing inwards. They are tender when touched. Sometimes painful and infective warts that occur on the soles of the feet are mistaken for corns.

Causes

Corns are usually formed as a result of pressure on the toes and skin surfaces of the feet, through incorrect footwear. The toes are malformed from the same cause. The modern craze for high-heeled shoes is the cause of an enormous amount of foot trouble, for the high heel pushes the toes forward into the front of the shoe, where owing to its narrowness, the toes are crammed together mercilessly and exposed to all the inconvenience to which it is possible for them to be subjected.

Treatment

For proper treatment of corns, it is essential to first stop wearing the shoes that caused it. In most cases, the corn will disappear when the pressure is removed.

One method for the removal of corns is to soften them by soaking the foot in the hot soap-suds, and then check them down with a sharp scalpel, and carefully dissect out the corn without causing bleeding. The resulting cavity should be filled in with vaseline adding a drop of lemon juice.

Another method of treating corns is to cut it off with a sharp knife or razor and apply the sap of the papaya tree over it. It should then be covered with a cut lemon and bandaged. It will subside. If the corn is formed again, the same treatment should be followed.

For soft corns, which usually occur between the toes, the feet should be bathed daily. This should be followed by the application of bland powder and the insertion of wool between the toes.

Several home remedies have been found beneficial in the treatment of corns. One of the most valuable of these is the use of liquorice (*mulethi*). A paste made by grinding liquorice sticks and mixing it with sesame oil or mustard oil should be rubbed into the hardened skin at bed time. The skin gradually softens and the corn decreases in size. This remedy is especially useful for corns which are just appearing.

Lemon (*bara nimbu*) is another valuable remedy for corns. A fresh slice of the lemon should be tied over the painful area at night and it should be allowed to remain there whole night. The juice of pineapple can also be applied externally over corns with beneficial results.

Raw papaya (*papita*) is beneficial in the treatment of corns. Its juice is an irritant and is therefore a useful application in this condition. The juice can be applied three times daily.

The skin of ripe bananas (*kela*) has been found valuable in treating corns. This skin should be applied to the corns, before retiring to bed. It should be kept covered for the whole night and removed in the morning. This treatment may have to be continued for three or four nights.

The miky juice of green figs (*anjeer*) is valuable for corns of long duration. It helps to soften them. This has a mild *nicrotic* action.

The pulp of raw potato is also useful in the treatment of this condition. It should be placed on the corn and secured with a bandage and allowed to remain for two or three hours.

The oil extracted from the outer shell of the cashewnut (*kaju*) being acrid and rubefacient, is valuable in corns. It should be applied externally over the affected parts in treating this condition.

The herb Indian Squill (*jungli piyaz*), botanically known as Urginea Indica, is useful in removing corns. A poultice of the roasted bulb should be applied over the affected areas in treating this disorder.

Epsom-salt bath is highly beneficial in the treatment of corns. About 100 gms. of epsom salt should be dissolved in bowl full of water. The feet should be bathed in the water for five to 10 minutes twice daily in the morning and night.

CHAPTER 54

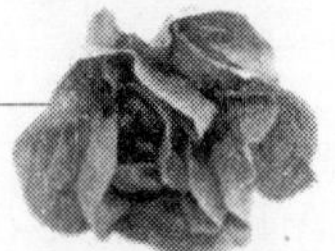

Cough

The air passage of the lungs are lined with cells secreting mucus, which normally traps particles of dust. When the membranes are infected and inflammed, the secretion of mucus increases and the lining of air passage is irritated. Coughing is the action by which excess mucus is driven out. In the process a dry hacking sound is produced. It is a very common condition affecting persons of all ages.

Coughing is a vital body defence mechanism. It ejects every thing from germs to foreign bodies from the lungs and windpipe. When a person is unable to cough which may happen, for instance, post surgery or a chest injury, pneumonia can become a serious threat.

Symptoms

First a person who is going to cough draws a deep breath in. He then closes his glottis and contracts his muscles. This builds up pressure in the chest. Then, he suddenly opens his glottis so that there is an explosive discharge of air which sweeps through the air passage and carries with it the excess secretions or, in some cases, foreign matter which has irritated the larynx, trachea or bronchi.

Causes

Cough may be caused by inflammation of the larynx or the pharynx. It may also be caused by digestive disturbance. A cough can develop in the chest due to weather condition or seasonal changes. The real cause of this disorder, however, is clogging of the bronchial tube with waste matter. This has been brought about by wrong feeding habits. The reason for higher incidence of cough during winter than in other seasons is that an average person usually eats more of the catarrh-forming foods such as white bread, meat, sugar, porridge, puddings, and pies in the colder months of the year. Over clothing with heavy-under-garments during this period also prevents proper aeration of the skin.

Treatment

In case of severe cough, the patient should fast on orange juice and water till the severity is reduced. The procedure is to take the juice of an orange diluted in warm water every two hours from 8 a.m. to 8 p.m. A warm water enema should be used daily to cleanse the bowels. After the juice fast, the patient should adopt an all-fruit diet for two or three days. In case of

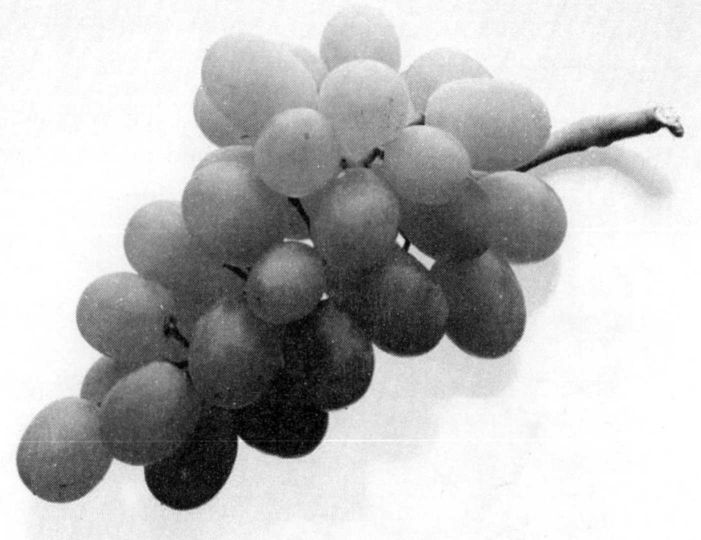

Grapes are beneficial for cough

mild cough, the patient can begin with an all-fruit diet for five to seven days, taking three meals a day of fresh fruit juice such as apples, pears, grapes, grape-fruit, oranges, pineapple, peaches and melon. For drinks, unsweetened lemon water or cold or hot plain water may be taken. After the all-fruit diet, the patient should follow a well-balanced diet, with emphasis on whole grain cereals, raw or lightly-cooked vegetables and fresh fruits.

The patient should avoid meats, sugar, tea, coffee, condiments, pickles, refined and processed foods. He or she should also avoid soft drinks, candies, ice-cream and all products made from sugar and white flour.

Several home remedies have been found beneficial in the treatment of cough. One of the most effective of these is the use of grapes. They tone up the lungs and act as an expectorant. Simple cold and cough are relieved through its use in a couple of days. A combination of honey with grape juice is a specific for cough.

Almonds (*badam*) are useful in dry coughs. They should be soaked in water for about an hour or so and the brown skin

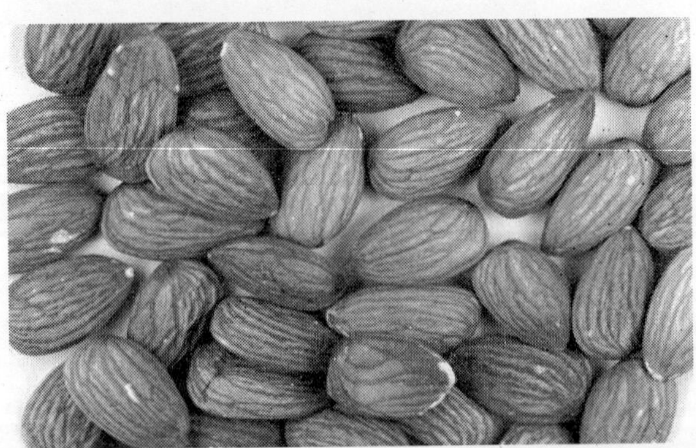

Almonds are one of the best protein foods, containing all the essential amino-acids.

removed. They should then be ground well to form a fine paste and 20 grams each of butter and sugar added to it. This paste should be given in the morning and evening.

Onion (*Piyaz*) is valuable in cough. This vegetable should be chopped fine and juice extracted from it. This juice mixed with honey and kept for four or five hours will make an excellent cough syrup. It is also useful in removing phlegm. A medium size onion should be crushed, the juice of one lemon should be added to it, and then one cup of boiling water should be poured on it. Some honey should be added for taste and it should be taken two or three times a day.

The root of turmeric (*haldi*) plant is useful in dry cough. The root should be roasted and powdered. This powder should be taken in three gram doses twice daily in the morning and evening.

The herb belleric myroblan (*bhaira*) is a household remedy for cough. A mixture of the pulp of the fruit, long pepper and honey should be administered for the treatment of this condition. The dried fruit covered with wheat flour and roasted, is another popular remedy for cough condition.

A sauce prepared from raisins (*munaqqa*) is also useful in cough. This sauce is prepared by grinding 100 grams of raisins with water. About 100 grams of sugar should be mixed with it and the mixture should be heated and preserved when the bulk has turned saucy. This sauce should be taken in 20 grams dose at bed time daily.

Aniseed (*vilaiti saunf*) is another effective remedy for hard dry cough with difficult expectoration. It breaks up mucus. A tea made from this spice should be taken regularly for treating this condition.

CHAPTER 55

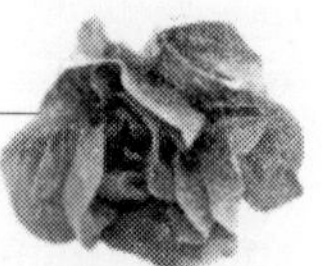

Cystitis

The term 'Cystitis' refers to 'inflammation of the bladder'. It is a most common complaint in women. *Escherichia coli* infections are considered the primary culprit in cystitis. The female anatomy makes it more convenient for *e. coli* bacteria, which normally inhabit the colon, to travel from the rectum to the vagina, up the urethra and into the bladder. This condition is rarely dangerous but it is generally a forerunner to more serious troubles. The reoccurrence of cystitis may in some cases be associated with kidney troubles.

The kidney and bladder are the principal structures in the urinary system. The kidneys are situated on the back of the abdomen, one on each side of the spine at about the level of the lowest rib. The bladder is situated in the lower abdomen, in the pelvis. The body is relieved of the greater part of the waste matter, resulting from the complex working of the whole body's vital processes by means of these two organs.

Symptoms

Cystitis is characterised by symptoms which may cause great discomfort. The patient complains of frequency and burning on urination as well as an almost continual urge to void. There may be a feeling of pain in the pelvis and lower abdomen. The urine may become thick, dark and may have an unpleasant smell and contain blood or pus. The 'scalding' sensation on passing urine indicates that the inflammation has spread to the urethra. Some pain in the lower back may also be felt in certain cases. In an acute stage there may be a rise in body temperature.

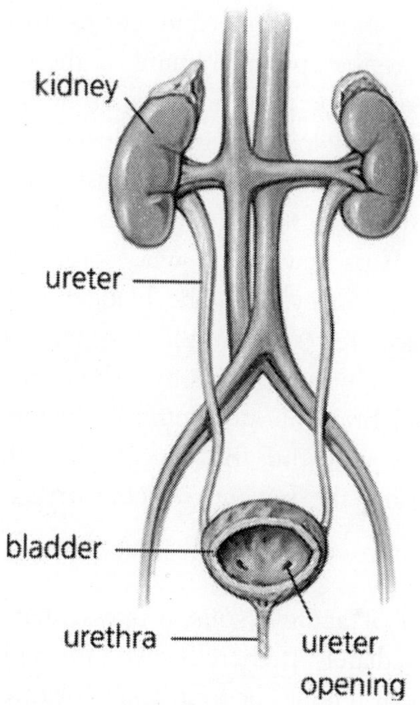

The organs which form the urinary tract

In the chronic form of cystitis, the symptoms are similar but generally less severe and without a rise in temperature. The persistence of the chronic form of the disease indicates a process of deterioration, almost invariably due to wrong treatment of the acute form by suppressive drugs.

Causes

Cystitis may result from infections in other parts adjacent to the bladder such as the kidneys, the urethra, and the vagina. Local irritation and inflammation of the bladder may be caused if urine is retained there for an unduly long time. It may also result from severe constipation.

Continual draining of pus and germs from an infected kidney may injure the epithelial lining of the bladder. Trouble may also arise from the presence of a stone in either bladder or kidney. Childbirth injuries and major surgical procedures within the pelvis may also lower the resistance of the bladder wall and predispose to the development of cystitis. There is also the problem of new brides who sometimes suffer from so-called honeymoon cystitis. The bladder wall may become swollen and ulcerated so that the bladder cannot hold the normal amount of urine. Germs may then find their way into the bladder and bring about chemical changes in the urine. Calcium or lime may thus be deposited in the wall of the bladder, increasing the patient's discomfort.

Treatment

At the onset of acute cystitis, it is essential to withhold all solid food immediately. If there is fever, the patient should fast either on water or tender coconut water for three or four days. If there is no fever, raw vegetable juices, especially carrot juice diluted with water, should be taken every two or three hours. By so doing the biochemical energy needed for digestion and metabolism of food is diverted to the process of eliminating toxins and promoting healing and repair. It is advisable to rest and keep warm at this time.

Pain can be relieved by immersing the pelvis in hot water, or alternatively by applying heat to the abdomen, using a towel wrung out in hot water, covering it with a dry towel to retain warmth. Care should be taken to avoid scalding. A little vegetable oil gently rubbed into the skin, will avoid too much reddening. This treatment may be continued for three or four days, by which time the inflammation should have subsided and the temperature returned to normal.

For the next two or three days, only ripe sub-acid fruits may be taken three or four times daily. These fruits may include grapes, pears, peaches, apples and melon, as available.

While the hot compresses are intended to relieve pain, the use of cold water compresses to the abdomen is most valuable, if correctly applied, in relieving pelvic congestion and increasing the activity of the skin. Care should, however, be taken to ensure that compresses do not cause chilling.

After the all-fruit diet, the patient may gradually embark upon a well-balanced diet, consisting of seeds, nuts, grains, vegetables and fruits. The patient should avoid refined carbohydrates and salt, both at table and in cooking. Salt disturbs the balance of electrolytes and tends to raise blood pressure, which is already raised in kidney troubles.

The prescribed dietary should exclude meat, fish and poultry. They produce uric acid. Most cases of food poisoning and infections, which may lead to gastritis and colitis, are also caused by the flesh foods.

In case of chronic cystitis, the patient should commence the treatment by strict adherence to the dietary programme, designed to cleanse the blood and other tissues and at the same time provide a rich source of natural vitamins and minerals in balanced proportions. The patient may adopt the following restricted diet for seven to ten days:

Upon arising: A glass of unsweetened apple juice or carrot juice.

Breakfast: Fresh fruits, selected mainly from apple, pear, grapes, melon, peach and pineapple, and a glass of buttermilk, sweetened with a little honey.

Mid-morning: Tender coconut water.

Lunch: A salad of raw vegetables such as carrot, beetroot

and cabbage, mixed with curd and a teaspoon of honey. This may be followed by a ripe apple.

Mid-afternoon: One cup of unsweetened grape juice.

Dinner: A salad of green leafy vegetables and a fresh fruit, preferably a portion of melon sweetened with a teaspoon of honey.

Before retiring: One glass of mixed raw carrot and beetroot juice.

After the restricted diet, the patient should gradually embark on a well-balanced diet consisting of seed, nuts, grains, vegetables and fruits. Even after recovery from the chronic condition, it would be advisable for the individual to live exclusively on vegetables or on tender coconut water or raw vegetable juices for a day or two, every month. The water treatment and other health building methods should, however, be continued to the greatest extent possible, so that the patient may stay cured.

CHAPTER 56

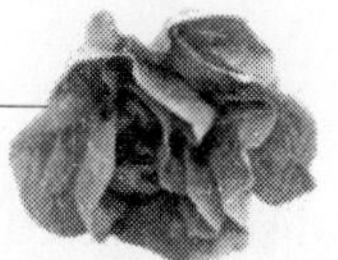

Dandruff

Dandruff refers to the flaking scalp which falls like snow flakes and settles on one's brows, shoulders and clothes, but assumes an unpleasant, irritating condition associated with bacteria, in the case of excessive formation of scales on the scalp. These scales are formed from the horny layer of the skin.

Symptoms

The scaliness increases whenever the hair is brushed or rubbed, it may also appear as lumps or crusts on the scalp. Often there is itching as well, and the scalp may become red from scratching.

Causes

The main causes of dandruff are—impairment of general health, toxic condition of the system brought on mainly by wrong feeding, constipation and lowered vitality due to infectious diseases. Other factors contributing to dandruff are emotional tension, harsh shampoos, exposure to cold and general exhaustion.

Treatment

Numerous medicated shampoos are available in the market for the treatment of dandruff. Most of these, however, in the process of curing the disorder, cause irreparable damage to the hair roots because of the synthetic ingredients contained in them. The treatment of dandruff has to be largely constitutional, if a permanent cure is desired.

The foremost consideration in the treatment of this disorder is to keep the hair and scalp clean so as to minimise the accumulation of dead cells. The hair should be brushed daily to improve the circulation and remove any flakiness. The most effective way to brush the hair is to bend forward from the waist with the head down towards the ground, and brush from the nape of the neck towards the top of the head. Short or shoulder-length hair can be brushed right from the roots to the ends in one stroke. In the case of long hair, two strokes would be best to avoid stretching the hair.

The scalp should also be thoroughly massaged every day, using one's finger tips and working systematically over the head. This should be done just before or after brushing the hair. Like brushing, this stimulates the circulation, dislodges dirt and dandruff and encourages hair growth. For a proper massage, spread your fingers fanwise and slip them through the hair. With your thumbs pressed behind your ears, press down on your scalp with your fingertips. Now rotate your fingers so that they move the scalp over the bony structure of the head. You will feel your skin move and the scalp tingle. Move up an inch at a time until you have covered the whole head. It is a very simple procedure, and takes only a few minutes to perform.

Several home remedies have been found useful in the treatment of dandruff. The use of fenugreek (*methi*) seeds is one such remedy. Two tablespoons of fenugreek seeds should be soaked overnight in water. The softened seeds should be ground into a fine paste in the morning. This paste should be applied all over the scalp and left for half-an-hour. The hair should then be washed thoroughly with soapnut (*ritha*) solution or shikakai.

The use of a teaspoon of fresh lime juice for the last rinse, while washing hair, is equally beneficial. This not only leaves the hair glowing but also removes stickiness and prevents dandruff. Washing the hair twice a week with green gram powder in curd is another useful prescription.

Dandruff can be removed by massaging one's hair for half-an-hour with curd which has been kept in the open for three days, or with a few drops of lime juice mixed with amla juice every night, before going to bed. Another measure which helps to counteract dandruff is to dilute cider vinegar with an equal quantity of water and dab this on to the hair with cotton wool in between shampooing. Cider vinegar added to the final rinsing water after shampooing also helps to disperse dandruff.

Diet plays an important role in the treatment of dandruff. To begin with, the patient should resort to an all-fruit diet for about five days. In this regimen, there should be three meals a day, consisting of fresh, juicy fruits, such as apples, pears, grapes, grapefruit, pineapple and peaches. Citrus fruits, bananas, dried, stewed or tinned fruits should not be taken. Only unsweetened, lemon or plain water, either hot or cold, should be drunk. During this period, a warm water enema should be taken daily to cleanse the bowels and all other measures adopted to eradicate constipation.

After the all-fruit diet, the patient can gradually adopt a well-balanced diet. Emphasis should be on raw foods, especially fresh fruits and vegetables; sprouted seeds, raw nuts and whole grain cereals, particularly millet and brown rice. Further short periods on the all-fruits diet for three days or so may be necessary at a monthly interval, till the skin's condition improves.

Strict attention to diet is essential for recovery. Starchy, protein and fatty foods should be restricted. Meats, sugar, strong tea or coffee, condiments, pickles, refined and processed foods—all these should be avoided, as also soft drinks, candies, ice cream and products made with sugar and white flour.

Exposure of the head to the rays of the sun is also a useful measure in the treatment of dandruff. Simultaneously, an attempt should be made to keep the body in good health. This also helps clear dandruff.

CHAPTER 57

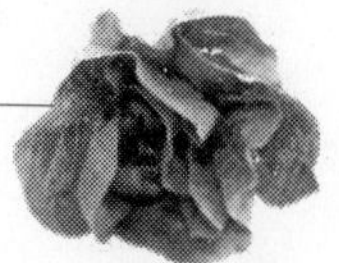

Defective Vision

Defective vision is a common problem nowadays. The main reasons for eye defects are reading in bad light (either too dim or excessively bright), excessive reading, reading in moving trains, buses or cars, watching too much television, seeing too many films, and eating artificial food. The popular belief that the use of spectacles can rectify all cases of defective vision is based on the assumption that such defects are caused by permanent changes in the eyes. This assumption is not correct as defective vision results from functional derangements which can be rectified by simple natural methods of treatment.

Persons who are prescribed glasses are told that they should avoid taking them off because of the danger of eye strain and that they should always look straight through the centre of the lens. So, when looking in other directions they do not move their eyeballs and eye muscles as is natural, but instead move the head up and down or sideways. Thus, constant use of glasses throws the whole natural process of vision out of gear and causes 'parking' of the eyes. Gradually, the muscles of the eyes degenerate through non-use. Moreover, the use of glasses results in a reduction of blinking which is a movement intended to assist and preserve eyesight. Wearing glasses for many years results in stiff, dull-looking eyes without any sparkle.

Causes

The three chief causes of defective vision are mental strain, wrong diet, and improper blood and nerve supply.

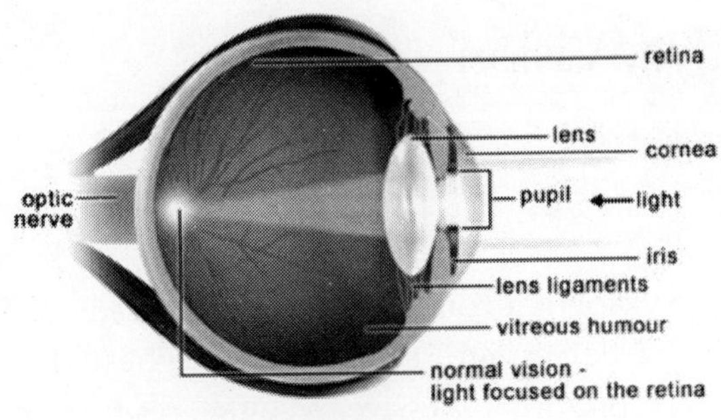

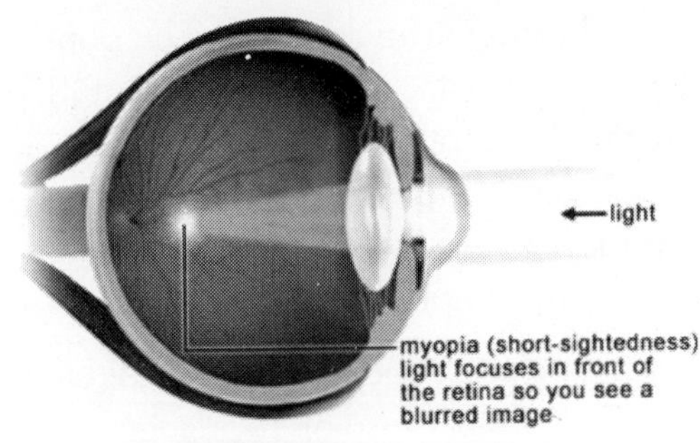

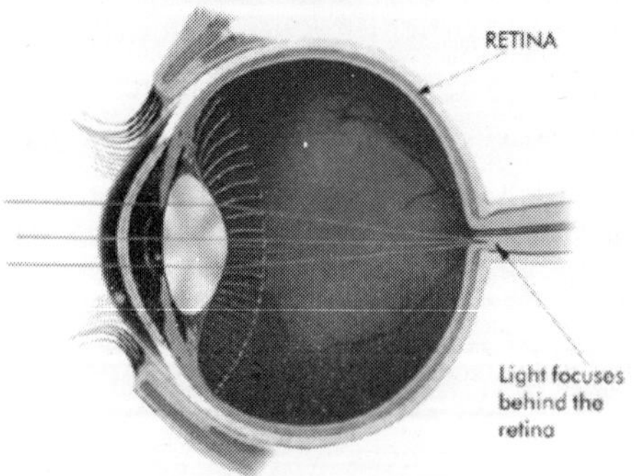

Defects of the Eye

(i) *Mental Strain*: Dr. W.H. Bates, the founder of revolutionary methods of eye treatment , considers mental strain to be the cause of all defects of vision, which puts corresponding physical strain on the eyes, their muscles and nerves. In his opinion the lesser defects are mainly due to mental strain owing to overwork, fear, anxiety, etc. In pursuance of this theory. Dr. Bates has concentrated his efforts on methods of treatment which will remove the condition of mental strain.

(ii) *Wrong Feeding*: The eye is a part of the body and as such must share in any condition affecting the system. Most of the diseases affecting the eyes are symptoms of a general toxemic condition of the body due mainly to excessive starch, sugar and protein ingestion. The muscles and blood vessels surrounding the eyes share in the clogging process taking place over the body due to improper metabolism caused by an imbalanced and too-concentrated diet.

(iii) *Improper blood and nerve supply*: The eyes need to be properly supplied with blood and nerve force for proper vision. Any factor capable of interfering either with the blood-vessels or with the nerves of the eyes could cause defective vision. The muscles covering the upper portion of the spine at the back of the neck are the main seat of mechanical interference with the blood and nerve supply to the eyes.

The Cure

Eye exercise: The following exercises will loosen the strained and contracted muscles surrounding the eyes:

(i) Keep your head still and relaxed. Gently move the eyes up and down six times. Repeat the same movement twice or thrice at two-second intervals. The eyes should move slowly and regularly as far down as possible and then as far up as possible.

(ii) Move the eyes from side to side as far as possible, without any force or effort six times. Repeat two or three times.

(iii) Hold the index finger of your right hand about eight inches in front of the eyes, then look from the finger to any other large object ten or more feet away—the door or window will do. Look from one to the other ten times. Do this exercise fairly rapidly.

(iv) Move the eyes up gently and slowly in a circle, then move them low in the reverse direction. Do this four times in all. Rest for a second and repeat the movements two or three times, using minimum effort. All eye muscle exercises should be performed while seated in a comfortable position.

Neck exercises: Rotate the neck

(a) in circles and semi-circles,

(b) move the shoulders clockwise and anti-clockwise briskly, drawing them up as far as possible several times,

(c) allow the head to drop forward and backward as far as possible,

(d) turn the head to the right and left as far as possible several times. These exercises help to loosen up contracted neck muscles which may restrict blood supply to the head.

Sun gazing: Sit on a bench facing the sun with your eyes closed and gently sway sideways several times for 18 minutes. Open the eyes and blink about 10 times at the sun and look at some greenery. This helps shortsight and is good for inflamed eyes.

Splashing: Splash plain, cold water several times on closed eyes. Rub the closed lids briskly for a minute with a clean towel. This cools the eyes and boosts blood supply.

Palming: Sit comfortably in an armchair or on a settee and relax with your eyes closed. Cover your eyes with your palms, right palm over the right eye and the left over the left eye. Do not, however, press down on the eyes. With your eyes completely covered in this manner, allow your elbows to drop to your knees, which should be fairly close together. With your eyes closed thus, try to imagine blackness, which grows blacker and blacker. Palming reduces strain and relaxes the eyes and its surrounding tissues.

Swinging: Stand with your feet 12 inches apart, hands held loosely at the sides, the whole body and mind relaxed. Gently sway your body from side to side, slowly, steadily with the heels rising alternatively but not the rest of the foot. Imagine you are the pendulum of a clock, and move just as slowly. Swinging should be done in front of a window or a picture. You will see the object moving in the opposite direction of your swing. This must be noted and encouraged. When you face one end of the window or object, blink once. This exercise has a very beneficial effect upon the eyes and nervous system.

Diet

Natural, uncooked foods are the best diet. These include fresh fruits such as oranges, apples, grapes, peaches, plums, cherries; green vegetables like lettuce, cabbage, spinach, turnip tops; root vegetables like potatoes, turnips, carrot, onions and beetroots; nuts, dried fruits and dairy products.

Cereals are also necessary, but they should only be consumed sparingly. Genuine wholemeal bread is the best and most suitable. *Nans,* cakes, pastries, white sugar, white bread, confectionery, tea, coffee, etc., together with meat, fish, or eggs, soon play havoc with the digestion and the body.

The value of vitamin A for improving vision must be stressed. The intake of sufficient quantities of this vitamin is essential as a safeguard against or treatment of defective vision or eye disease of any kind. The best sources of this vitamin are cod liver oil, raw spinach, turnip tops, cream, cheese, butter, egg yolk, tomatoes, lettuce, carrot, cabbage, soya beans, green peas, wheat germ, fresh milk, oranges and dates.

Yogic Exercises

The four yogic exercises prescribed for strengthening the optic nerve known as 'trataka' as explained in chapter 7 on yoga therapy should be practised daily. Certain yogasanas such as bhujangasana, shalabhasana, yogamudra, paschimottan asana and kriyas like jalneti are also beneficial for the eyes.

CHAPTER 58

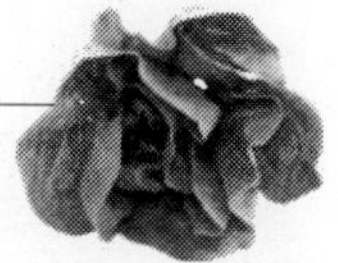

Dental Caries

Dental caries or tooth decay is the most important cause of tooth loss. It is characterised by a bacteria-induced progressive destruction of the mineral and organic components of the enamel and dentine, the two outer layers of the tooth. It is considered to be one of the most common diseases of modern age caused, in large measure, by eating denatured foods of today, which are too soft and too sweet.

The teeth are an amazing balance of form and function, aesthetic beauty and engineering. Good teeth are an important part of one's health and appearance. They play a very important role in the digestion. One can look one's best with a good smile, which emanates from good teeth.

Symptoms

At first, the tooth may be merely sensitive to hot and cold substances in the mouth and also to pressure from biting. Later, an abcess forms at the base of the tooth and the pain becomes severe. It may be sharp, throbbing, shooting or constant. If the tooth is not properly treated, it will eventually have to be extracted.

Causes

Dental caries results from faulty diet. The most common cause of this disease is the consumption of soft drinks, cakes, pasteries, refined carbohydrates and sugar in all forms. Lack of balance between carbohydrates and proteins and insufficient intake of vitamins and minerals also contribute to this disease.

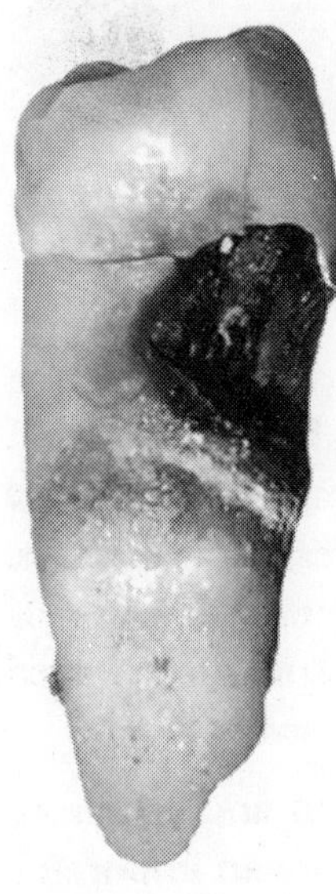

It is commonly prevalent where refined, devitalised, processed and demineralised food, grown on soils deficient in minerals, are eaten.

Food particles lodged in the mouth may provide a suitable place for the growth of bacteria. These, in turn, produce a local acid reaction which then attacks the surface of the tooth. Minute cracks or defects in the enamel, or hard outer coverings of the tooth may also lead to this process. Once the enamel has been eroded away, the body of the tooth is more easily damaged.

Treatment

The treatment of dental caries consists of the removal of decayed regions of the tooth and filling the cavities. If the cavities have reached the pulp, it may become necessary to extract the affected tooth.

Proper cleaning is the most important step towards healthy and sparkling teeth. Ideally, teeth should be cleaned after every meal, but one thorough cleansing each day will be far better than any number of hurried brushings. A quick brushing is a waste of time. The teeth may appear clean, but they will still be coated with a layer of plaque, a sticky, transparent substance. It is invisible, but it can be felt as a fuzzy coating on teeth. It is this substance which leads to decay. In fact, even with a normal brushing, one can still miss removing as much as 80 per cent of the plaque.

There are many theories on how best to clean the teeth. The consensus of dental opinion, however, seems to back using a circular motion with the brush, so as to ensure that all dental surfaces are cleaned. One should not be afraid to touch the gums with the brush, as this gentle stimulation improves the blood circulation, in the gums.

Toothpaste is not in fact essential for the removal of plaque, although most people prefer to use it. It does help to keep the mouth fresh. The fluoride, which is now being added to an increasing number of pastes, also helps to strengthen the outer enamel and this renders it less susceptible to decay.

The mineral fluorine is essential for tooth-building. Studies on dental caries in human beings have shown that the incidence is high in areas where the drinking water contained less than 0.5 ppm. fluorine and low in areas where the water contains 1 to 2 ppm. fluorine. It has further been shown that the addition of 1 ppm. fluorine to drinking water significantly reduces the incidence of dental caries.

Diet plays a vital role in dental health. The condition of the teeth, after they are formed, depends on the food one eats. Dental decay, the destruction of the bone around the teeth, and infections of the gums can be prevented with an appropriated diet. In fact, with proper diet, the teeth and jaw-bones can be made harder and healthier as the years go by.

All sweets and refined foods and all products made with white flour, and white sugar should be avoided as fibreless refined foods allow particles to accumulate on the teeth. It is important to ensure that the diet includes plenty of raw vegetables and whole meal bread. Whole foods are ideal. They are good for the teeth. The gums need friction to keep them firm and whole foods also help remove plaque. They are therefore called 'detergent foods' by some dentists. Millet and sesame (*til*) seeds are extremely rich in calcium.

Onions are considered beneficial in the prevention of tooth decay. Latest research by Russian doctors have confirmed the bactericidal properties of onion. According to these findings, if a person consumes one raw onion every day through mastication, he will be protected from a host of tooth disorders. The Russian doctor, B.P. Tohkin, who has contributed to this research, has expressed the opinion that chewing raw onions for three minutes is sufficient to kill all the germs in the mouth. Toothache is often allayed by placing a small piece of onion on the bad tooth or gum.

Tooth decay can be prevented by regular consumption of apples, as they possess a mouth cleansing property. Dr. T.T. Hanks in his books 'Dental Survey' says, 'Apples have a mouth cleansing property that no other fruit possesses, and taken after meal, they have the same effect as a tooth brush in cleansing the tooth, with the added advantage that the acid content, aside from its nutritive value, is of assistance in promoting the flow of saliva in the mouth, which is also beneficial to the teeth'. The acids of the apple also exerts an antiseptic influence upon the germs present in the mouth and teeth when it is thoroughly chewed. Apples are thus regarded as natural preserves of teeth and should be taken during tooth troubles.

Lemon and lime also promote healthy teeth and gums, due to their high Vitamin C content. They strengthen the gums and teeth and are very effective in preventing and curing acute inflammation of the gum margins. They should therefore form a part of children's diet.

In preventing tooth decay, what one eats is no doubt important, but equally important is when one eats. Frequent small snacks are very harmful to teeth, as they produce an acid medium in which the bacteria thrive. The number of times one eats sugar is one of the most important factor in determining the rate of decay. For this reason, it is better to eat sweets at the end of a meal rather than between meals.

CHAPTER 59

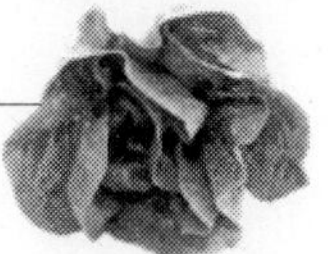

Depression

Depression is the most prevalent of all the emotional disorders. This may vary from feelings of slight sadness to utter misery and dejection. It brings together a variety of physical and psychological symptoms which together constitute a syndrome.

Depression is the most unpleasant experience a person can endure. It is far more difficult to cope with than a physical ailment. The growing complexities of modern life and the resultant crisis, as well as mental stress and strain in day to day living, usually leads to this disorder. It also arises out of the monotony and drudgery of a daily routine, without any meaningful variation in urban life. Suicide is the major risk in extreme cases of depression.

Symptoms

It is not always easy to diagnose depression clinically. The most striking symptoms of depression are feelings of acute sense of loss and inexplicable sadness, loss of energy and loss of interest. The patient usually feels tired and lacks interest in the world around him. Sleep disturbance is frequent. Usually the patient wakes up depressed at 4 or 5 in the morning and is unable to return to sleep. Other disturbed sleep patterns are difficulty in getting sleep on going to bed at night, nightmares and repeated waking from midnight onwards.

The patient often suffers from guilt, oppressive feelings and self-absorption. Other symptoms of depression are: loss of appetite, giddiness, itching, nausea, agitation, irritability, impotence or frigidity, constipation, aches and pains all over the body, lack of concentration and lack of power of decision. Some persons may lose interest in eating and suffer from rapid loss of weight while others may resort to frequent eating and as a result gain weight.

Cases of severe depression may be characterised by low body temperature, low blood pressure, hot flushes and shivering. The external manifestations represent a cry for help from the tormented mind of the depressed persons. The severely depressed patient feels worthless and is finally convinced that he himself is responsible for his undoing and his present state of hopeless despair.

Causes

Depleted functioning of the adrenal glands is one of the main causes of mental depression. Irregular diet habits cause digestive problems and lead to the assimilation of fats. An excess of carbohydrates like cereals, white sugar, coffee, tea, chocolates and comparatively less quantities of vegetables and fruits in the diet may result in indigestion. Due to indigestion, gases are produced in the digestive tract, causing compression over the diaphragm in the region of the heart and lungs. This in turn, reduces the supply of oxygen to the tissues, which raises the carbon dioxide level, causing general depression.

The excessive and indiscriminate use of drugs also leads to faulty assimilation of vitamins and minerals by the body and ultimately causes depression. The use of aspirin leads to deficiencies of vitamin C and antacids can cause deficiencies of calcium and vitamin B. Diabetes, low blood sugar (hypoglycaemia) and weakness of the liver resulting from the use of refined or processed foods, fried foods and an excessive intake of fats may also lead to depression.

The Cure

The modern medical system treats depression with anti-depression drugs which provide temporary relief but have harmful side-effects and do not remove the causes or prevent its recurrence. The harmful side-effects include gross liver damage, hypersensitivity, insomnia, hallucinations, a confused state, convulsions, a fall in blood pressure which brings on headaches and dizziness, blurred vision, difficulty in inhaling and urine retention. The plan of action for self-treatment of depression consists of regulating the diet, exercise, scientific relaxation and meditation.

Diet has a profound effect on the mental health of a person. Even a single nutritional deficiency can cause depression in susceptible people. Dr. Priscilla, associate clinical professor at the University of California, prescribes nutritional therapy to build up brain chemicals, such as serotonin and norepinephrine, that affect mood and are often lacking in depressed people. She recommends eating foods rich in B vitamins, such as whole grains, green vegetables, eggs and fish.

The diet of persons suffering from depression should completely exclude tea, coffee, alcohol, chocolate and cola, all white flour products, sugar, food colourings, chemical additives, white rice and strong condiments. The diet should be restricted to three meals. Fruits can be taken in the morning for breakfast with milk and a handful of nuts and seeds. Lunch may consist of steamed vegetables, whole wheat chappatis and a glass of butter-milk. For dinner, green vegetable salad and all available sprouts such as alfalfa seeds, mung, cottage cheese or a glass of butter-milk would be ideal.

Activity and Exercise

The depressive mood can be overcome by activity. Those

who are depressive will forget their misery by doing something. They should turn away from themselves and consider others, At home they can take to decorating, repairing or constructing something new. The pleasure of achievement overcomes the distress of misery.

Exercise also plays an important role in the treatment of depression. It not only keeps the body physically and mentally fit but also provides recreation and mental relaxation. It is nature's best tranquiliser. According to Dr. Robert Brown, a clinical associate professor at the University of Virginia School of Medicine, "Exercise produces chemical and psychological changes that improves your mental health. It changes the levels of hormones in blood and may elevate your betaendorphins (mood-affecting brain chemicals). Exercise may also improve the function of the autonomic nervous system."

Exercise also gives a feeling of accomplishment and thus reduces the sense of helplessness. Some form of active exercise, must be undertaken each day at a regular hour. To be really useful, exercise should be taken in such a manner as to bring into action all the muscles of the body in a natural way. Walking is one such exercise. It is, however, so gentle in character that one must walk several kilometres in a brisk manner to constitute a fair amount of exercise. Yogic asanas such as vakrasana, bhujangasana, shalabhasana, halasana, paschimottanasana, sarvangasana and shavasana and pranayamas like kapalbhati, anuloma-viloma and bhastrika are highly beneficial in the treatment of depression.

Relaxation and Meditation

The patient must gain control over his nervous system and channelise his mental and emotional activities into restful harmonius vibrations. This can be achieved by ensuring sufficient rest and sleep under right conditions. He must also learn the art of scientific relaxation and meditation which will go a long way in curing depression.

Relaxation enables the muscles to work more efficiently and eliminates fatigue by promoting venous blood circulation throughout the body. The best method of relaxation is to

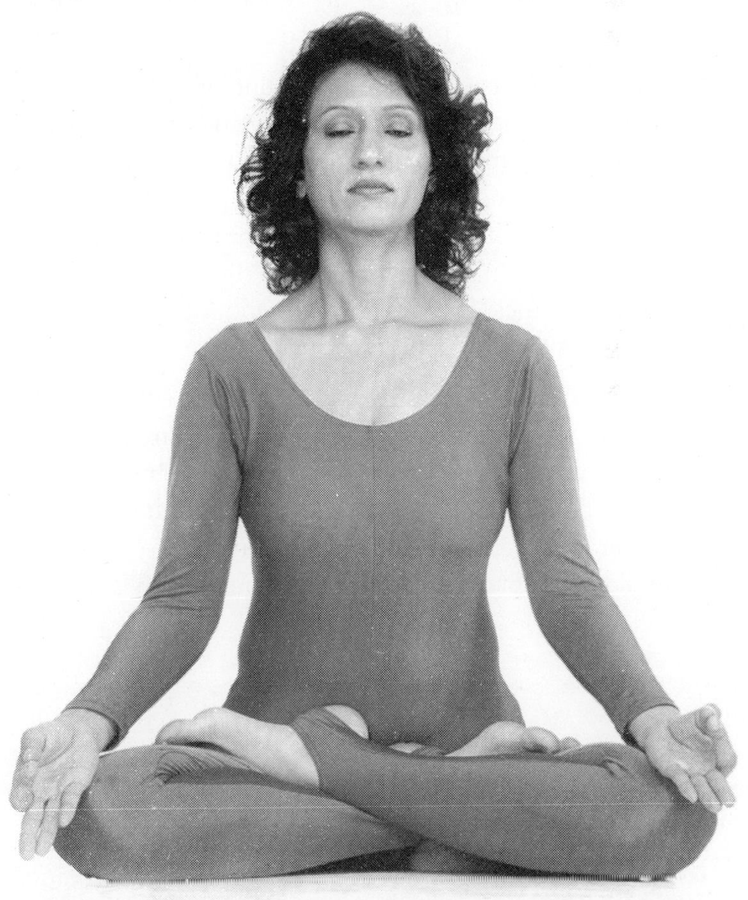

Meditation is a simple and effective technique for mental depression.

practice shavasana or the 'dead pose'. The procedure for this asana has been outlined in chapter 7 on yoga therapy.

Meditation involves training the mind to remain fixed on a certain external or internal location. All the mental faculties should be directed, without cessation, towards the object of meditation. It can be achieved by constant practice. It will be advisable to meditate on God or Atman as one becomes imbued with the quality of the object on which one meditates.

Meditation will help create an amount of balance in the nervous system. This would enable the glands to return to a correct state of hormonal balance and thereby overcome the feeling of depression. Regularity of time, place and practice are very important in meditation. Regularity conditions the mind to slowing down its activities with a minimum delay. The most effective times are early dawn and dusk, when the atmosphere is serene and peaceful.

A neutral immersion bath for one hour daily is also helpful in the treatment of depression. This bath is administered in a bath tub which should be properly fitted with hot and cold water connections. The patient should lie in the tub after filling it with water at a temperature ranging from 92° to 98°F. The head should be kept cold with a cold compress.

CHAPTER 60

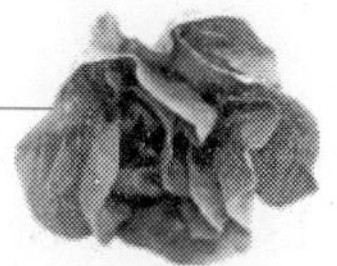

Dermatitis

Dermatitis refers to an inflammation of the skin, both external and internal. It is characterised by redness, swelling, heat and pain or itching. Any part of the body may be affected by this disease. The genital areas and exposed areas such as the eyelids, forearms, face and neck are more prone to it.

The cells of the epidermis (the surface layer of the skin) are normally protected from damage by the tightly-packed squamae of keratin of the horny layer. The elasticity of keratin varies with its water content. This water content can be reduced by evaporation or by removal of the lipid with which it retains moisture. Substances which produce inflammation of

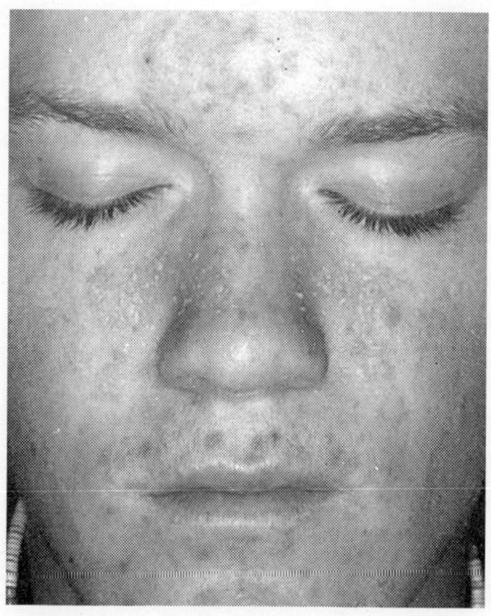

Dermatitis venenata (Rhus toxicodendron)

the epidermis or dermatitis by mechanical or chemical disruption of the horny layer are called irritants. Degreasing agents like soaps, if used too frequently over a short time, will cause dryness, redness, fissuring and irritation of the skin in almost everyone.

Symptoms

The appearance of dermatitis varies according to its severity and the stage of its evolution. The first symptom is erythema or redness. This is usually followed by swelling of the skin due to oedema (excessive fluid retention). Vesicles may appear thereafter. In case of their rupture, their bases exude serum. This condition is known as weeping dermatitis. Later, the serum dries up to form crusts. In some people, the disease seems to come and go without making any great change in the skin itself.

Causes

Chemical substances usually give rise to dermatitis. They may reach the skin from outside or from inside through the blood-stream. About 100 different plants are known to be capable of causing dermatitis in susceptible persons. The onset is usually acute and begins an hour or two after contact. Dermatitis may be caused by external contact with mineral irritants. This includes most cases of industrial dermatitis which arise on the hands or forearms which actually come in contact with the irritant.

Certain drugs applied externally such as atropine, belladona, carbolic acid, iodine, mercury, penicillin, sulphonamides, sulphurs, tars and turpentine sometimes cause dermatitis. Other substances causing this disease include hair dyes, bleaches, skin tonics, nail polish, perfume, wool, silk, nylon, floor-wax, and various detergents. Other causes of this disease are indiscretion in diet, deficiency of vitamin A, pantothenic acid, nervous and emotional strains.

Treatment

As dermatitis may appear due to varied causes, treatment also varies accordingly. If, however, the trouble is constitutional arising from internal causes, the patient should commence the treatment by adopting an all-fruit diet for at least a week. In this regimen, he should take three meals a day of juicy fruits such as orange, grapes, apple, pineapple and papaya at five hourly intervals.

After an exclusive fruit diet, the patient may adopt a restricted diet, for 10 days. In this regimen, breakfast may consist of orange juice or grapefruit. Raw salad, consisting of vegetables available in season, with raisins, figs or dates may be taken for lunch and dinner may consist of steamed vegetables such as spinach, cabbage, carrots, turnips, cauliflower, along with a few nuts or fresh fruit. Milk puddings and desserts such as jellies, jams and pastries, all condiments, spices, white sugar, white flour products, tea, coffee and other stimulating drinks should all be avoided.

After the restricted diet, the patient should gradually embark upon a well-balanced diet, consisting of seeds, nuts and grains, vegetables and fruits. The emphasis should be on fresh fruits and raw vegetables. In case of a severe condition, the patient should undertake a fast of fruit or vegetable juices for three to five days. This may be followed by a restricted diet for 10 to 15 days. Further fasts and a period of restricted diet at intervals may be adopted after the resumption of a normal diet.

The warm water enema should be used daily to cleanse the bowels during the first week of the treatment and thereafter as necessary. Epsom-salts baths may be taken two or three times a week. The affected areas may also be bathed twice daily in hot water with Epsom salts. About 100 grams of Epsom salts should be added to a bowlful of hot water for this purpose. A little olive oil should be applied after Epsom salt bathing.

The patient should avoid white sugar, refined carbohydrates, tea, coffee and other denatured foods. He should make liberal use of fruits and vegetable juices. The combined juice from apple, carrot and celery is especially beneficial in the treatment of dermatitis. About 175 ml. each of these juices should be mixed to prepare 525 ml. of combined juice.

No medicines of any kind should be used. In case of trouble due to external causes, the most effective treatment consists of applying a mixture of baking soda (bicarbonate of soda) and olive oil. The alkaline sodium neutralises the poisonous acids formed in the sores and oil keeps the flesh in a softened condition.

The patient should undertake moderate physical exercise, preferably simple yoga asanas after the fast is completed and the start of the restricted diet. Exercise is one of the most valuable means for purifying the blood and for preventing toxaemia. The patient should also have adequate physical and mental rest and fresh air. He should avoid exposure to cold, and adopt regular hours of eating and sleeping.

CHAPTER 61

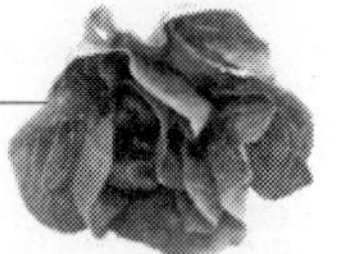

Diabetes

Diabetes mellitus is a nutritional disorder, characterised by an abnormally elevated level of blood glucose and by the excretion of the excess glucose in the urine. It results from an absolute or relative lack of insulin which leads to abnormalities in carbohydrate metabolism as well as in the metabolism of protein and fat.

Diabetes is a disease known to the medical world since time immemorial. Its incidence is, however, much higher at present than ever in the past. This is especially true in case of more advanced countries of the world due to widespread affluence and more generous food supply.

The most commonly used screening tests are the determination of the fasting blood glucose level and the two-hour postprandial, that is after a meal. The normal fasting blood sugar content is 80 to 120 mg. per 100 ml. of blood and this can go up to a level of 180 mg. per 100 ml. of blood two hours after meals. Anything above these norms can be termed diabetic levels.

Diabetes occurs in all age groups, from young infants to the elderly. The greatest incidence occurs in middle or older aged persons. It is estimated that 80 to 85 per cent of all individuals with diabetes mellitus are 45 years of age or older.

Symptoms

The word diabetes is derived from the Greek word meaning 'to siphon; to pass through', and mellitus comes from the Latin word 'honey'. Thus two characteristic symptoms, namely, copious urination and glucose in the urine give the name to the disease. The normal volume of urine passed daily is about one and a half litre, but in the diabetic condition it can vary from four to twenty litres. The urine is of a pale colour, has an acidic reaction and sweetish odour. The quantity of sugar present in it varies from one-and-a-quarter decigram to two and-a-half grams the total per day in many cases reaching as much as one kg in 15 litres of urine.

A diabetic feels hungry and thirsty most of the time, does not put on weight, though he eats every now and then, and gets tired easily, both physically and mentally. He looks pale, may suffer from anaemia, constipation, intense itching around the genital organs, palpitations and general weakness. He feels drowsy and has a lower sex urge than a normal person.

Causes

Diabetes has been described by most biological doctors as a "prosperity" disease, primarily caused by systematic over-eating and consequent obesity. Not only the overeating of sugar and refined carbohydrate but also of proteins and fats, which are transformed into sugar if taken in excess, is harmful and may result in diabetes. Too much food taxes the pancreas and eventually paralyses its normal activity. It has been estimated that the incidence of diabetes is four times higher in persons of moderate obesity and 30 times higher in persons of severe obesity.

Grief, worry and anxiety also have a deep influence on the metabolism and may cause sugar to appear in the urine. The disease may be associated with some other grave organic disorders like cancer, tuberculosis and cerebral disease. Heredity is also a major factor in the development of the

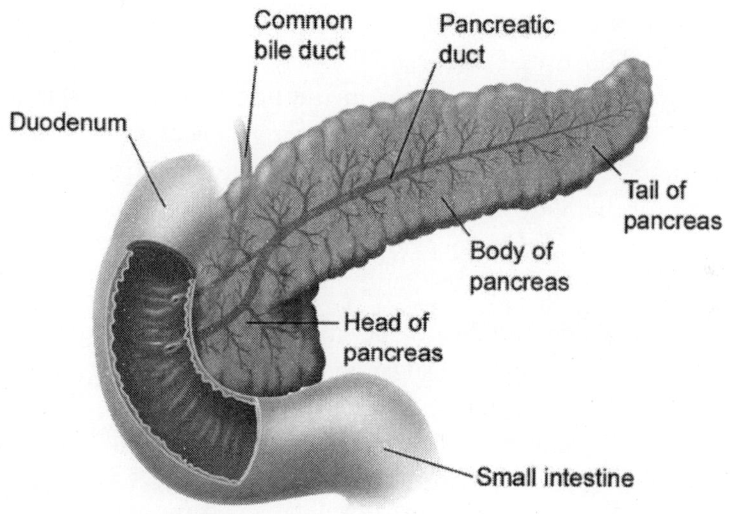

Sketch showing parts of Pancreas

disease. It has been rightly said, "Heredity is like a cannon and obesity pulls the trigger."

Treatment

Any successful method of diabetes treatment should aim at removal of the actual cause of the disease and building up of the whole health-level of the patient. Diet plays a vital role in such a treatment. The primary dietary consideration for a diabetic patient is that he should be a strict lacto-vegetarian and take a low-calorie, low-fat, alkaline diet of high quality natural foods. Fruits, nuts and vegetables, whole wheat bread and dairy products form a good diet for the diabetic. These foods are best eaten in as dry a condition as possible to ensure thorough salivation during the first part of the process of digestion.

Cooked starchy foods should be avoided as in the process of cooking the cellulose envelops of the starch granules burst and, consequently, the starch is far too easily absorbed in the system. The excess absorbed has to be got rid of by the kidneys and appears as sugar in the urine. With raw starchy foods, however, the saliva and digestive juices in the small intestine regulate the quantities required to be changed into sugar for the body's needs. The unused and undigested portion of raw starchy foods does not become injurious to the system, as it does not readily ferment.

The diabetic should not be afraid to eat fresh fruits and vegetables which contain sugar and starch. Fresh fruits contain sugar fructose, which does not need insulin for its metabolism and is well tolerated by diabetics. Fats and oils should be taken sparingly, for they are apt to lower the tolerance for proteins and starches. Emphasis should be on raw foods as they stimulate and increase insulin production. For protein, home-made cottage cheese, various forms of soured milks and nuts are best. The patient should avoid overeating and take four or five small meals a day rather than three large ones.

The following diet should serve as a guideline.

Upon arising: A glass of lukewarm water with freshly squeezed lemon juice.

Breakfast: Any fresh fruit with the exception of bananas, soaked prunes, a small quantity of whole wheat bread with butter and fresh milk.

Lunch: Steamed or lightly cooked green vegetables such as cauliflower, cabbage, tomatoes, spinach, turnip, asparagus and mushrooms, two or three whole wheat chappatis according to appetite and a glass of butter-milk or curd.

Mid-afternoon: A glass of fresh fruit or vegetable juice.

Dinner: A large bowl of salad made up of all the raw vegetables in season. The salad may be followed by a hot course, if desired, and fresh home-made cottage cheese.

Bedtime snack: A glass of fresh milk.

Flesh foods find no place in this regimen, for they increase the toxaemic condition underlying the diabetic state and reduce the sugar tolerance. On the other hand, a non-stimulating vegetarian diet, especially one made up of raw foods, promotes and increases sugar tolerance.

Celery, cucumbers, string beans, onion and garlic are especially beneficial. String bean pod tea is an excellent natural substitute for insulin and highly beneficial in diabetes. The skin of the pods of green beans are extremely rich in silica and certain hormone substances which are closely related to insulin. One cup of string bean tea is equal to one unit of insulin. Cucumbers contain a hormone needed by the cells of the pancreas for producing insulin. Onion and garlic have proved beneficial in reducing blood sugar in diabetes.

Recent scientific investigations have established that bitter gourd (*karela*) is highly beneficial in the treatment of diabetes. It contains an insulin-like principle, known as plant-insulin which has been found effective in lowering the blood and urine sugar levels. It should, therefore, be included liberally in the diet of the diabetic. For better results, the diabetic should take the juice of about four or five fruits every morning on an empty stomach. The seeds of bitter gourd can be added to food in a powdered form. Diabetics can also use bitter gourd in the form of decoction by boiling the pieces in water or in the form of dry powder.

Another effective home remedy is jambul fruit known as *jamun* in the vernacular. It is regarded in traditional medicine as a specific against diabetes because of its effect on the pancreas. The fruits as such, the seeds and fruit juice are all useful in the treatment of this disease. The seeds contain a glucoside 'jamboline' which is believed to have the power to check the pathological conversion of starch into sugar; in cases of increased production of glucose they should be dried and powdered. This powder should be taken mixed in milk, curd or water.

The patient should avoid tea, coffee and cocoa because of their adverse influence on the digestive tract. Other foods which should be avoided are white bread, white flour products, sugar, tinned fruits, sweets, chocolates, pastries, pies, puddings, refined cereals and alcoholic drinks.

The most important nutrient in the treatment of diabetes is manganese which is vital in the production of natural insulin. It is found in citrus fruits, in the outer covering of nuts, grains and in the green leaves of edible plants. Other nutrients of special value are zinc, B-Complex vitamins and poly-unsaturated fatty acids.

Exercise is also an important factor in the treatment of diabetes. Light games, jogging and swimming are recommended. Yogic asanas such as bhujangasana, shalabhasana, dhanurasana, paschimottanasana, sarvangasana, halasana, ardhamatsyendrasana and shavasana, yogic kriyas like jalaneti and kunjal and pranayamas such as kapalbhati, anuloma-viloma and ujjai are highly beneficial.

Hydrotherapy and colonic irrigations form a very important part of treatment. The colon should be thoroughly cleansed every second day or so, until the bowel discharge assumes normal characteristics. Bathing in cold water greatly increases the circulation and enhances the capacity of the muscles to utilise sugar.

The diabetic patient should eliminate minor worries from his daily life. He must endeavour to be more easy-going and should not get unduly worked up by the stress and strain of life.

CHAPTER 62

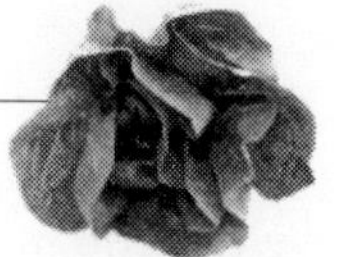

Diarrhoea

Diarrhoea refers to the frequent passage of loose or watery unformed stools. As a rough guide it can be said that three or four loose or watery stools a day can be considered as diarrhoea. The disease may be acute or chronic. Commonly known as 'loose motion', it is perhaps the most common disease in India.

The intestine normally gets more than 10 litres of liquid per day which comes from the diet and from secretion of the stomach, liver, pancreas and intestines. In the case of diarrhoea, water is either not absorbed or is secreted in excess by the organs of the body. It is then sent to the colon where water-holding capacity is limited. Thus the urge to defecate comes quite often.

Causes

There are many and varied causes of diarrhoea. The chief causes are overeating or eating of wrong foods, putrefaction in intestinal tract, fermentation caused by incomplete carbohydrate digestion, nervous irritability, use of antibiotic drugs and excessive intake of laxatives. Other causes include parasites, germs, virus, bacteria or a poison which has entered into the body through food, water or air; allergies to certain substances or even common foods such as milk, wheat, eggs and sea foods and emotional strain or stress in adults and fright in children.

Diarrhoea may be a prominent feature of organic disease

affecting the small or large intestine such as the sprue syndrome, malignant disease and ulcerative colitis. It may also result from operations on the gastro intestinal tract. Diarrhoea may alternate with constipation. This may result from the irritation of the mucous membrane by impacted hard faeces.

Diarrhoea for prolonged periods can lead to certain complications. These may include (i) weakening, due to loss of vitamins like A, D, E and K and other nutrients as food is rushed through the body without giving the nutrients a chance of being absorbed, (ii) dehydration, due to loss of body fluids and washing out of minerals from the body and nervous conditions.

Treatment

In severe cases of diarrhoea, it is advisable to observe a complete fast for two days to provide rest for the gastro-intestinal tract. Hot water only may be taken during the period to compensate for the loss of fluids. Juices of fruits may be taken after the acute symptoms are over. After the condition improves, meals can be enlarged gradually to include cooked vegetables, whole rice, soured milks. Raw foods should be taken only after the patient completely recovers.

An effective remedy for diarrhoea is the use of buttermilk. It is the residual milk left after the fat has been removed from yogurt by churning. It helps overcome harmful intestinal flora and re-establish the benign or friendly flora. The acid in the buttermilk also fights germs and bacteria. It may be taken and mixed with a pinch of salt three or four times a day for controlling diarrhoea.

Carrot soup is another effective home remedy for diarrhoea. It supplies water to combat dehydration, replenishes sodium, potassium, phosphorus, calcium, sulphur and magnesium, supplies pectin and coats the intestine to allay inflammation. It checks the growth of harmful intestinal bacteria and prevents vomiting. One pound of carrot may be cooked in five ounces of water until it is soft. The pulp should be strained and boiled water added to make a quart. Three-quarter tablespoon of salt may be mixed. This soup should be given in small amounts to the patient every half an hour.

The pomegranate has proved beneficial in the treatment of diarrhoea on account of its astringent properties. If the patient develops weakness due to profuse and continuous purging, he should be given repeatedly about 50 ml. of pomegranate juice to drink. This will control the diarrhoea.

Mango seeds are also valuable in diarrhoea. The seeds should be collected during the mango season, dried in the shade and powdered and kept stored for use as medicine when required. It should be given in doses of about one and a half gram to two grams with or without honey.

Turmeric has proved another effective home remedy for diarrhoea. It is a very useful intestinal antiseptic. It is also a gastric stimulant and a tonic. Turmeric rhizome, its juice or dry powder are all very helpful in curing chronic diarrhoea. In the form of dry powder, it may be taken in buttermilk or plain water.

In case of diarrhoea caused by indigestion, dry or fresh ginger is very useful. A piece of dry ginger is powdered along with a crystal of rock salt. A quarter teaspoonful of this powder should be taken with a small piece of jaggery. It will bring quick relief as ginger, being carminative, aids digestion by stimulating the gastrointestinal tract.

Starchy liquids such as arrowroot water, barley water, rice gruel and coconut water are highly beneficial in the treatment of diarrhoea. They not only replace the fluid lost but also bind the stools. Other home remedies include bananas and garlic. Bananas contain pectin and encourage the growth of beneficial bacteria. Garlic is a powerful, effective and harmless antibiotic. It aids digestion and routs parasites.

The best water treatment for diarrhoea are the abdominal compress (at 60°F) renewed every 15 to 20 minutes and cold hip bath (40°–50°F). If the patient is in pain, abdominal fomentations for 15 minutes should be administered every two hours.

CHAPTER 63

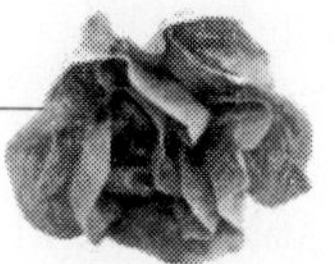

Diphtheria

The term diphtheria is derived from a Greek word meaning leather. It refers to a severe infection, generally affecting the upper respiratory passages. It is essentially a disease of children and occurs very rarely in adult life.

Diphtheria is highly contagious and is caused by certain germs occasionally found in the throat of apparently normal persons. The highest incidence of this disease occurs in cool season, but it can occur at any time. The incubation period is usually from four to six days.

Symptoms

The onset of diphtheria is mild and often uncertain. The disease often looks like tonsillitis in the early stages. There may be fever ranging from 101° to 104° F and soreness of the throat. The patient feels weak and depressed. A membrane appears generally on one tonsil and in rare cases, on both of the tonsils. This gradually increases in size. It may be thick or thin, grey or brownish in colour and is surrounded by a zone of red inflammation.

The membrane may be restricted to tonsils, or it may involve the whole of the back of the throat and soft palate. It may extend upward into the nose or downward into the larynx. Diphtheria can also occur without the false membrane with tissues being red and swollen and the bacilli being present. The glands of the neck are usually enlarged, and when the nose is involved, they increase rapidly in size.

The patient is very low in spirits and rapidly become anaemic and pale. Unless treated properly, he may die from steadily increasing debility or from rapid weakening of the heart due to toxins of diphtheria. In favourable cases, the symptoms gradually subside and the membranes slowly disappear. The duration of the disease ranges from a few days to two or three weeks.

Causes

Diphtheria is caused by an organism known as Corynebacterium diphtheria. This bacterium multiplies in the throat or nose. Droplets and discharges from the throat of an infected person spread the disease to susceptible persons. This is the major mode of spread of the infection. Sometimes, milk and similar substances also serve as vehicles for the spread of this disease.

Thus, the immediate cause of diphtheria, according to medical views, is germ infection. However, no person can catch this disease if he does not have the basis for its propagation in his system, in the form of morbid matter and toxic wastes, brought about by wrong feeding and unhygienic living.

Complications

Children with large tonsils and adenoids are more susceptible to diphtheria, especially if they have not been given the DPT shots in infancy. Greatest danger arises from blockage of the windpipe due to the infection in the throat. This causes strangling. The disease may also damage the heart, the brain and the kidneys. Diphtheria germs produce powerful toxins or poisons which damage the nearby cells and even affect distant organs, such as the kidneys. The toxins are carried to these areas by the blood stream. Heart failure may occur due to weakened muscle fibres which are unable to contract as they should.

Treatment

The use of anti-toxins for the treatment of diphtheria may sometimes prove apparently successful. The real treatment for this disease, however, as with all other fevers, is constitutional. The patient should be given only orange juice and water in small quantities. This will provide energy, increase urinary output and promote body resistance against infection, thereby facilitating recovery. A warm-water enema should be administered daily during this period to cleanse the bowels.

The patient of diphtheria should be kept in bed and isolated from others for four to six weeks. To avoid the swallowing of the secretion constantly forming in the mouth during the fever, the patient should sleep on his sides and not allowed to lie on his back. Some absorbent cotton may be arranged in the mouth to absorb much of this matter. This can be renewed several times a day as required.

The moist hot inhalation will be beneficial in the treatment of this condition. It will aid greatly in maintaining the resistance of the tissues and facilitates the separation of the membranes. Another valuable application is the wet pack to the throat. This pack should be applied at two-hourly intervals. The procedure is to wring out some linen material in cold water, wrap it two or three times round the affected part and cover it with flannel material, duly secured. Similar packs may also be applied to the whole trunk.

If the above treatment is faithfully carried out, the fever will run its course without any trouble and complications or serious after-effects. The patient can then be placed on an all-fruit diet for few days. Thereafter, he may be allowed to gradually embark upon a well-balanced diet. The emphasis should be on whole grain cereals, fresh fruits and raw or lightly-cooked vegetables.

An excellent home remedy for diphtheria is the use of garlic (lahasoon). Its constant application by chewing a clove of garlic removes the membranes, reduces temperatures and relieves the patient. About 30 gms. of garlic can be used in this way in three or four hours for a week. After the membrane disappears, the same quantity of garlic should be chewed daily. The diphtheric patient has no taste or smell and merely finds the garlic hot.

The juice of fresh pineapple (ananas) is considered another valuable remedy. This juice can be given to the patient in small quantities at frequent intervals. This will help remove the diphtheric membrane as well as deposits on the throat so that the patient will feel better.

CHAPTER 64

Diverticulosis

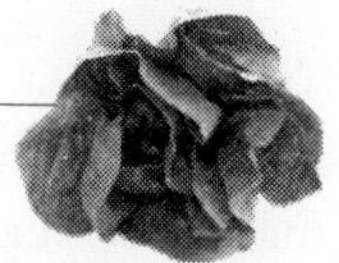

Diverticulosis is a condition of the colon, in which the muscular wall gives way in places and allows the mucous membrane lining the large intestine to form pouches. These pouches are known as a diverticula, a name which comes from the word "diverted". They become lodging places for decaying particles of food or faecal matter.

The disease by itself is of no consequence. Sometimes, however, diverticula become inflammed, as they do not have muscles in their walls and cannot empty themselves. This condition is known as diverticulitis. This disease is usually established by means of X-rays. It usually occurs in the middle and later years.

Symptoms

The main symptoms of diverticulitis are pain in the left lower side of the abdomen, diarrhoea or constipation or alternation of the two, and bleeding. Attacks may recur over a long time.

Severe complications may arise from the tendency of obstructed diverticula to perforate and thus give rise to pericolic abcess, peritonitis or fistula to bladder, vagina or other parts of the guts. Inflammatory masses may form and may result in obstructive symptoms which closely resemble carcinoma of the colon. Such complications may require surgical treatment.

Persons with diverticulosis frequently develop anaemia. The

bacteria in the diverticula, caused by stagnant food and faecal matter, appear to grab all the B vitamin and folic acid from the food and prevent it from reaching the blood. This condition is corrected when these putrefactive bacteria are destroyed by a generous intake of yogurt oracidophilus milk provided the diet contains folic acid. The patient may also develop other intestinal and general problems due to the increase of toxins generated by this condition.

Causes

The prime cause of diverticulosis or diverticulitis is low-residue diet of highly refined foods. The disease is rare in primitive tribes, who consume high-roughage diet. It is thus, primarily a deficiency disease caused by deficiency of 'high-residue' foods like whole, unrefined, natural and bulky foods.

Another cause of this disease is severe mental tension. When tension is great, gas cannot be expelled normally and is forced against the intestinal walls. This may sometimes lead to the formation of diverticula and ultimately result in diverticulosis or diverticulitis.

Treatment

Modern medical system in most cases prescribes surgery to remove the diverticula. But the surgical removal of old diverticula does not prevent the formation of new ones. The best way to treat the disease is through natural methods. The treatment should aim at improving digestion, decreasing gas formation, building stronger intestinal walls to resist the formation of diverticula and relieving stress to avoid tension building up in the body.

Diet plays an important role in this treatment. The emphasis should be on high roughage diet consisting of seeds, nuts and whole grains, vegetables and fruits. Seeds may be consumed in the sprouted form. Cooked cereals like millet, brown rice and oats are beneficial. Sour milk like yogurt and buttermilk, potatoes and flax seeds should be taken daily in adequate quantities.

The patient should take small, frequent meals, rather than few large ones. He should avoid refined and processed foods, tea, coffee, condiments, pickles and animal foods.

If the disease is accompanied by constipation, all measures should be adopted for its eradication through natural methods. Purgatives should not be used. If constipation occurs despite the patient adhering to the diet of natural foods, warm water enema should be used to cleanse the bowels. If the patient is over-weight, he should take a diet of natural foods aimed at reducing the weight.

The use of bran is considered highly beneficial in the treatment of diverticulosis or diverticulitis. Unprocessed wheat bran has five times the fibre of ordinary whole wheat. The quality of bran to be used varies from one table spoon daily to three table spoons three times a day, depending on the severity of the disease. Most of the patients, however, need two spoons of bran three times a day, to render the stools soft and easy to pass. The quantity can be increased, if necessary, after two weeks until the patient can move his bowels once or twice a day without straining. As it is difficult to eat bran dry, it may be sprinkled on cereals, or mixed with porridge, or added to soup or taken with milk or water.

Certain vegetable juices have been found beneficial in the treatment of diverticulosis. These include juices extracted from carrot, beet and green vegetables. The best fruit juices are those extracted from papaya, apple, pineapple and lemon.

The use of vitamins can also help in diverticulosis. Vitamin E is a well known muscle strengthener and should be used liberally by the patient. Vitamins of group B are needed, not only to provide the folic acid but to prevent stress and strengthen nerves. Vitamin C can help greatly in removing toxic matter from the body. Minerals are also needed in diverticulosis. Potassium, manganese, calcium and magnesium, all can help strengthen the muscular and nervous systems.

Diverticulosis and diverticulitis can be treated successfully through natural methods as outlined above. Surgery may be resorted to in rare cases where there is severe obstruction, perforation or abscess formation or where there is severe involvement of the intestine.

CHAPTER 65

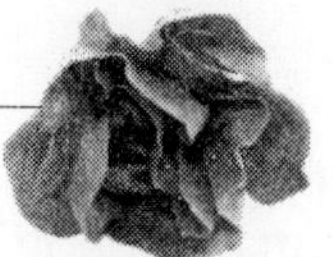

Dropsy

Dropsy, technically known as oedema, refers to the abnormal accumulation of fluids in the body. It causes a type of swelling called oedema. It is a typical 'impurities' disease caused by an accumulation of waste products in the blood. This swelling may be localized, as with ascites (the distended abdomen that develops in cases of liver disease and some types of cancer), or generalised, occurring throughout the body, as with progressive kidney failure. It is a feature of many diseases, specially those relating to heart and kidneys.

Symptoms

In case of kidney disease, dropsy is first noticed beneath the eyes and face and is worse in the morning. In case of heart disease, the swelling tends to be worse in the evening and begins in the lower parts of the body such as the ankles. In liver disease, the swelling is in the legs and abdomen.

Causes

The main cause of this disease is the obstruction to the free circulation of blood and lymph and consequent impaired elimination. The localized oedema with pain may be due to interference with the circulation. When it is associated with itching, allergy is likely to be the cause.

Hormonal factors can also produce oedema. This is evident from two examples of swelling that occurs during pregnancy and the pre-menstrual phase of a woman's monthly cycle.

Other causes include heart failure, advanced kidney disease, malnutrition, and thyroid disorders.

The real cause of dropsy, however, is abnormal accumulation of morbid matter in the system. This accumulation is so great that the kidneys and liver become overloaded and unable to perform their purifying tasks properly. The stagnation of unhealthy fluid in the tissues can also be aggravated by the heart muscle being too weak to pump the blood with sufficient force through the veins and arteries to carry the necessary oxygen and nourishment to the cells of the vital organs. This can result in the poisoning of the whole system.

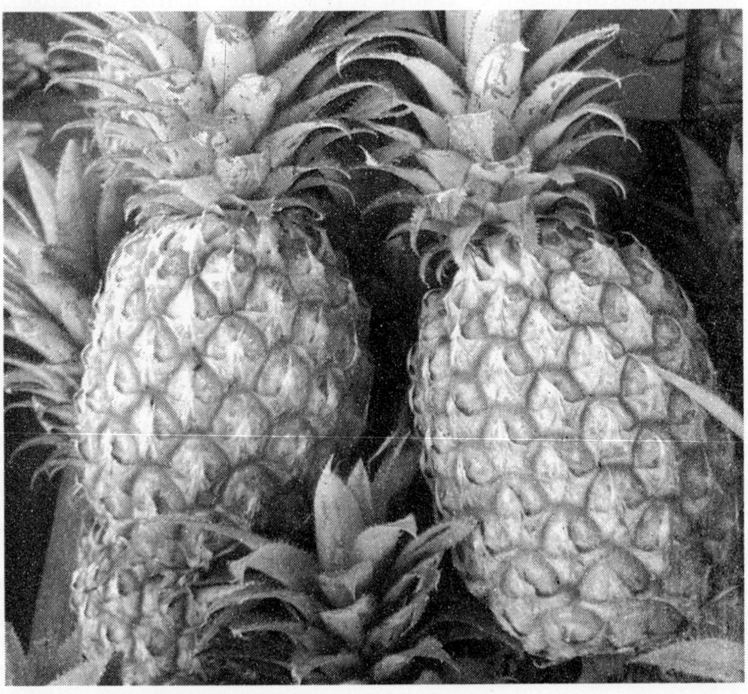

Pineapple is an effective home remedy for Dropsy

Treatment

To begin with, the patient should adopt an exclusive diet of fresh fruits for five days. In this regimen, he should take three meals a day of juice fruits, such as apple, pear, peach, grapes, pineapple and papaya, at five-hourly intervals. He should take warm water enema during this period to cleanse the bowels. Thereafter, he may adopt a restricted diet. In this regimen, the breakfast may consist of a glass of fresh juice of lemon or apple or grapes, and the lunch may comprise one or two potatoes cooked with their skins, French beans as often as possible, a mixed salad of raw vegetable with lemon juice and olive oil dressing, one or two whole wheat bread or chappatis, and a little cottage cheese. Dinner may be repetition of the lunch.

After the restricted diet, the patient may gradually embark upon a well-balanced diet, with emphasis on fresh fruits and raw vegetables. A hot water bath taken daily will be beneficial in the treatment of dropsy.

Certain home remedies have been found beneficial in the treatment of dropsy. Of these, the use of pineapple is very effective. It contains sufficient chlorine which stimulates the activity of the kidneys and helps remove much of the waste products from the body. It also relieves the body of a water-logged condition.

The use of Garlic is another effective remedy for this disease. Two or three cloves of this vegetable should be chewed early in the morning. This will bring good results. The juice of bitter gourd (karela) can also be taken, with beneficial results.

The leaves of margosa (*neem*) are considered useful in

dropsy. A tea made from these leaves can be taken with advantage. The leaves of bael (*bel*) tree are also valuable in dropsy. The juice of these can be taken for treating this condition.

Another useful remedy of dropsy is the use of the herb arjuna (*Kahu*). This herb has been employed successfully by practitioners of indigenous system of medicine in the treatment of this condition. It can be used in the form of decoction of the thick bark, made with milk, every morning on an empty stomach.

CHAPTER 66

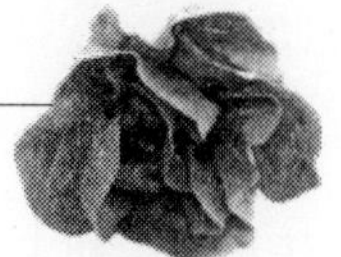

Dysentery

Dysentery is a serious condition affecting the large intestine. It is characterised by inflammation and ulceration of the bowel, a colic pain in the region of the abdomen and passing of liquid or semi-formed stools with mucus and blood.

The pathological condition of dysentery is caused by two organisms, protozoa and bacilli. The former is generally known as amoebic dysentery and the latter as bacillary dysentery. An attack of amoebic dysentery is milder in comparison with bacillary dysentery. But while bacillary dysentery can respond quickly to treatment, amoebic dysentery does not leave the patient easily, unless he is careful.

Dysentery is prevalent all over the world except in very cold countries. Places where insanitary conditions prevail are particularly affected. The disease strikes both sexes equally. Similarly, no age is immune, though children are more prone.

Symptoms

Dysentery may be acute and chronic. The acute form is characterised by pain in the abdomen, diarrhoea and dysenteric motions. Yellowish white mucus and sometimes only blood from the intestinal ulcers passes with stools. The evacuations are preceded by pain and tenesmus. The patient feels a constant desire to evacuate, although there may be nothing to throw off except a little mucus and blood. There is a feeling of pain in the rectum and along the large intestine. With the advance of the disease the quantity of mucus and blood increases.

Occasionally casts or shreds of skinlike mucous membrane, from small fragments to 12 inches or so long and an inch wide, are seen to pass out with motions. Sometimes pus is also thrown out with motions and often the smell of the stools becomes very foetid. All the digestive processes are upset and secretions are changed or stopped. The saliva becomes acid instead of being alkaline and the gastric juice itself may become alkaline. The stomach loses power to digest and absorb food.

The bacilli create toxins and the foetid matters formed also augment further manufacture of toxins and their consequent absorption in blood.

Chronic cases are after-effects of acute attacks. The patient does not recover completely. Stool remains putrid and may contain blood, while diarrhoea and constipation may alternate, and general health is disturbed. In severe cases, the temperature may rise to 104-105°F. It may occasionally become subnormal.

Causes

The cause of dysentery, according to modern medical system, is germ infection. The germs, which are supposed to cause dysentery only develop in the colon as a result of putrefaction of excessive quantities of animal protein food, fried substances, over-spiced foods and hard to digest fatty substances. The real cause of dysentery is thus dietary indiscretion and eating of excessive amounts of flesh food in hot weather or tropical climate unsuited to the digestion of such foods. Other causes include debility, fatigue, chill, lowered vitality, intestinal disorders and overcrowding under insanitary conditions.

Treatment

The treatment of dysentery should aim at removing the offending and toxic matter from the intestines and for alleviating painful symptoms, stopping the virulence of the bacteria and promoting healing of the ulcer.

Fasting is the only correct remedy for dysentery to begin with. The patient should fast as long as acute symptoms are present. During the period of fasting, only orange juice and water should be taken. In the alternative, the patient should subsist on buttermilk till the acute symptoms are over. Butter-milk combats offending bacteria and helps establishment of helpful micro-organisms in the intestines.

The patient may be given small doses of castor oil in the form of emulsion. This acts as a mild aperient and facilitates quicker removal of offensive matter, minimises the strain during motion and also acts as a lubricant to the ulcerated surfaces. In addition to administration of castor oil, the mechanical removal of accumulated poisonous matter should be attempted by giving very low pressure enema, admitting as much water as the patient can tolerate. This can be done twice or thrice daily. The patient should take complete bed rest as movement induces pain and aggravates distressing symptoms. A hot water bag may be applied over the abdomen.

After the acute symptoms are over, the patient may be allowed rice, curd, fresh ripe fruits, especially bael, banana and pomegranate and skimmed milk. Solid foods should be introduced very carefully and gradually according to the pace of recovery. Flesh foods of all kinds should be avoided in future as far as possible. Other foods which should be avoided are tea, coffee, white sugar and white flour and products made from them as well as alcohol in all forms.

Among specific food remedies, bael fruit is, perhaps, the most efficacious in the treatment of dysentery of both the varieties. Pulp of the fruit mixed with jaggery should be given thrice daily. To deal with a chronic case of dysentery, unripe bael fruit is roasted over the fire and the pulp is mixed with water. Large quantities of the infusion so made should be administered with jaggery. The pulp of the unripe fruit mixed with an equal quantity of dried ginger can also be given with butter-milk.

The use of pomegranate rind is another effective remedy for dysentery. About 60 grams of the rind should be boiled in 250 grams of milk. It should be removed from the fire when one third of the milk has evaporated. It should be administered to the patient in three equal doses at suitable intervals. It will relieve the disease very soon.

Lemon juice is very effective in dealing with ordinary cases of dysentery. A few lemons, peeled and sliced, should be added to 250 ml. of water and boiled for a few minutes. The strained infusion should be administered thrice daily.

Other remedies considered useful in the treatment of dysentery are the use of small pieces of onions mixed with curd and equal parts of tender leaves of the peepal tree, coriander leaves and sugar chewed slowly.

CHAPTER 67

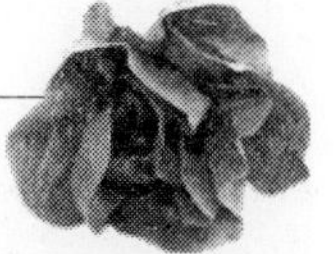

Eczema

The term 'eczema' is derived from a Greek word meaning 'to boil'. It refers to an inflammation of the skin which results in the formation of vesicles or pustules. It is the most common and most troublesome of all skin diseases.

Eczema is essentially a constitutional disease, resulting from a toxic condition of the system. The disease covers a wide variety of forms, the majority of them being of a chronic variety.

Symptoms

Eczema in its acute form is indicated by redness and swelling of the skin, the formation of minute vesicles and severe heat. If the vesicles rupture, a raw, moist surface is formed. From this, a colourless discharge oozes, which forms skin crusts when it accumulates. The disease is usually worse at night when the heat of the body is retained by the bed-clothes.

The skin itches at all stages. In the wet stage, it may become infected with bacteria. The healing of the condition is affected by scratching in response to the irritation. Scratching not only spreads infection but also lengthens the stage of dryness and scaling.

Causes

Allergies play an important part in causing eczema. Some women get eczema on their hands due to an allergy to soap

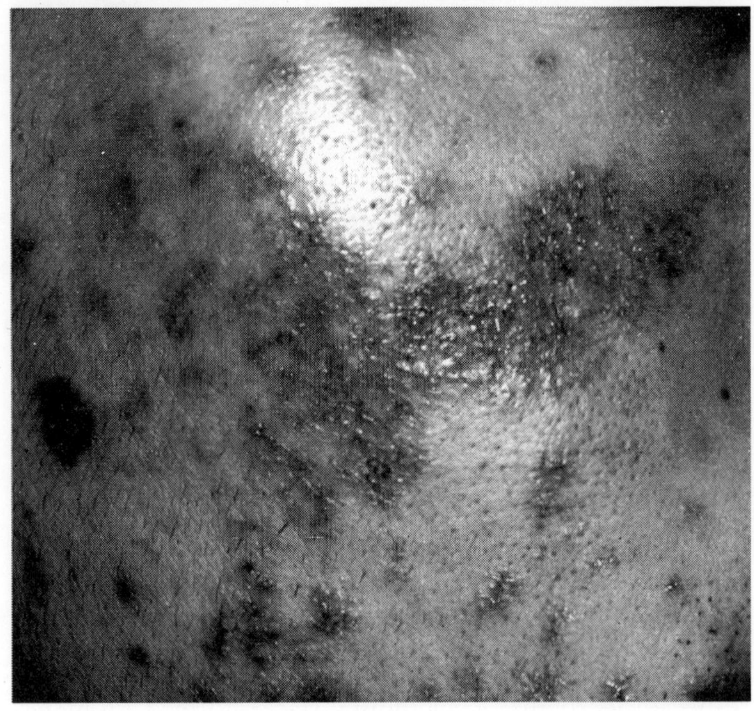

Eczema

or detergents used to wash clothes or dishes. Some persons develop it around the fingers when they wear rings because of allergy to metals. Researchers at the University of Texas Health Science Centre at San Antonio, in a recent study of children with atropic eczema, found that 75 per cent were allergic to a number of foods. The most common triggers for sensitive persons are eggs, peanuts, chocolate, wheat, cow's milk, chicken and potato.

The real cause of eczema however is the failure of the human system to excrete the poisons from the various orifices of the body. Waste matter is excreted from the rectum through stools, from the bladder through urine, from the lungs through breath and from the pores of the skin through sweat. Sometimes the pores of the skin are overworked as waste matter is not properly eliminated from the other orifices. If the pores are not given the chance to perform their normal function, the sweat will be full of morbid matter and this gives rise to skin diseases like eczema, acne, boils, and other eruptions.

Other causes include faulty metabolism, constipation, nutritional deficiencies and stress brought about by nagging spouses, jealousy, frustration and a host of other emotions. Suppressive drug treatment of a former disease is also a most potent subsidiary causative factor in many cases.

The Cure

Skin applications to cure eczema may give temporary relief. If the exudation is suppressed, some other more serious disease may develop. The best way to deal with eczema is to cleanse the bloodstream and the body.

The treatment should start with a fast on orange juice and water from five to 10 days, depending on the severity and duration of the trouble. Juice fasting will help eliminate toxic waste from the body and lead to substantial improvement. In some cases, the condition may worsen in the beginning of the fast due to the increased elimination of waste matter through the skin. But as fasting continues, improvement will manifest itself.

Fruits, salt-free, raw or steamed vegetables with whole meal bread or chappatis may be taken after the juice fast. Carrot and musk melon are particularly beneficial. Coconut oil may be used instead of ghee. After a few days, curd and milk may be added to the diet. The patients may thereafter gradually embark upon a well-balanced diet of three basic food groups, namely (i) seeds, nuts and grains, (ii) vegetables and (iii) fruits. The large proportion of the diet should consist of raw foods. Seeds and beans such as alfalfa, mung and soyabeans can be sprouted. This diet may be supplemented with cold-pressed vegetable oils, honey and yeast. Juice fasting may be repeated at intervals of two months or so, depending on the progress being made. In chronic and more difficult cases of eczema, the patient should fast at least once a week till he is cured.

The patient should avoid tea, coffee, alcoholic beverages and all condiments and highly flavoured dishes. He should also avoid sugar, white flour products, denaturated cereals like polished rice and pearled barley and tinned or bottled foods. He should eat only pure and wholesome foods.

Raw vegetable juices, especially carrot juice in combination with spinach juice, have proved highly beneficial in the treatment of eczema. The formula proportions considered helpful in this combination are carrot 300 ml. and spinach 200 ml. to make 500 ml. or half a litre of juice.

The patient should get as much fresh air as possible. Restrictive clothing should not be worn. Two or three litres of water should be taken daily and the patient must bathe twice or thrice a day. The skin, with the exception of the parts affected with eczema, should be vigorously rubbed with the palms of the hands before taking a bath.

Coconut oil may be applied to the portions with eczema. It will help the skin to stay soft. Walking or jogging should be resorted to in order to activate the bowels. Sunbathing is also beneficial as it kills the harmful bacteria and should be resorted to early in the morning, in the first light of dawn. A light mud-pack applied over the sites of the eczema is also helpful.

The pack should be applied for an hour at a time and should be repeated twice or thrice a day.

Water Treatment

In cases of acute eczema, cold compress or cold wet fomentations are beneficial. The affected part should be wrapped with a thick soft cloth. The cloth should be moistened with cold water (55°-60°F) every 15 to 30 minutes for two hours at a time. The bandage should be left intact, keeping the cloth cold. There may be intensification of itching or pain initially but this will soon subside. A cold compress may be applied twice daily for a week or so.

CHAPTER 68

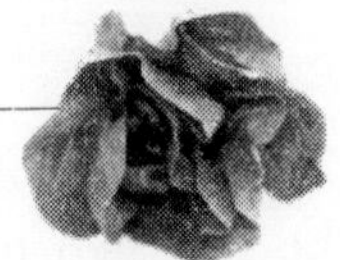

Emphysema

Emphysema is a serious and debilitating lung disease. In this condition, alveoli, the tiny air sacs in the lungs and bronchioles, the narrow passages leading to the air sacs, become permanently distended with air. The lung tissues lose their elasticity and the number of blood vessels is reduced. It is essentially a chronic disease, which generally occurs after the age of 40. It is less frequent in women.

Symptoms

The main symptoms of emphysema is breathlessness followed by coughing. It goes worse with the lapse of time. Eventually the patient is breathless at rest, as the alveoli become so damaged that the exchange of gases between the blood and the air is much impaired. The patient feels difficulty in chewing and swallowing due to breathlessness. There may be discomfort after a meal because the lungs have expanded, pushing the diaphragm into the stomach. Other symptoms include loss of appetite and weight loss.

In severe cases, the chest itself may get enlarged and the movement of the ribs may diminish. The volume of air passed in and out of the lungs at each breath becomes very much less than normal.

Causes

Emphysema is frequently found in association with asthma and chronic bronchitis. Obstruction of the air passages and infection are thus the main factors which bring about this disease. This weakens the elastic tissues of the lungs. Other causes of emphysema are continuous exposure to dust and high levels of air pollution. Smoking is also an important contributory factor.

Treatment

To begin with, the patient should undertake a fast on fruit or vegetable juice for five to seven days. During this period, a warm-water enema should be used daily to cleanse the bowels. The juice fast may be followed by an exclusive diet of fresh juicy fruits, such as apple, pineapple, peach, pear, orange and papaya, for further five days or so.

The patient may thereafter gradually adopt a well-balanced diet consisting of seeds, nuts and grains, vegetables and fruits. The diet should be supplemented with vegetable oil, honey and goat's milk, preferably in sour form like curd and buttermilk. The emphasis should be on fresh fruits and raw vegetables, as well as fruit and vegetable juices. The short juice fast followed by an all-fruit diet may be repeated at intervals of two months or so, depending on the condition.

Certain home remedies have been found beneficial in the treatment of emphysema. The most remarkable of these remedies is the use of garlic. Two or three cloves of this vegetable should be chewed daily. A small amount of garlic juice can also be added to vegetable juices.

The use of lemon or lime is another valuable home remedy for emphysema. A teaspoon of fresh juice of either of the two fruits should be taken several times a day before or between meals.

Amaranth (*chaulai-ka-saag*) has proved beneficial in the treatment of this disease. Fresh juice should be extracted from this green leafy vegetable. This juice should be mixed with honey and drunk liberally by the patient.

The aniseed (*saunf*) has also been found valuable in emphysema due to its expectorant properties. Five to ten drops of aniseed oil should be mixed with one teaspoon of brown sugar. This mixture can be taken with beneficial results in treating this disease. It is old emphysema 'cure' in folk medicine.

The patient should live in a place, with least air pollution and smog-free environment. The chronic bronchitis, which is associated with emphysema must be kept under control as far as practicable through natural methods of treatment. Smoking, if habitual, should be given up completely. Breathing pure oxygen from a cylinder will allow enough of the gas to enter the blood.

Weight loss can be overcome by taking frequent small meals consisting of high energy foods.

The patient should undertake mild exercises which help maintain muscle tone and prevent them from becoming rigid. Walking is especially beneficial and the patient should walk atleast five kms. morning and evening daily. He should also undertake deep breathing exercises in fresh air.

CHAPTER 69

Epilepsy

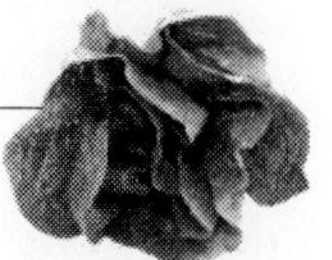

Epilepsy refers to a chronic condition in which repeated fits or attacks of unconsciousness occur with or without convulsions. It is a serious disorder of the central nervous system. It occurs in both children and adults. Most attacks, however, occur in childhood and in early adult life. Attack rates show a progressive decline in frequency with age.

Epilepsy is a very ancient disease which afflicted some of the world's greatest personalities, including Napoleon, Alexander and Julius Caesar. The actual word "epilepsy" comes from the Greek word which means "to seize upon". The ancient people believed that evil spirits entered the body of the person afflicted, seized upon his soul and threw his body into convulsions. The Greeks believed that the gods induced this disease. The early Christians blamed the devil for these convulsions.

One of the main problems that a person with epilepsy has to face is continual uncertainty about whether or not he or she will have an attack on any particular occasion. Patients may find themselves increasingly inhibited from engaging in social events because of the understandable fear that they might embarrass themselves by having another attack. Such people also encounter difficulties in employments and other relationships.

Symptoms

Epilepsy is recognised by recurrent sudden attacks at

irregular intervals. The patients twitch convulsively and fall unconscious to the ground during these attacks which cause tremendous nervous upheaval. There are two main types of epilepsy known as petit mal and grand mal. Each follows its own specific pattern.

In petit mal, which is a less serious form of epilepsy, an attack comes and goes within a few seconds. The patient has a momentary loss of consciousness, with no convulsions except sometimes a slight rigidity, or there may be slight attack of convulsion such as a jerk, or movement of the eyes, head, trunk or extremities, with no perceptible loss of consciousness. The patient may not fall. He may suddenly stop what he is doing and then resume it when the attack is over, without even being aware of what has happened. Petit mal attacks may occur at any time in life but are most frequent in children.

The attack in case of grand mal comes with a dramatic effect. There are violent contractions of the arms, legs and body, accompanied by a sudden loss of consciousness. Before the onset of an attack, some patients have a warning or aura in the form of strange sensations such as a current of air or a stream of water flowing over the body, noises, odours and flashes of light. In a typical attack, the patient cries out, falls to the ground, loses consciousness and develops convulsions. With the convulsions may come foaming at the mouth, twitching of the muscles, biting of the tongue, distorted fixation of limbs, rotation of the head and deviation of the eyes. The patient may lose control of his urine and faeces. The attack may last several minutes and is usually followed by a deep sleep. On waking up, he may remember nothing of what happened to him.

People who suffer from epilepsy are not abnormal in any other way. They usually know that fits can be triggered off by particular stimuli. Between epileptic attacks, their brain functions normally.

Causes

Epilepsy denotes electrical malfunctioning within the brain due to damage of brain cells or some inherited abnormality. There are many causes of epilepsy. Digestive disturbances, intestinal toxaemia and a strained nervous condition are very often the main cause of petit mal. Grand mal usually results from hereditary influences, serious shock or injury to the brain or nervous system. Meningitis, typhoid and other diseases with prolonged high temperature can also lead to grand mal.

Epilepsy may be caused by several other factors. It may result from allergic reaction to certain food substances, especially some particular form of protein which is the main constituent of meat. Circulatory disorders such as hardening of arteries leading to the brain may also cause epileptic seizures. This type is rare and occurs only in very aged people. Chronic alcoholism, lead poisoning, cocaine and other such habits can also lead to this disease. Other causes of epileptic seizure include mental conflict, deficient mineral assimilation, particularly of magnesium and calcium and wrong vitamin metabolism. According to some researchers, hypoglycemia or low blood sugar is also involved in most cases of epilepsy.

Treatment

In the natural form of treatment, the sufferer from epilepsy has to follow a rigorous regimen consisting of a strict dietary, complete relaxation and optimum exercise in the open air. He must adhere to a simple and correct natural life. He must assume a cheerful, optimistic attitude, refrain from mental and physical overwork and worry.

The most important aspect of the treatment is the diet. To begin with, the patient should be placed on an exclusive fruit diet for first few days. During this period, he should have three meals a day of fresh juicy fruits such as oranges, apples, grapes, grapefruit, peaches, pears, pineapple and melon. Thereafter, he may gradually adopt a well balanced diet of three basic food groups, namely, (i) seeds, nuts and grains, (ii) vegetables and (iii) fruits with emphasis on sprouted seeds such as alfalfa seeds and mung beans, raw vegetables and fruits. The diet should include a moderate amount of raw milk preferably goat's milk and milk products such as raw butter and homemade cottage cheese.

The diet should eliminate completely all animal proteins, except milk, as they not only lack in magnesium but also rob the body of its own magnesium storage as well as of vitamin B_6. Both these substances are needed in large amounts by epileptics. The best food sources of magnesium are raw nuts, seeds, soyabeans, green leafy vegetables such as spinach, kale, beet-tops, etc. The patient should avoid all refined foods, fried and greasy food, sugar and products made with it, strong tea, coffee, alcoholic beverages, condiments and pickles.

The patient should avoid overeating and take frequent small meals rather than a few large ones. He should not eat large meals before going to bed.

Mud packs on the abdomen twice daily help remove toxaemic conditions of the intestines and thereby hasten removal of epileptic conditions. The application of alternate hot and cold compresses to the base of the brain, that is at the back of the head will be beneficial. The procedure is to dip the feet in a bucket of hot water and apply first a hot towel and then a cold to the base of the brain. The alternate hot and cold towels should be kept for two or three minutes about four times. The process should be repeated twice every day. Full Epsom-salt baths, twice a week are also beneficial.

If the sufferer from epilepsy has taken strong drugs for many years, he should not leave off entirely all at once. The dosage may be cut to half to begin with and then gradually reduced further until it can be left off completely.

An epileptic should strictly observe all the natural laws of good health and build and maintain the highest level of general health. He should remain active mentally but avoid all severe mental and physical stress. And above all, he should avoid excitements of all kinds.

CHAPTER 70

Falling of Hair

Loss of hair at a very tender age has become a common disorder these days. It causes a great deal of concern to persons affected by loss of hair, especially Indian women who regard good hair growth, with thick long hair as a sign of beauty.

Hair is formed in minute pockets in the skin, called follicles. An upgrowth at the base of the follicle, called the papilla, actually produces hair, when a special group of cells turn amino acids into keratin, a type of protein of which hair is made. The rate of production of these protein 'building blocks' determines hair growth. The average growth rate is about 1.2 cm per month, growing fastest on women between the ages 15 and 30.

Causes

The most important cause of loss of hair is inadequate nutrition. Even a partial lack of almost any nutrient may cause hair to fall. Persons lacking vitamin B_6 lose their hair and those deficient in folic acid often become completely bald. But the hair grows normally after the liberal intake of these vitamins.

Another important cause of falling of hair is stress such as worry, anxiety and sudden shock. Stress leads to a severe tension in the skin of the scalp. This adversely affects the supply of essential nutrition required for the healthy growth of the hair. General debility, caused by severe or long standing illnesses like typhoid, syphilis, chronic cold, influenza and anaemia, also gives rise to this disorder. It makes the roots of the hair weak, resulting in the falling of hair. Unclean condition of the scalp can also cause loss of hair. It weakens the hair roots by blocking the pores with the collected dirt. Heredity is another predisposing factor which may cause hair to fall.

Treatment

The healthy condition of the hair depends, to a very large extent, on the intake of sufficient amounts of essential nutrients in the daily diet. Hair is made of protein and adequate protein is necessary for luxuriant hair. Women require 60 grams, men 80 to 90, adolescent boys and girls 80 to 100 grams of protein. It is supplied by milk, buttermilk, yogurt, soyabean, eggs, cheese, meat and fish. A lack of vitamin A may cause the hair to be coarse and ugly. A deficiency of some of the B vitamins, of iron, copper and iodine may cause hair disorders like falling of hair and premature greying.

Lack of inositol causes loss of hair. Any person having trouble with his or her hair should eat foods rich in inositol such as yeast, liver and molasses. Research has, however, shown that women have a low requirement of inositol. Although this vitamin may help to stimulate the growth of a woman's hair, its lack is probably not a major cause of slow growth. Women are generally deficient in iodine and vitamin B_1, either of which can slow down circulation to the scalp to such an extent that hair may fall out and new hair grow in very slowly. Women who keep their diets adequate in iodine, the B vitamins and iron have a better growth of hair.

According to Adelle Davis, a world famous nutritionist, "Increasing the intake of protein, particularly of liver, wheat germ and yeast, and supplementing the diet with a teaspoon of inositol daily usually stops a man's hair from falling, and I have seen three or four persons whose hair became thick after these improvements were made."

Persons with a tendency to lose hair should thus take a well balanced and correct diet, made up of foods which in combination should supply all the essential nutrients. It has been found that a diet which contains liberal quantities of (i) seeds, nuts and grains, (ii) vegetables, and (iii) fruits would provide adequate amounts of all the essential nutrients. Each food group should roughly form the bulk of one of the three principal meals. These foods should, however, be supplemented with certain special foods such as milk, vegetable oils, honey, wheat germ, yeast and liver.

Home Remedies

Several home remedies have been found useful in the prevention and treatment of the loss of hair. The most effective among these remedies is a vigorous rubbing of the scalp with fingers after washing the hair with cold water. The scalp should be rubbed vigorously till it starts to tingle with the heat. It will activate the sebaceous glands and energise the circulation of blood in the affected area, making the hair grow healthy.

Amla oil, prepared by boiling dry pieces of amla in coconut oil, is considered a valuable hair tonic for enriching hair growth. A mixture of equal quantity of fresh amla juice and lime juice used as a shampoo stimulates hair growth and prevents hair loss.

Lettuce (salad-ka-patta) is useful in preventing hair loss through deficiencies. A mixture of lettuce and spinach juice is said to help the growth of hair if it is drunk to the extent of half a litre a day. The juice of alfalfa (lucerne) in combination with carrot and lettuce juice, taken daily also helps the growth of hair to a remarkable extent. The combination of these juices is rich in elements which are particularly useful for the growth of hair. While preparing alfalfa juice, the leaves of the plant only may be used when it can be obtained fresh.

Daily application of refined coconut oil mixed with limewater and lime juice on the hair, prevents loss of hair and lengthens them. Application of the juice of green coriander leaves on the head is also considered beneficial. Amaranth, known as chaulai-ka-saag in the vernacular, is another valuable remedy. Application of its fresh leaf-juice helps the growth of the hair and keeps them soft.

Mustard oil, boiled with henna leaves, is useful in healthy growth of hair. About 250 grams of mustard oil should be boiled in tinned basin. A little quantity of henna leaves should be gradually put in this oil till about 60 grams of these leaves are thus burnt in the oil. The oil should then be filtered through a cloth and stored well in a bottle. A regular massage of the head with this oil will produce abundant hair.

Another effective home remedy for loss of hair is the application of coconut milk all over the scalp and massaging it into the hair roots. It will nourish the hair and promote hair growth. The coconut milk is prepared by grinding the coconut shavings and squeezing it well.

Washing the hair with a paste of cooked black gram dal, (*urad dal*) and fenugreek (*methi*) lengthens the hair. A fine paste made from pigeon pea or red gram (*arhar dal*) can also be applied regularly with beneficial results on bald patches. Regular use of castor oil as hair oil helps the luxuriant growth of the hair.

Certain home remedies have also been found useful in case of patchy loss of hair. The seeds of lime and black pepper seeds, ground to get a fine paste, is one of the valuable remedies. This paste applied on the patches, has mildly irritant action. This increases blood circulation in the affected area and stimulates hair growth. The paste should be applied twice a day for a few weeks.

Another useful remedy for patchy loss of hair is the paste of liquorice (mulethi) made by grinding the pieces in milk with a pinch of saffron. This paste should be applied over the bald patches in the night before going to bed.

CHAPTER 71

Fatigue

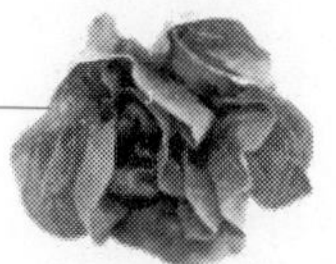

Fatigue refers to a feeling of tiredness or weariness. It can be temporary or chronic. Almost every person has to work overtime on certain occasions, sacrificing rest and sleep, which may cause temporary fatigue. This condition can be remedied by adequate rest. Chronic or continuous fatigue is, however, a serious problem which requires a comprehensive plan of treatment.

Chronic fatigue can result from a variety of factors. A specific character trait, compulsiveness, can lead to continuous fatigue. Many persons constantly feel that they cannot take rest until they finish everything that needs to be done at one time. These persons are usually perfectionists, tense and cannot relax unless they complete the whole job, no matter how tired they may be.

Causes

The chief cause of fatigue is lowered vitality or lack of energy due to wrong feeding habits. Fatigue is an indication that the cells of the body are not getting sufficient live atoms in the food to furnish them with a constant flow of needed energy. The habitual use of refined foods such as white sugar, refined cereals and white flour products as well as processed, tinned and preserved foods have a very bad effect on the system in general. Foods 'denatured' in this way are deprived, to a very great extent, of their invaluable vitamins and minerals. Such foods lead to nervousness, tiredness, obesity and a host of other complaints prevalent today.

Certain physical conditions can cause fatigue. Anaemia is a very common ailment leading to tiredness. It is known as 'tired blood' disturbance. In anaemia, very little oxygen reaches the tissues with the result energy cannot be produced normally. This causes constant tiredness and mental depression. Anaemia usually results from deficiencies of iron and vitamin B_{12}.

Sometime deficiencies of vitamin B_6 and folic acid are also involved.

Insomnia or lack of sleep can be a cause of fatigue. Sleep induced by sleeping pills and other drugs does not banish fatigue. Intestinal parasites can also lead to fatigue as they rob the body of good nourishment and gorge themselves on rich red blood. Other ailments which can cause fatigue are low blood pressure, low blood sugar, any kind of infection in the body, liver damage, a sluggish thyroid and allergy in foods and drugs caused by additives including artificial flavours, colours and preservatives.

Mental tension is one of the major causes of fatigue. A person who is tense and cannot relax has all the muscles of his body more or less contracted. This leads to needless waste of unusually large amounts of energy. Food is continuously burnt, lactic acid accumulates more rapidly than it can be carried to liver for conversion to body starch. Persons who are high-strung, nervous and irritable usually suffer from this type of fatigue.

Treatment

Nutritional measures are most vital in the treatment of fatigue. Studies reveal that people who eat small mid-meals suffer less from fatigue and nervousness, think more clearly and are more efficient than those who eat only three meals daily. These mid-meals should consist of fresh or dried fruits, fresh fruit or vegetable juices, raw vegetables or small sandwich of whole grain bread. The mid-meal should be small and less food should be consumed at regular meals. They should be taken at specified time such as 11 a.m., 4 p.m. and before retiring to bed.

The patient should eat health foods which supply energy to the body. Charles De Coti Marsh of London in his book 'Prescription for Energy' prescribes foods to relieve fatigue and gain energy. He says, "Regenerating must begin with foods .... They must be taken in their natural state. These cereals are corn seeds, wheat seeds, rye seeds, maize seeds, barley seeds and oat seeds. They must be freshly milled. In uncooked cereals, we do have one perfect food for perfect health which contains the essential vitamins and energy creators." In addition to cereal seeds, Marsh recommends fresh raw nuts taken directly from the shell and root vegetables. He says, "Any seed or root vegetable that will grow again will renew human vitality."

The patient should take an optimum diet made up of (i) seeds, nuts and grains, (ii) vegetables, and (iii) fruits. Roughly, each food group should supply the bulk of one of the three meals. Sprouting is an excellent way to eat seeds, beans and grains in raw form. Sprouting increases the nutritional value of foods and many new vitamins are created or multiplied in seeds during sprouting. The patient should supplement the three health-building food groups with special protective foods such as milk, high quality cold-pressed unrefined vegetable oil and honey.

The patient should also take natural vitamin and mineral supplements as an effective assurance against nutritional deficiencies, as such deficiencies have been found to be a factor in fatigue. Lack of pantothenic acid, B vitamin in particular, leads to extreme fatigue as deficiency of this vitamin is associated with exhaustion of the adrenal glands. In fact the entire B-complex protect nerves and increases energy by helping to nourish and regulate glands. The vegetarian foods rich in vitamin B are wheat and other whole grain cereals, green leafy vegetables, rice polishings, milk, nuts, banana, yeast, pulses and peas.

Minerals are also important. Potassium is especially needed for protection against fatigue. Raw green vegetables are rich in this mineral. Calcium is essential for relaxation and is beneficial in cases of insomnia and tension both of which can lead to fatigue. Sodium and zinc are also beneficial in the treatment of fatigue.

Raw vegetable juices, especially carrot juice, taken separately or in combination with juices of beets and cucumbers, is highly valuable in overcoming fatigue. The formula proportions considered helpful in the combination juice of 500 ml. are carrot 300 ml. and beet and cucumber 100 ml. each.

The patient should avoid depending for an energy lift, on crutches such as taking aspirin, tranquilizers and other drugs, drinking coffee or alcohol, smoking, eating some sugar or sweets. They give only a temporary boost and this is soon followed by a downward plunge of energy, leaving a person worse than before.

CHAPTER 72

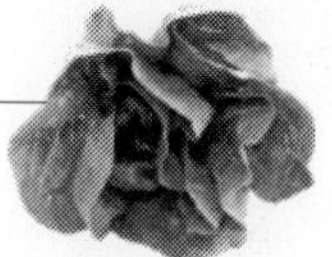

Gall-bladder Disorders

The gall-bladder is a pear-shaped organ, 10 cm. long and three to five cm. wide, attached to the under-surface of the liver on the right side. The main function of the gallbladder is to store the bile secreted by the liver. Bile is an excretion composed mainly of bile salts and acids, colour pigments and cholesterol. Bile assists in the digestion and absorption of fats and the absorption of fat-soluble vitamins A, D, E and K, minerals and calcium.

The gall-bladder is usually full and relaxed between meals. During the process of digestion, when food reaches the duodenum, the hormone cholecystokinin begins to be produced in the internal mucosa. When this hormone reaches the gall-bladder through the bloodstream, it causes the gallbladder to contract, thereby releasing the bile concentrate into the duodenum via a common duct.

The main problems which afflict the gall-bladder are an inflammatory condition known as cholecystitis and gallstones. Gall-stones are usually caused by disturbances in the composition of the bile. A change in the ratio of cholesterol and bile salts may result in the formation of deposits. At the start, these may be in the form of fine gravel. But these fine particles constitute the nucleus for further deposits, ultimately leading to the formation of larger stones. An irritation of the lining of the gall-bladder due to inflammation may also lead to the formation of particles. The incidence of gall-stones is higher in females than males, particularly in those who are obese.

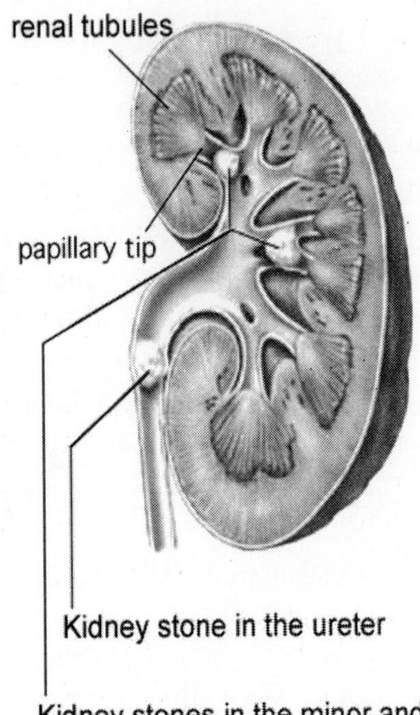

Kidney Stones

Symptoms

Indigestion, gas, a feeling of fullness after meals, constipation, nausea and disturbed vision are the usual symptoms of gallbladder disorders. Other symptoms are intolerance to fats, dizziness, jaundice, anaemia, acne and other lesions. Varicose veins, haemorrhoids and breakdown of capillaries are also disorders associated with gall-bladder troubles.

Causes

The main causes of gall-bladder disorders are digestive disturbances due to a regular excessive intake of fats and carbohydrates in the diet. They can also be brought on by disturbances of the liver and gall-bladder. Meals rich in fats may cause an attack of gall-bladder pain or gall-stone colic. Often the disorder is caused by a diet rich in refined carbohydrates such as white flour and white sugar. Poor health, hereditary factors, stress, spinal displacements, bad posture and muscular tension may also cause gall-bladder disorders.

Types of gall stones

There are three types of gall-stones, depending on the cause of their formation. These are: cholesterol stones caused by a change in the ratio of cholesterol to bile salts; pigment stones (composed of bile pigment) caused by the destruction of red blood cells due to certain blood diseases, and mixed stones consisting of layers of cholesterol, calcium and bile pigment (bilirubin) resulting from stagnation of the bile flow.

The Cure

Surgery becomes necessary if the gall-stones are very large or in cases in which they have been present for long. Smaller gallstones can, however, be cleared through nature cure methods. Diet is the basic factor in the treatment of gall bladder disorders. In cases of acute gall-bladder inflammation, the patient should fast for two or three days, until the acute condition clears. Nothing but water should be taken during the fast. After the fast, the patient should take carrot, beet, grapefruit, lemon or grape juice for a few days. Ensure that the diet contains an adequate amount of all the essential nutrients. Ideally, the diet should be lacto-vegetarian, consisting of raw and cooked vegetables, vegetable juices, and a moderate amount of fruit and seeds. Yogurt, cottage cheese and a tablespoon of olive oil twice a day should also be taken. Oil serves as a stimulant for the production of bile and lipase, the fat digesting enzymes. All meats, eggs, animal fats and processed and denatured fats as well as fried foods should be avoided. The diet should also exclude refined carbohydrates, especially sugar, sugar products, alcohol, soft drinks, cakes, puddings, ice-cream, coffee and citrus fruits.

The patient should eat small meals at frequent intervals, rather than three large meals. The following is the suggested menu for those suffering from gall-bladder disorders:

On rising: A glass of warm water mixed with lemon juice and honey or fresh fruit juice.

Breakfast: Fresh fruit, one or two slices of whole meal toast and a cup of skimmed powder milk.

Mid morning: Fresh fruit juice.

Lunch: Vegetable soup, a large salad consisting of vegetables in season with dressing of lemon or vegetable oil. Fresh fruit for dessert, if desired.

Dinner: Vegetable juice, one or two lightly cooked vegetables, baked potato, brown rice or whole wheat chappati and a glass of buttermilk.

Water Treatment

Regular applications of hot and cold fomentations to the abdomen improve the circulation of the liver and gall-bladder. They also induce contractions of the gall-bladder, thereby improving the flow of bile. A cold hip bath improves the general abdominal tone. The pain of gall-stone colic can be relieved by the application of hot packs or fomentation to the upper abdominal area. A warm water enema at body temperature will help eliminate faecal accumulations if the patient is constipated.

Exercise is essential as physical inactivity can lead to lazy gall-bladder type indigestion which may ultimately result in the formation of stones. Yogic asanas which are beneficial in toning up the liver and gall-bladder are: sarvangasana, paschimottanasana, shalabhasana, dhanurasana and bhujangasana.

CHAPTER 73

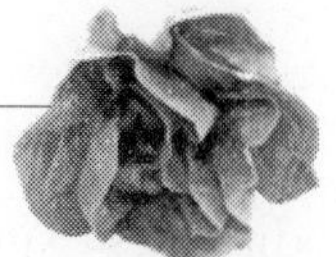

Gastritis

Gastritis is an inflammation of the lining of the stomach. It is a troublesome condition which may lead to many complications, including ulcers if not treated in time. Constipation aggravates the condition more than any other disorder.

The inflammatory lesions may be either acute erosive gastritis or chronic atrophic gastritis. The latter type has been found to be present in half the patients suffering from severe iron deficiency anaemia.

Symptoms

The main symptoms of gastritis are loss of appetite, nausea, vomiting, headache and dizziness. There is also pain and a feeling of discomfort in the region of the stomach. In more chronic cases, there is a feeling of fullness in the abdomen, especially after meals. The patient complains of heartburn. Prolonged illness often results in the loss of weight, anaemia and occasional haemorrhage from the stomach. There may be an out-pouring of mucus and a reduction in the secretion of hydrochloric acid during acute attacks and also in most cases of chronic gastritis.

Causes

The most frequent cause of gastritis is a dietetic indiscretion such as habitual overeating, eating of badly combined or improperly cooked foods, excessive intake of strong tea, coffee or alcoholic drinks, habitual use of large quantities of condiments, sauces, etc. It may sometimes follow certain diseases such as measles, diphtheria, influenza, virus pneumonia, etc. Most often it also results from worry, anxiety, grief and prolonged tension. Use of certain drugs, strong acids and caustic substances may also give rise to gastritis.

Treatment

The patient should undertake a fast in both acute and chronic cases of gastritis. In acute cases, the patient will usually recover after a short fast of two or three days. In chronic condition, the fast may have to be continued for a longer period of seven days or so. In the alternative, short fasts may be repeated at an interval of one or two months, depending on the progress being made.

The fast may be conducted on fruit juices. By fasting, the intake of irritants is at once effectively stopped, the stomach is rested and the toxic condition, causing the inflammation, is allowed to subside. Elimination is increased by fasting and the excess of toxic matter accumulated in the system is thrown out.

After the acute symptoms subside, the patient should adopt an all-fruit diet for further three days. Juicy fruits such as apple, pear, grapes, grapefruit, orange, pineapple, peach and melon may be taken during this period at five-hourly intervals. The patient can thereafter gradually embark upon a well-balanced diet of three basic food groups, namely: (i) seeds, nuts and grains, (ii) vegetables and (iii) fruits on the following lines:

Upon arising: A glass of lukewarm water with freshly squeezed lemon and a spoonful of honey.

Breakfast: Fresh fruits, such as apple, orange, banana, grapes, grapefruit or any available berries, a handful or raw nuts and a glass of milk.

Mid-morning snack: One apple, banana or any other fruit.

Lunch: Steamed vegetables, two or three slices of whole wheat bread or whole wheat chappatis, according to appetite and a glass of butter-milk.

Mid-afternoon: A glass of fresh fruit or vegetable juice or sugarcane juice.

Dinner: A large bowl of fresh salad of green vegetables such as tomatoes, carrots, red beets, cabbage, cucumber with dressing of lemon juice and cold-pressed vegetable oil, all available sprouts such as alfalfa seeds, mung beans, fresh butter and fresh home-made cottage cheese.

Bed time snack: A glass of fresh milk or one apple.

The patient should avoid the use of alcohol, nicotine, spices and condiments, flesh foods, chillies, sour things, pickles, strong tea and coffee. He should also avoid sweets, pastries, rich cakes and aerated waters. Curds and cottage cheese should be used freely.

Carrot juice in combination with the juice of spinach is considered highly beneficial in the treatment of gastritis. 200 ml. of spinach juice should be mixed with 300 ml. of carrot juice in this combination.

Too many different foods should not be mixed at the same meal. Meals should be taken at least two hours before going to bed at night. Eight to 10 glasses of water should be taken daily but water should not be taken with meals as it dilutes the digestive juices and delays digestion. And above all, haste should be avoided while eating and meals should be served in a pleasing and relaxed atmosphere.

Coconut water is an excellent food remedy for gastritis. It gives the stomach necessary rest and provides vitamins and minerals. The stomach will be greatly helped in returning to its normal condition if nothing except coconut water is given during the first 24 hours.

Rice gruel is another effective remedy in acute cases of gastritis. In chronic cases where the flow of gastric juice is meagre, such foods require prolonged vigorous mastication which will be beneficial as this induces a greater flow of gastric juices.

From the commencement of the treatment, a warm water enema should be used daily, for about a week, to cleanse the bowels. If constipation is habitual, all steps should be taken for its eradication. The patient should be given daily a dry friction and sponge bath. Application of heat, through hot compressor or hot water bottle twice in the day either on an empty stomach or two hours after meals, should also prove beneficial.

The patient should not undertake any hard physical and mental work. He should, however, undertake breathing and other light exercises like walking, swimming and golf. He should avoid worries and mental tension.

CHAPTER 74

Gastroenteritis

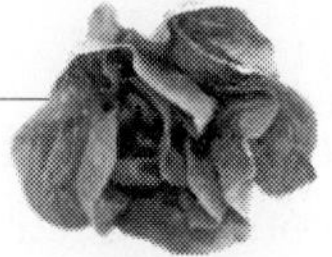

Gastroentritis is an acute inflammation of the lining of the stomach and small bowel. It usually results from infection from contaminated food or water. The disease affects both children and adults alike.

Symptoms

Gastroentritis usually begins suddenly with a feeling of nausea and abdominal cramps, followed by vomiting, diarrhoea, fever and weakness. There may be intense rectal burning and the stools may contain blood and mucus. The patient may pass loose or watery motions several times a day. All this loss of fluid from the bowel may result in severe dehydration which is characterised by sunken eyes, dry skin, dry tongue, thirst, excessive weakness and occasionally muscle cramps. This may lead to a condition known as acidosis, which is indicated by deep rapid respiration as the body tries to get rid of carbondioxide. There may be pain in the abdomen, with some distention, especially in the lower areas. It is a sign of potassium deficiency. The course of disease may last from few hours to a week.

Causes

There are many and various causes of gastroenteritis. The worst attacks of this disease are caused by germs. Foods prepared at home and sold in restaurants are easily contaminated either by toxins or poisonous substances, produced by different types of germs. These germs multiply and form colonies in the contaminated food. Foods most frequently contaminated with these germs are various meats, fish, custards, cream-filled pastry, milk and different kinds of desserts. The trouble usually arises from the infected nails, skin infections on the hands of those who handle food and perhaps by coughing. Some persons are allergic to certain foods, which may act as poison to them. Others react poorly to various drugs, cathartics and chemicals.

Gastroenteritis attacks occur within two to four hours after taking the contaminated foods. Most of these attacks only last a few hours and are followed by complete recovery. In outbreaks of gastroenteritis, a number of people are usually involved, all of whom have eaten the same food at the same time. The disease is also spread by contamination of water supply with sewage in the rains.

Treatment

The patient should be kept in bed. He should not be given any food as long as nausea and vomiting persist. Application of gentle heat to the abdomen will help relieve spasm or pain. To treat dehydration, the patient should be given plenty of boiled water to drink with electrolyte formulation. An oral rehydration solution can be made at home by extracting the juice of one lemon in a glass of water and adding a pinch of salt and five teaspoons of sugar. This solution should be given to the patient several times a day.

To check vomiting, ice-bag should be applied over stomach, throat and spine. Cold compresses can also be applied over the abdomen with beneficial results. They should be changed every 15 or 20 minutes.

When the vomiting subsides, the patient should be given sips of some warm drink, such as barley or rice water. After the acute symptoms are over, he should be given a bland diet like rice, curd, apple and ripe bananas. Oily and spicy foods should be avoided. After complete recovery, the patient should be allowed to gradually embark upon a well-balanced diet. The emphasis should be on whole grain cereals, raw or lightly-cooked vegetables and fresh fruits.

Prevention

Gastroenteritis can be prevented by not taking uncooked foods outside or stale food at home, especially in the monsoon or summer. Water should not be drunk outside the house and water should always be boiled before drinking during monsoon. All fruits and vegetables should be washed in a solution of potassium permanganate before eating them. Hands should be thoroughly washed before taking food. Nails must be cut at least once a week. Foods must be stored in a cool place free from flies and well-ventilated. All persons, who handle food, plates and containers used in cooking and serving, should strictly observe the rules for personal cleanliness. The kitchen must be kept thoroughly clean and no rubbish should be allowed to remain in or near it. It should be ensured that there is no sewage drain near water supply.

CHAPTER 75

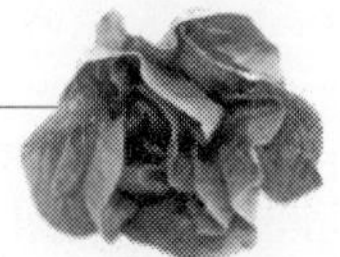

Glaucoma

Glaucoma is a serious eye condition characterised by an increase of pressure within the eye ball, called intraocular pressure. It is similar to high blood pressure in the body. The condition is, therefore, also known as hypertension of the eye.

A certain amount of intraocular pressure is considered necessary, but too much can cause damage to the eye and may result in vision loss. Glaucoma is the major cause of blindness among adults today. One out of every eight blind persons is a victim of glaucoma. Far sighted persons are more prone to develop this disease than near sighted ones.

Symptoms

The first symptom of glaucoma is the appearance of halos or coloured rings round distant objects, when seen at night. In this condition, the iris is usually pushed forward, and the patient often complains of constant pain in the region of the brow, near the temples and the cheeks. Headaches are not uncommon. There is gradual impairment of vision as glaucoma develops, and this may ultimately result in blindness if proper steps are not taken to deal with the disease in the early stages.

Causes

Medical science regards severe eye-strain or prolonged working under bad lighting conditions as the chief causes of glaucoma. But, In reality, the root cause of glaucoma is a highly toxic condition of the system due to dietetic errors, a faulty life style and the prolonged use of suppressive drugs for the treatment of other diseases. Eye-strain is only a contributory factor.

Glaucoma is also caused by prolonged stress and is usually a reaction of adrenal exhaustion. The inability of the adrenal glands to produce aldosterone results in excessive loss of salt from the body and a consequent accumulation of fluid in the tissues. In the region of the eyes, the excess fluid causes the eyeball to harden losing its softness and resilience. Glaucoma has also been associated with giddiness, sinus conditions, allergies, diabetes, hypoglycemia, arteriosclerosis and an imbalance of the autonomic nervous system.

Treatment

The modern medical treatment for glaucoma is through surgery which relieves the internal pressure in the eye due to excess fluid. This, however, does not remove the cause of the presence of the excess fluid. Consequently, even after the operation, there is no guarantee whatsoever that the trouble will not recur, or that it will not affect the other eye. The natural treatment for glaucoma is the same as that for any other condition associated with high toxicity and is directed towards preserving whatever sight remains. If treated in the early stages, the results are encouraging. Though cases of advanced glaucoma may be beyond a cure, even so certain nutritional and other biological approaches can prove effective in controlling the condition and preserving the remaining sight.

Certain foodstuffs should be scrupulously avoided by patients suffering from glaucoma. Coffee in particular, should be completely avoided because of its high caffeine content. Caffeine causes stimulation of vasoconstrictors, elevating blood pressure and increasing blood flow to the eye. Beer and tobacco, which can cause constriction of blood vessels, should also be avoided. Tea should be taken only in moderation. The patient should not take excessive fluids, whether it is juice, milk or water at any time. He may drink small amounts several times with at least one hour intervals.

The diet of the patient suffering from glaucoma should be based on three basic food groups, namely, seeds, nuts and grains; vegetables and fruit, with emphasis on raw vitamin C-rich foods; fresh fruits and vegetables. The breakfast may consist of oranges or grapes or any other juicy fruit in season and a handful of raw nuts or seeds. A raw vegetable salad with olive oil and lemon juice dressing, two or three whole wheat chappatis and a glass of buttermilk may be taken for lunch. The dinner may comprise of steamed vegetables, butter and cottage cheese.

Certain nutrients have been found helpful in the treatment of glaucoma. It has been found that the glaucoma patients are usually deficient in vitamins A, B, C, protein, calcium and other minerals. Nutrients such as calcium and B-complex have proved beneficial in relieving the intraocular condition. Many practitioners believe that intraocular pressure in glaucoma can be lowered by vitamin C therapy. Dr. Michele Virno and his colleagues reported recently at a meeting of the Roman Opthalmological Society in Rome, Italy, that the average person weighing 150 pounds be given 7000 mg of ascorbic acid, five daily, acquired acceptable intraocular pressure within 45 days. Symptoms such as mild stomach discomfort and diarrhoea from the large doses of Vitamin C were temporary and soon disappeared. It has also been suggested that some calcium should always be taken with each dose of ascorbic acid to minimise any side effects of the large dose.

The patient should undertake various methods of relaxing and strengthening the eyes. He should avoid emotional stress and cultivate a tranquil, restful life style. He should also avoid prolonged straining of the eyes such as occurs during excessive T.V. or movie watching and excessive reading. The use of sunglasses should be avoided.

CHAPTER 76

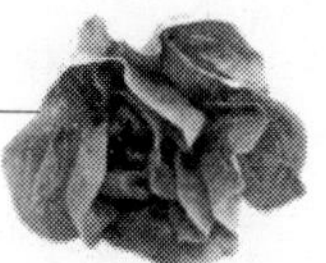

Goitre

Goitre is a disease of the thyroid gland. It generally refers to a swelling of the thyroid gland in the neck. The disease can however, also occur without any swelling of the neck.

The thyroid gland is best known for its ductless glands. Through its secretions, it regulates the day-to-day activities, maintains homeostatis through periods of stress and strain and provides a fine balance to the regulatory systems of the body. No part of the body seems to escape its influence.

Women are more prone to this serious disease. It is more common in women who are over worked and who do not get sufficient rest and relaxation. The periods in a woman's life when she is more likely to be affected by goitre are at puberty, during pregnancy, at menopause or when there is any extra physical strain on the body.

Symptoms

It is difficult to recognise the first symptoms of goitre because they are of a very short duration. They usually appear as emotional upsets and can pass almost unnoticed. These spells of emotional upsets gradually increase in duration, when other symptoms also appear. These include loss of power of concentration, depression and weeping. The patient appears to be very easily irritated. The approach of a nervous breakdown is often suspected.

The thyroid gland may swell but this has no relation to the severity of the ailment, because many serious cases have

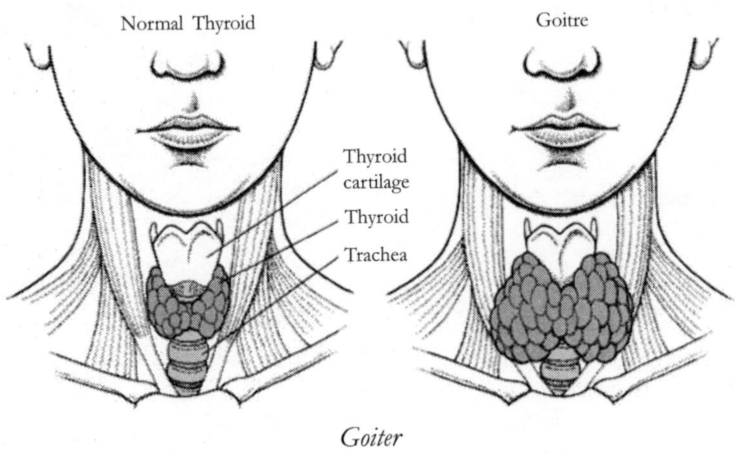

Goiter

practically no visible swelling. There is always a rapid though regular heart beat and any undue excitement increases this to a quick pulsation which may even be conveyed to the thyroid gland. There is, in most cases, a tremor of the hands and a feeling of extreme tiredness, together with a lack of power to make any real muscular effort. The eyes may incline to protrude although this does not appear in all patients.

A most alarming symptom of goitre is the weight loss which no treatment seems to check, and this can persist till the patient feels extremely weak. All the symptoms appear very gradually and that is why so many women do not complain until the trouble has reached serious proportions.

Whenever goitre occurs, it must not be assumed that it is sudden flaring up because disease is not an abrupt derangement of a healthy system nor a sign that there has been a gradual loss of health. In practically every instance the bowel is clogged and there has been a slow poisoning of the entire system over a period of years.

Causes

Deficiency of iodine in the diet is the most common cause of goitre. The thyroid gland makes use of organic iodine in its secretion; and a diet deficient in organic iodine is a predisposing factor towards the appearance of this disease in certain cases, especially if other physical and emotional disturbances are present. People living near the sea rarely contract goitre, because all seafoods are rich in organic iodine. It should not, however, be concluded from this that fish and other sea-foods are essential to the diet to avoid goitre, or that people who eat plenty of fish are necessarily immune from this disease. In fact, organic iodine is present in practically all foods which come from the earth as well as from the sea. Goitre gradually affects those who habitually live on denatured, that is cooked and refined foods, and not those who eat much of their food in the raw or uncooked state.

Treatment

The only real treatment for goitre is cleaning of the system and adoption of a rational dietary thereafter, combined with adequate rest and relaxation. To begin with, juices of fruits such as orange, apple, pineapple, and grapes may be taken every two or three hours from 8 am to 8 pm for five days. The bowels should be cleansed daily with lukewarm water.

After the juice fast, the patient may spend a further three days on fruits and milk, taking three meals a day of juicy fruits such as apple, pineapple, grapes, papaya, with a glass of milk, at five hourly intervals. Thereafter, a balanced diet on the following line may be adopted.

Breakfast: Fresh acid fruits such as apples, grapefruit, oranges, pears, grapes, a glass of whole milk and a handful of raw nuts.

Mid-morning: A glass of fruit or vegetable juice to which a tablespoon of yeast has been added.

Lunch: Steamed vegetables, whole wheat chappatis and a glass of buttermilk.

Mid-afternoon: A glass of milk or fruit juice.

Dinner: Vegetable soup, a large bowl of salad of raw vegetables in season such as lettuce, tomato, cabbage, carrot, turnips, and celery, sprouts such as alfalfa seeds and mung beans and home made cottage cheese or nuts.

Before retiring: Milk or fruit juice.

The patient should take plenty of rest and spend a day in bed every week for the first two months of the treatment. More and more exercise should be taken after the symptoms subside.

The appetite of the thyroid patient is usually very large and the weight reduction cannot be prevented for some time. This is because until the heart beat slows down and the tremors stop, there will be incomplete assimilation of food. But as soon as the balance is restored, weight will slowly increase. To help the absorption of food, a narrow waist compress and, later, a neck compress should be worn for five nights a week.

As weight increases, the almost constant hunger will gradually disappear; on no account should any stimulants be administered to create an appetite.

Certain foods and fluids are extremely injurious for the goitre patient and these should be avoided by them. These include white flour products, white sugar, flesh foods, fried or greasy foods, preserves, condiments, tea coffee and alcohol.

No drugs should be taken as they cause irritation in the tissues, iodine is undoubtedly most helpful in many cases, but it should be introduced in organic form. All foods containing iodine should be taken liberally. These are asparagus, cabbage, carrots, garlic, onion, oats, pineapple, whole rice, tomatoes, watercress and strawberries.

Great care must be taken never to allow the body to become exhausted and any irritation likely to cause emotional upset should be avoided. The cure of goitre is not a speedy one and there is often a recurrence of symptoms but these should gradually become less pronounced. Strict adherence to a suitable diet is essential for complete cure.

Half the daily intake of food should consist of fresh fruits and vegetables, and the starch element should be confined to whole wheat products and potatoes. Potatoes are the most valuable form of starch. They should preferably be taken in their jackets. The protein foods should be confined to egg, cheese, peas, beans, lentils and nuts. Milk and all flesh proteins must be avoided.

The diet outlined here should be strictly adhered to for a year, and the compresses on the neck and the waist applied for five consecutive nights in a week for two months and discontinued for one month. Water treatments should be taken to increase skin elimination. Application of sponge to the entire body before retiring and a cold sponge on rising will be very helpful. It is most important that the bowels are kept working efficiently to avoid danger of a toxic condition of the blood arising from that source.

All efforts should be made to prevent emotional stress. There may be a light recurrence of this extremely nervous complaint for some time, but the attacks will become less severe and of shorter duration as the treatment progresses. And above all, there must be no lessening of the woman's efforts to help herself because success can only be attained by assiduous effort.

CHAPTER 77

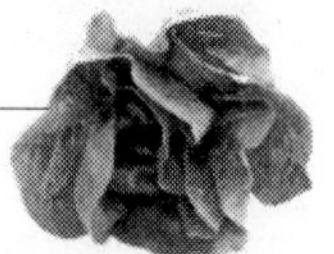

Gout

Gout refers to a certain form of inflammation of the joints and swellings of a recurrent type. Although chronic in character, it breaks in acute attacks. It is a disease of the wealthy and chiefly affects middle-aged men. Women, after menopause, are also sometimes affected by this disease.

Gout was known to the physicians of ancient Greece and Rome. The classical description was written in 1663 by Sydenham, himself a life-long sufferer, who clearly differentiated it from other joint disorders. It was recognised in the 18th century that large enjoyable meals and the consumption of alcoholic drinks were often the prelude to an attack of gout. This disease affected many famous men in history, including Alexander the Great, Luther, Newton, Milton, Dr. Johnson, Franklin and Louis XIV.

Symptoms

An attack of gout is usually accompanied by acute pain in the big toe, which becomes tender, hot and swollen in a few hours. Usually, it is almost impossible to put any weight on the affected foot during the acute stage of the disease. It may also similarly affect other joints such as the knees and the wrists, and sometimes more than one joint may be affected at a time. The attack usually occurs at midnight or in the early hours of the morning, when the patient is suddenly awakened. The acute attack generally lasts for a week or so. During this period the patient may run a slight fever, and feel disinclined to eat. His general health generally remains unaffected.

The attack may occur again after several weeks or months. The interval becomes shorter if the disease is not treated properly. The joint generally becomes damaged by arthritis. This is chronic gout, in which chalky lumps of uric acid crystals remain in the joint and also form under the skin.

Another serious complication of gout is kidney stones containing uric acid, causing severe colic pains in the stomach. In some cases the kidneys become damaged and do not function properly. This is a serious condition as the poisonous waste products which are normally removed by the kidneys accumulate in the blood.

Causes

The chief cause of gout is the formation of uric acid crystals in the joints, skin and kidneys. Uric acid is an end product of the body's chemical processes. Those affected by gout have a higher level of uric acid than the normal, either due to the formation of increased or reduced amounts of acid being passed out by the kidneys in the urine. This uric acid usually remains dissolved in the blood. But when the blood becomes too full of it, the uric acid forms needle-shaped crystals in the joints which bring about attacks of gout.

Heredity is an important factor in causing this disease and certain races are prone to gout. Other causes include excessive intake of alcoholic drinks, regular eating of foods rich in protein and carbohydrate and lack of proper exercise. Stress is also regarded as an important cause of gout. During the alarm reaction, millions of body cells are destroyed and large quantities of uric acid freed from these cells enter the tissues after being neutralised by sodium.

Treatment

For an acute attack, there is no better remedy than a fast. The patient should undertake a fast for five to seven days on orange juice and water. Sometimes the condition may worsen in the early stages of fasting when uric acid, dissolved by juices, is thrown into the bloodstream for elimination. This usually clears up if fasting is continued. In severe cases, it is advisable to undertake a series of short fasts for three days or so rather than one long fast. A warm water enema should be used daily during the period of fasting to cleanse the bowels.

After the acute symptoms of gout have subsided, the patient may adopt an all-fruit diet for a further three or four days. In this regimen, he should have three meals a day of juicy fruits such as grapes, apples, pears, peaches, oranges and pineapple. After the all-fruit diet, the patient may gradually embark upon the following diet:

Breakfast: Fruits such as oranges, apples, figs, apricot, mangoes, whole wheat bread or *dalia* and milk or butter-milk.

Lunch: Steamed vegetables such as lettuce, beets, celery, water-cress, turnips, squash, carrots, tomatoes, cabbage and potatoes, chappatis of whole wheat flour, cottage cheese and butter-milk.

Dinner: Sprouts such as alfalfa and mung beans, a good-sized salad of raw vegetables such as carrots, cabbage, tomatoes, whole wheat bread and butter.

The patient should avoid all purine and uric acid producing foods such as all meats, eggs, and fish. Glandular meats are especially harmful. He should also avoid all intoxicating liquors, tea, coffee, sugar, white flour and its products, and all canned and processed foods. Spices and salts should be used as little as possible.

The cherry, sweet or sour, is considered an effective remedy for gout. This was discovered by Ludwig W. Blan Ph. D. some 35 years ago. Himself a gout sufferer, Blan found the use of cherries to be miraculously effective in his own case and published his own experience in a medical journal. Subsequently, many people with gout used this simple therapy with great success. To start with, the patient should consume about 15 to 25 cherries a day. Thereafter, about 10 cherries a day will keep the ailment under control. While fresh cherries are best, canned cherries can also be used with success.

Foods high in potassium such as potatoes, bananas, leafy green vegetables, beans and raw vegetable juices are protective against gout. Carrot juice, in combination with juices of beet and cucumber, is especially valuable. 100 ml. each of beet and cucumber juices should be mixed in 300 ml. of carrot juice to make 500 ml. of combined juice.

The juice of French or string beans has also proved effective in the treatment of gout. About 150 ml. of this juice should be taken by the patient suffering from this disease. Raw potato juice and fresh pineapple juices are also beneficial.

The feet should be bathed in Epsom salt foot baths twice daily. Half a pound to one pound of salt may be added to a foot bath of hot water. Full Epsom salt baths should also be taken three times a week. The baths may be reduced to two per week later. Cold packs at night, applied to the affected joints, will be beneficial. Fresh air and outdoor exercise are also essential. The patient should eliminate as much stress from his life as possible.

CHAPTER 78

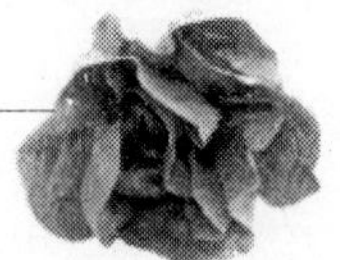

Halitosis

Halitosis refers to bad breath which is not only a sign of ill-health but it is also a social stigma. It is common in many people. Unfortunately, most people are completely unaware of their problem and the discomfort they cause to others.

Causes

The most common cause of halitosis is bad teeth and gum conditions. Dental decay at the roots of the teeth may result in abscesses in the gums with foul-smelling pus giving an objectionable odour to the breath. Even small holes in the teeth may provide a place where germs can multiply and release foul odours.

Other causes of halitosis are any conditions of the nose, throat, respiratory tract, or stomach which are associated with chronic infection or local upsets of one sort or another, such as chronic tonsillitis, lung diseases like chronic bronchitis and bronchiectasis, chronic gastritis and sinuses which cause a discharge at the back of the throat. Most cases of bad breath, however, are caused by gastro-intestinal disorders, intestinal sluggishness and particularly by chronic constipation. The unpleasant odour results from an exceptionally large amount of waste matter expelled through the lungs. Chewing pan, tobacco and smoking are other causes of bad breath. Diseases like anaemia may also lead to unpleasant breath.

Treatment

If halitosis is caused by tooth and gum conditions,

tonsillitis, sinusitis, smoking or anaemia, these conditions must be treated. Once they are eliminated the bad breath will disappear. Similarly, bad breath resulting from gastro-intestinal disorders can be successfully treated by correcting these disorders and cleansing the system of morbid matter.

The patients suffering from halitosis should take a well-balanced diet consisting of seeds, nuts, grains, vegetables and fruits, with emphasis on raw and cooked vegetables and fruits.

In case of constipation, all measures should be adopted for its eradication. The patient should avoid refined carbohydrate foods, such as white sugar, white bread and products made from them as well as flesh foods and egg. Even whole grain bread should be eaten sparingly.

The patient should also avoid overeating of any kind of foods. He should eat six to eight soaked prunes and a few dried and soaked figs with breakfast. He must also drink the water in which these fruits were soaked. He should also take plenty of liquids and drink six to eight glasses of water daily. This will help eliminate bad breath.

The teeth should be cleaned regularly twice a day especially before going to bed at night. Meat particles should be removed carefully with toothpicks. In case of decaying teeth and swollen and bleeding gums, a dentist should be consulted. Munching a raw apple or guava after lunch removes most of the trapped particles. The use of twigs of the margosa (*neem*) tree as toothbrush is the best method of cleaning the teeth.

Home Remedies

Among the several home remedies for halitosis, the use of fenugreek (*methi*) has proved most effective. A tea made from the seeds of the vegetable should be taken regularly for correcting the condition. This tea is prepared by putting a teaspoon of seeds in half a litre of cold water and allowing to simmer for 15 minutes over a low flame. It should then be strained and used as tea.

Another effective remedy for bad breath is the use of avocado (*kulu naspati*) which is far superior to any mouth lotion or remedies for this condition. It effectively removes intestinal putrefaction or decomposition which is one of the most important causes of bad breath.

The unripe guava (*amrud*) is useful in halitosis. It is rich in tannic, malic, oxalic and phospheric acids as well as calcium, oxalate and manganese. Chewing it is an excellent tonic for the teeth and gums. It helps cure bleeding from gums due to styptic effect and stops bad breath. Chewing tender leaves of guava tree also stops bleeding from gums and bad breath.

Parsley (*prajmoda*) is valuable in the treatment of bad breath. Two cups of water should be boiled and several sprigs of parsley, coarsely chopped, should be steeped in this water along with two or three whole cloves or a quarter spoon of ground cloves. This mixture should be stirred occasionally while cooling. It should then be strained and used as a mouth wash or gargle several times a day.

All fruit and vegetable juices are beneficial in the treatment of halitosis and should be taken liberally by those suffering from this disorder. Juices from fruits like apple, grapefruit (*chakatora*), lemon, pineapple and vegetables like tomato, carrot and celery are especially beneficial.

The person suffering from bad breath should take plenty of exercise as lack of sufficient exercise is one of the main causes of constipation leading to halitosis.

CHAPTER 79

Headaches and Migraine

Headaches afflict almost everyone at some time or the other. Most headaches are functional, caused by temporary upsets and are not related to any organic changes in the brain. A headache is often nature's warning that something is wrong somewhere in the body. The actual pain, however, arises from irritation to nerve endings in the shoulder, neck and scalp muscles and also in the smooth muscles encircling the blood vessels which serve these areas.

There are several types of headaches, with as many ways of treating them. Taking an aspirin or a tranquiliser may provide temporary relief but it does not remove the cause. Moreover, the frequent use of pain-relievers causes nervous debility, weakens the heart and brings on other complications.

The common causes of headaches are allergy, emotional reasons, eyestrain, high blood pressure, hangover, infection, low blood sugar, nutritional deficiency, tension, the presence of poisons and toxins in the body, and migraine. Allergies, an often unsuspected cause of headache, vary in different individuals. The foods to which some people are allergic and which can trigger headaches are milk and milk products, chocolates, chicken liver, alcohol and strong cheese. Sneezing and diarrhoea are further indications of an allergy.

Intense emotion often cause headaches. Many people who outwardly appear to have a pleasant disposition may actually be simmering about a job, or may bear resentment towards a person or something. This hidden hostility may manifest itself as headache. It is important, therefore, that negative feelings should not be bottled up, but should find some safe means of expression.

Eye-strain is a common cause of headache. In such cases, an eye specialist should be consulted and proper treatment taken. Simple eye exercises such as moving the eyes up and down and from side to side, palming, rotating the head, with neck outstretched, forward and backward three times, then thrice clockwise and thrice anti-clockwise, can relieve eye-strain.

High blood pressure can cause pounding headaches. The headache usually starts at the back of the head on getting up in the morning. A safe method of treatment for this is to immerse your legs to calf-level in a tub of hot water for 15 to 20 minutes. This draws the blood away from the head and down to the feet, giving relief from the headache.

Many people get a severe headache after consuming alcohol in excess. Alcohol causes the blood vessels to swell, resulting in a painful headache. The best treatment for this is to avoid excessive consumption of alcohol. A hangover headache can be avoided by taking a vitamin B-1 (thiamine) tablet with the drink.

Headaches may occur if there is an infection, such as a cold, virus and fever. Here, it is the infection that should be tackled. Vitamin C therapy is the best all-round method. For a cold high doses of vitamin C should be taken at hourly intervals with the appearance of the first symptoms like a sore throat, runny nose, etc. Vitamin C has worked miracles, and is considered a natural antibiotic.

Low blood sugar is one of the causes of irritability and headache. Sugar is not a cure for low blood sugar, though it may raise the blood sugar temporarily and make one feel better for a while. Low blood sugar is the result of an abused pancreas which overstimulates the production of insulin in the body. It can be controlled by eating smaller meals at short intervals rather than the standard three large meals daily. The intake of carbohydrates should be cut down to the minimum and coffee should be eliminated as it overstimulates the pancreas.

A lack of iron, resulting in anaemia, is a common cause of headache. The headache sometimes appears before the onset of anaemia, due to a chronic iron deficiency. Brewer's yeast is an excellent source of iron and anaemia can easily be prevented by taking a few teaspoons daily. Headache can also be brought on due to the deficiency of B vitamins, namely pantothenic acid, B-1 (thiamine), B-12 and B-6 (pyridoxine) and can be cured by taking these vitamins.

When taking any of the B vitamin factors separately, it is absolutely essential to add the entire B complex range to one's diet in some form such as Brewer's yeast, liver, wheat germ, etc., otherwise too much of one factor can throw the other factors into imbalance, resulting in other problems. Actually, the entire B complex group itself serves as protection against headaches, including migraine.

Tension headaches are probably the most common of all, and are caused by emotional conflicts which result in stress. Stress causes the muscles of the shoulder, neck and scalp to tense unconsciously. Persons who are irritable, tense and lose their temper quickly usually get this type of headache. It increases gradually and passes off with the release of tension. One should try to relieve the stress which produces headache.

Poisons and toxins admitted into the body through food, beverages and water, as well as through breathing polluted air, can cause any number of disturbances. A headache may be the first warning that a poison has entered the body. Additives in foods and in many cases, cosmetics, skin and hair products are also serious offenders in bringing on headaches. In addition, there are toxic air contaminants which are too numerous to mention.

Migraine Headache

Migraine is an ancient and formidable malady. It bothered such distinguished persons as Caesar and Freud. It has assumed alarming proportions under modern conditions of living and is now believed to afflict about 10 per cent of the world's population.

Migraine can be defined as a paroxysmal affection, accompanied by severe headache, generally on one side of the head and associated with disorders of the digestion, the liver and the vision. It usually occurs when a person is under great mental tension or has suddenly got over that state.

Migraine is also known as "sick headache" because nausea and vomiting occasionally accompany the excruciating pain which lasts for as long as three days. Migraine usually gives warning before it strikes: black spots or a brilliant zig-zag line appear before the eyes or the patient has blurring of vision or has part of his vision blanked out. When the headache occurs, the patient may feel tingling, numbness, or weakness in an arm or leg.

Migraine sufferers have what is known as a "migrainous personality". They are compulsive workers and perfectionists, who feel that they have to do everything right away. When they complete a task, they are suddenly let down from a state of temporary tension to a feeling of utmost relief. Then comes the migraine. It is a purely physiological process. The head and neck muscles, reacting to continuous stress, become over-worked. The tightened muscles squeeze the arteries and reduce blood flow. When a person relaxes suddenly, the constricted muscles expand, stretching the walls of the blood-vessel. With every heart beat, the blood being pushed through these vessels expands them further and causes incredible pain.

When a headache strikes, one should stay on one's feet in the daytime and do simple chores which do not require too much concentration, or walk, move around and get some fresh air.

The best remedy to prevent headaches is to build up physical resistance through proper nutrition, exercise and constructive thinking. As a first step, the patient should undertake a short fast. During the fast, citrus fruit juices diluted with water may be taken six times daily. By taking the load off the digestion the patient will at once save nervous energy which can be utilised for more important purposes. The blood and lymph will also be relieved of a great burden. After a short fast, the diet should be fixed in such a way as to put the least possible strain on the digestion. Breakfast should consist of fruits, both fresh and dried. Lunch should consist largely of protein foods. Starchy foods such as whole wheat bread, cereals, rice, or potatoes should be taken at dinner along with raw salads. Spices tomatoes, sour buttermilk and oily foodstuffs should be avoided. Drinking a glass of water (warm water in winter and cool water in summer) mixed with a teaspoonful of honey the first thing in the morning, is also a good remedy.

Water Treatment

There are certain water applications which help relieve headaches. Copious drinking of water can help, as do the cleansing enema with water temperature at 98.6°F, the hot foot bath, a cold throat pack, frequent applications of towels wrung out from very hot water to the back of the neck, a cold compress at 40° to 60°F applied to the head and face or an alternate spinal compress. Hot fomentations over the abdominal region just before retiring relieve headaches due to stomach and liver upsets.

Yogic kriyas like jalneti and kunjal, pranayamas like anuloma-viloma, shitali and sitkari and asanas such as uttanpadasana, sarvangasana, paschimottanasana, halasana and shavasana are useful in the treatment of headaches.

CHAPTER 80

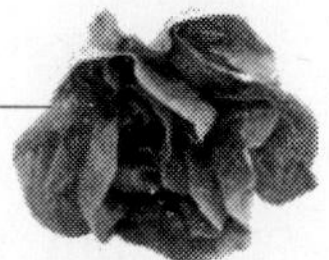

Head Lice

Head lice, known as pediculus humanus in medical parlance, are tiny, flat, wingless insects which often find their way into the scalp as parasites. They suck the blood by biting the skin. This results in an irritation which, in chronic cases, causes thickening and pigmentation of the skin. Head lice occurs more frequently in children than in adults.

Symptoms

Itching is the main symptom of head louse infection. The adult female louse lays eggs, known as nits, close to the surface of the scalp. They hatch before the hair has grown more than few millimetres. The eggs are fresh-coloured and are difficult to see, but once the female louse has emerged, the nits can be easily seen.

Occasionally flakes of dandruff or keratin casts may be mistaken for nits, but a microscopic examination of the material will reveal the distinction. At times, insects can be seen crawling on the hair. Their favourite haunts are on the scalp, around the ears or underneath hair grown at the back of the head.

Causes

Head lice are very infectious and can be easily acquired by head-to-head contact with a person harbouring the parasite. They are common in persons who are crowded together and live in poor sanitary condition. They spread rapidly during disasters.

Treatment

As with any other unhealthy condition, the first step towards treatment of head lice is thorough cleanliness. This should be observed by all members of the household. They should not share towels, pillows, combs and hair-brushes. The comb and hair brushes of infected person should be disinfected daily by scrubbing with soap and water, and boiling them after they are used. A special comb with close-knit, teeth, which is easily available, should be used. This will help remove the lice from the hair.

However, lice cannot be got rid of only with the help of a comb. They can be destroyed by certain effective methods. One of these methods is to soak the scalp and hair for 24 hours with a mixture of equal parts of kerosene and vinegar. The head should then be shampooed thoroughly with soap and hot water and dried with a towel. The nits should be removed with a fine comb dipped in hot vinegar. The kerosene kills the lice and the vinegar loosens the eggs or nits, so that they can be repeated two or three times and the hair should be combed with a fine-toothed comb many times between each treatment to remove the loosened eggs. Great caution must be exercised in keeping away from a heated stove or a flame because of the danger of igniting the hair.

Another method to destroy the head lice is to dust five per cent DDT powder in 95 per cent of inert talc into the hair and scalp. Care should be taken to keep the powder out of the eyes by protecting them with gauze squares. The entire head should be wrapped in a scarf or clean towel. The scarf should be removed after several hours, preferably at bed-time. The next morning, the hair should be carefully combed with a fine tooth comb to get rid of the nits and dead lice. On the seventh day of the treatment, the hair should be washed with soap and warm water and allowed to dry. Thereafter, the DDT powder should be applied again in the same manner as before. On the 14th day, the hair should be given a final shampoo. Normally, two courses of treatment are sufficient. In some cases, it may be necessary to repeat this treatment, for the third time.

The third effective method is to thoroughly cleanse the whole body from the scalp to the toes, using plenty of soap and water. Next, five per cent benzyl benzoate emulsion should be applied to all the itching areas. This should be rubbed well into the scalp at night, especially if the hair has been invaded by the parasites.

As the person affected with head lice can infect other members of the family, it is essential to examine the heads of all of them and treat them if lice and nits are found. Any head-dress worn by a person with lice should be sterilised by spraying with five per cent of DDT solution.

Prevention

The condition can be prevented by the maintenance of personal cleanliness, the clothing of individuals suffering from pediculosis should be soaked in boiling water and washed. As children are more likely to suffer from this problem, it would be advisable to keep their hair short.

CHAPTER 81

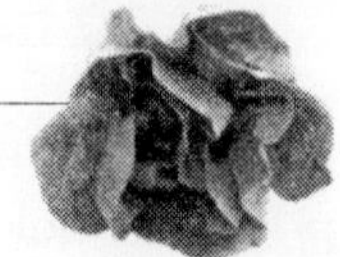

Heart Disease

The term coronary heart disease covers a group of clinical syndromes arising particularly from failure of the coronary arteries to supply sufficient blood to the heart. They include angina pectoris, coronary thrombosis or heart attack and sudden death without infarction.

There has been a marked increase in the incidence of heart disease in recent years. Heart attacks have become the number

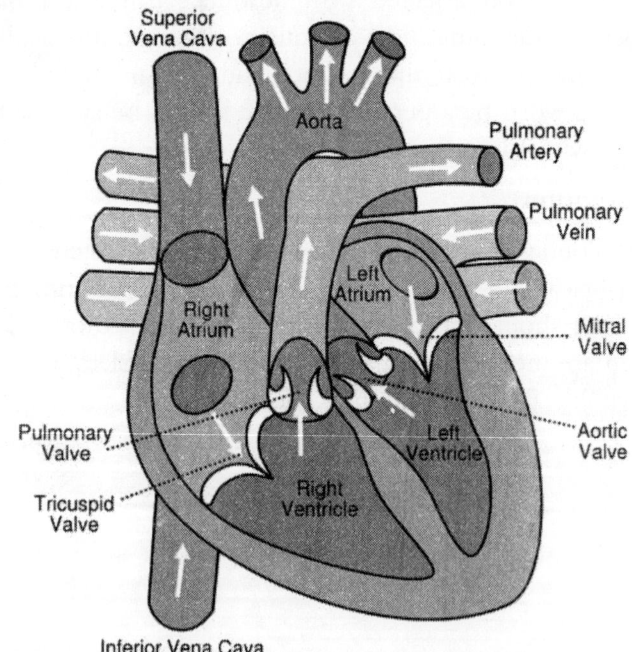

The interior of the heart

one killer in Western countries. They rank third in India, after tuberculosis and infections. The disease affects people of all ages and both sexes, although it is more common in men than in women, especially among those aged 40-60 years.

The heart, the most vital organ in the body, is a muscle about the size of a clenched fist. It starts working even before birth inside the womb. Weighing less than 350 grams, it pumps about 4,300 gallons of blood per day through the body and supplies oxygen and nourishment to all the organs. It beats 1,00,000 times a day, continuously pumping the blood through more than 60,000 miles of tiny blood vessels. The heart, in turn, needs blood for its nourishment which is supplied by coronary arteries. Coronary arteries are so called because they are arranged rather like a crown or carona. In case of strain, etc., the heart needs more blood and the arteries, under normal conditions, adjust themselves to the increased flow.

In the event of narrowing or hardening of the arteries on account of their getting plugged with fatty substances, the flow of blood is restricted. The heart then does not get sufficient oxygen. This condition is known as ischaemia of the heart or angina pectoris. In this condition, exercise or excitement provokes severe chest pain and so limits the patient's physical activity. It serves as a warning to slow down and prompt preventive measures will prevent a heart attack.

If the narrowed arteries get blocked due to a clot or thrombus inside them, causing death of that portion of the heart which depends upon the choked arteries, it is called a heart attack or coronary thrombosis. It may lead to death or heal, leaving a scar. Patients with healed lesions may be severely disabled or may be able to resume normal life with restrictions in their physical activities.

Symptoms

A common symptom of heart disease is shortness of breath, which is caused by the blood being deprived of the proper amount of oxygen. Another common symptom is chest pain or pain down either arm. Other symptoms are palpitation, fainting, emotional instability, cold hands and feet, frequent perspiration and fatigue. All these symptoms may be caused by many other disorders. Appropriate tests and studies are, therefore, essential to establish the true nature of these symptoms.

Causes

The basic causes of heart disease are wrong dietary habits, faulty style of living and various stresses. The famous Framingham Heart Study of the National Heart and Lung Institute identified seven major risk factors in coronary heart disease. These are: (i) elevated blood levels of cholesterol, triglycerides and other fatty substances, (ii) elevated blood pressure, (iii) elevated blood uric acid levels (mainly caused by high protein diet), (iv) certain metabolic disorders, notably diabetes, (v) obesity, (vi) smoking, and (vii) lack of physical exercise. Each or a combination of these risk factors can contribute to heart disease. Most of them are of dietary origin. These risk factors can be controlled by changing one's life style and readjusting the diet. Constant worry and tension stimulates the adrenal glands to produce more adrenaline and cartisons. This also contributes to constricted arteries, high blood pressure and increased work for the heart.

Treatment

The fundamental conditioning factor in all heart diseases is the diet. A corrective diet designed to alter body chemistry and improve the quality of general nutritional intake can, in many cases, reverse the degenerative changes which have occurred in the heart and blood vessels.

The diet should be lacto-vegetarian, low in sodium and calories. It should consist of high quality, natural organic foods, with emphasis on whole grains, seeds, fresh fruits and vegetables. Foods which should be eliminated are all white flour products, sweets, chocolates, canned foods in syrup, soft drinks, squashes, all hard fats of animal origin such as butter, cream and fatty meats. Salt and sugar should be reduced substantially. The patient should also avoid tea, coffee, alcohol and tobacco.

The essential fatty acids which reduce serum cholesterol levels and minimise the risk of arteriosclerosis can be obtained from sunflower seed oil, corn oil or safflower oil. Several studies have indicated that garlic can reduce the cholesterol level in persons whose body normally cannot regulate the cholesterol fractions. Other important cholesterol lowering foods are alfalfa and yogurt. Lecithin helps prevent fatty deposits in arteries. Best food sources are unrefined, raw, crude vegetable oils, seeds and grains.

Fruits and vegetables in general are highly beneficial in the treatment of heart disease. Seasonal fruits are quite effective heart tonics. Apples especially contain heart stimulating properties and the patients suffering from the weakness of heart should make liberal use of apples and apple jams. Fresh grapes, pineapples, oranges, custard apples, pomegranate and coconut water also tone up the heart. Grapes are effective in heart pain and palpitation of the heart and the disease can be rapidly controlled if the patient adopts an exclusive grapes diet for few days. Grape juice, especially will be valuable when one is actually suffering from a heart attack.

Indian gooseberry or *amla* is considered an effective home remedy for heart disease. It tones up the functions of all the organs of the body and builds up health by destroying the heterogeneous elements and renewing lost energy.

Another excellent home remedy for heart disease is onions. They are useful in normalising the percentage of blood cholesterol by oxidising excess cholesterol. One teaspoon of raw onion juice first thing in the morning will be highly beneficial in such cases.

Honey has marvellous properties to prevent all sorts of heart disease. It tones up the heart and improves the circulation. It is also effective in cardiac pain and palpitation of the heart. One tablespoonful daily after food is sufficient to prevent all sorts of heart troubles.

Patients with heart disease should increase their intake of foods rich in vitamin E, as this vitamin promotes the functioning of the heart by improving oxygeneration of the cells. It also improves the circulation and muscle strength. Many whole meal products and green vegetables, particularly outer leaves of cabbage are good sources of vitamin E. The vitamin B group is important for heart and circulatory disorders. The best sources of vitamin B are whole grains.

Vitamin C is also essential as it protects against spontaneous breaches in capillary walls which can lead to heart attacks. It also guards against high blood cholesterol. The stress of anger, fear, disappointment and similar emotions can raise blood fat and cholesterol levels immediately but this reaction to stress can do little harm if the diet is adequate in vitamin C and pantothenic acid. The richest sources of vitamin C are citrus fruits.

The following is the suggested diet for persons suffering from hypertension or some disorder of the heart:

On rising: Warm water with lemon juice and honey or fresh fruit juice of apple, grapes, orange, pineapple.

Breakfast: Fresh fruit such as apples, grapes, pears, peaches, pineapple, orange, melons, one or two slices whole meal toast, yogurt, skimmed milk or soya milk.

Mid-morning: Fresh fruit juice or coconut water.

Lunch: Combination salad of vegetables such as lettuce, cabbage, endive, carrots, cucumber, beetroot, tomato, onion and garlic. One or two slices of whole meal bread or chappatis, curd, fresh grapes and other fruits in season.

Mid-afternoon: One or two wholemeal biscuits and fruit juice.

Dinner: Fresh fruit or vegetable juice or soup, two lightly cooked vegetables, one or two whole wheat chappatis.

The patient should also pay attention to other laws of nature for health building such as taking moderate exercise, getting proper rest and sleep, adopting the right mental attitude and getting fresh air and drinking pure water.

Water Treatment

The use of an ice bag on the spinal area between the second and tenth thoracic vertebrae for 30 minutes three times a week, a hot compress applied to the left side of the neck for 30 minutes every alternate day and massage of the abdomen and upper back muscles are water treatments which are beneficial in cases of heart disease.

Hot foot and hand baths are excellent for relieving the pain of angina pectoris. To this may be added hot packs on the chest over the heart for one minute and a cold pack applied alternately for five minutes.

Asanas such as shavasana, vajrasana and gomukhasana, yogic kriyas like jalaneti and pranayamas such as shitali, sitkari and bhramari are also helpful in providing relief to heart patients.

CHAPTER 82

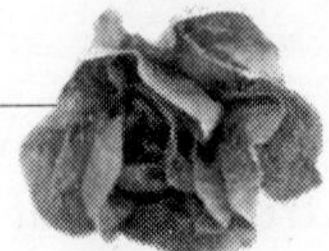

Hiatus Hernia

Hiatus hernia can be defined as displacement of a portion of the stomach through the opening in the diaphragm through which the oesophagus passes from the chest to the abdominal cavity. In this disease, a part of the upper wall of the stomach protrudes through the diaphragm at the point where the gullet passes from the chest area to the abdominal area.

The diaphragm is a large dome-shaped muscle dividing the chest from the abdominal cavity. It is the muscle concerned with breathing, and it is assisted by the muscles between the ribs during exertion. It has special openings in it to allow the passage of important blood vessels and for the food channel, the oesophagus. Hiatus hernia occurs at the oesophageal opening.

This disease is quite common after middle age. It is estimated that about half the people above 60 years of age suffer from it, although most of them may not have any symptoms. The correct diagnosis of hiatus hernia can be arrived at by means of barium meal x-ray test.

Symptoms

Hiatus hernia is characterised by pain in certain areas. The most common areas are behind the breast bone at the nipple level and lower, at the end of the breast bone. Pain may also occur on the left chest and this is often mistaken for angina.

Other areas of pain are the base of the throat, right lower ribs and behind the right shoulder blade. The pain increases when the patient stoops with effort and lies down. Other symptoms of this disease are heart-burn, especially after a meal, a feeling of fullness and bloatedness, flatulence and discomfort on swallowing.

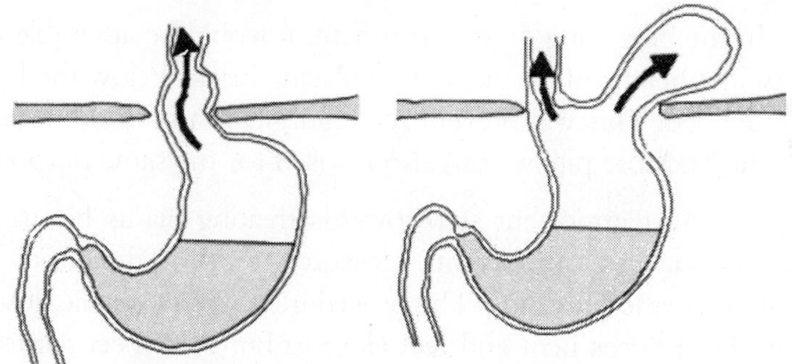

Types of hiatus hernia: 1. Sliding hiatus hernia, 2. Rolling hiatus hernia

Causes

The chief cause of the mechanical defect associated with hiatus hernia is faulty diet. The consumption of white flour, refined sugar and products made from them, such as cakes, pastries, biscuits and white bread as well as preservatives, and flavourings devitalise the system and weaken the muscle tone. As a consequence, the muscles become less resilient, and connective and fibrous tissue suffers through poor nourishment, and thus become more prone to decomposition and damage. This ultimately leads to diseases like hiatus hernia.

Drinks like tea, coffee, alcohol also affect the mucous lining of the stomach and irritate the digestive tract. These drinks, when taken with meals, encourage fermentation and produce gas. This increases the distension of the stomach, causing pressure against the diaphragm and the oesophageal opening and greatly increasing the risk of herniation. Other causes of hiatus hernia include sedentary occupations, without sensible exercise, over-weight resulting from overeating, smoking, shallow breathing and mental and emotional tensions.

Treatment

In the beginning of the treatment, it would be advisable to raise the head end of the bed by placing bricks below the legs of the bed. This will prevent the regurgitation of food during the night. More pillows can also be used for the same purpose.

The next important step towards treating hiatus hernia is relaxation. An important measure in this direction is diaphragmatic breathing. The procedure is as follows: lie down with both knees bent and feet close to buttocks. Feel relaxed. Put both the hands lightly on the abdomen and concentrate the attention on this area. Now breathe in, gently pushing the abdomen up under the hands at the same time, until no more air can be inhaled. Then relax, breathing out through the mouth with an audible sighing sound and allow the abdominal wall to sink back. The shoulders and chest should, remain at rest throughout.

It is important to be able to relax at any time and thereby prevent building up of physical and mental tensions which may cause actual physical symptoms. The best method for this is to practise shavasana or 'dead body' pose. The procedure for this asana has been explained in chapter 7 on yoga therapy.

The patient of hiatus hernia should observe certain precautions in their eating habits. The foremost amongst these is not to take water with meals, but half an hour before or one hour after a meal. This helps the digestive process considerably and reduces the incidence of heart-burn. Drinking water with meals increases the overall weight in the stomach, slows down the digestive process by diluting the digestive juices and this increases the risk of fermentation and gas formation, which distends the stomach and causes discomfort and pain. Another important factor in the treatment of this disease is to take frequent small meals instead of three large ones. Thorough mastication of food is also essential, both to break up the food into small particles and to slow down the rate of intake.

The diet of the patient should consist of seeds, nuts, whole cereal grains, vegetables and fruits, with emphasis on fresh fruits, raw or lightly cooked vegetables and sprouted seeds. The foods which should be avoided are over-processed foods like white bread and sugar, cakes and biscuits, rice puddings and overcooked vegetables. At least 50 per cent of the diet should consist of fruits and vegetables, and the remaining 50 per cent of protein, carbohydrates and fat.

Raw juices extracted from fresh fruits and vegetables are valuable in haitus hernia, and the patient should take these juices half an hour before each meal. Carrot juice is specially beneficial as it has a very restorative effect, and is rich in vitamin A and calcium. It is an alkaline, food, which soothes the stomach. All juices should be diluted with water on a 50 : 50 basis as they are concentrated.

The hot drinks should always be allowed to cool a little before taking. Extremes in temperature, in both food and drink should be avoided, drinks should not be taken hurriedly, but sipped slowly. The patient should avoid condiments, pickles, strong tea, coffee, alcoholic beverages and smoking.

CHAPTER 83

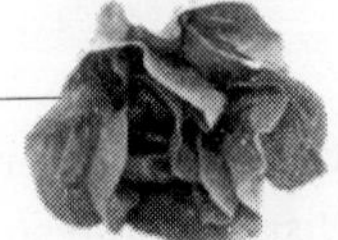

High Blood Cholesterol

Cholesterol, a yellowish fatty substance, is one of the essential ingredients of the body. Although it is essential to life, it has a bad reputation, being a major villain in heart disease. Every person with a high blood cholesterol is regarded as a potential candidate for heart attack, a stroke or high blood pressure.

Cholesterol is a building block of the outer membrane of cells. It is the principal ingredient in the digestive juice bile, in the fatty sheaths that insulate nerves and in sex hormones, namely, estrogen and androgen. It performs several functions such as transportation of fat, providing defence mechanism, protecting red blood cells and muscular membrane of the body.

Most of the cholesterol found in the body is produced in the liver. However, about 20 to 30 per cent generally comes from the foods we eat. Some cholesterol is also secreted into the intestinal tract in bile and becomes mixed with the dietary cholesterol. The percentage of ingested cholesterol absorbed seemed to average 40 to 50 per cent of the intake. The body excretes extra cholesterol from the system through bowels and kidneys.

The amount of cholesterol is measured in milligrams per 100 millimetres of blood. Normal level of cholesterol varies between 150–250 mg per 100 ml. Persons with atherosclerosis have uniformly high blood cholesterol usually above 250 mg. per 100 ml.

In blood, cholesterol is bound to certain proteins-lipoproteins which have an affinity for blood fats, known as lipids. There are two main types of lipoproteins; a low density one (LDL) and a high density one (HDL). The low density lipoprotein is the one which is considered harmful and is associated with cholesterol deposits in blood vessels. The higher the ratio of LDL to the total cholesterol, the greater is the risk of arterial damage and heart disease. The HDL on the other hand plays a salutary role by helping remove cholesterol from circulation and thereby reduce the risk of heart disease.

Cholesterol has been the subject of extensive study by researchers since 1769, when French chemist, Polutier de La Salle purified the soapy-looking yellowish substance. The results of the most comprehensive research study, commissioned by the National Heart and Lung Institute of the U.S.A. were announced. The 10-year study, considered most elaborate and most expensive research project in medical history, indicates that heart disease is directly linked to the level of cholesterol in the blood and that lowering cholesterol level significantly reduces the incidence of heart attacks. It has been estimated that for every one per cent reduction in cholesterol, there is a decrease in the risk of heart attack by two per cent.

Causes

Hypercholesterolemia or increase in cholesterol is mainly a digestive problem caused by rich foods such as fried foods, excessive consumption of milk and its products like ghee, butter and cream, white flour, sugar, cakes, pastries, biscuits, cheese, ice cream as well as non-vegetarian foods like meat, fish and eggs. Other causes of increase in cholesterol are irregularity in habits, smoking and drinking alcohol.

Stress has been found to be a major cause of increased level of cholesterol. Adrenaline and cortison are both released in the body under stress. This, in turn, produces a fat metabolising reaction. Adrenal glands of executive type aggressive persons produce more adrenaline than the easy going men. Consequently they suffer six to eight times more heart attacks than the relaxed men.

The Cure

To reduce the risk of heart disease, it is essential to lower the level of LDL and increase the level of HDL. This can be achieved by improving the diet and changing the life style. Diet is the most important factor. As a first step, foods rich in cholesterol and saturated fats, which lead to increase in LDL level, should be reduced to the minimum. Cholesterol-rich foods are eggs, organ meats and most cheese. Butter, bacon, beef, whole milk, virtually all foods of animal origin as well as two vegetable oils, namely coconut and palm, are high in saturated fats and these should be replaced by polyunsaturated fats such as corn, safflower, soyabeans and sesame oils which tend to lower the level of LDL. There are monosaturated fats such as olive and peanut oils which have more or less neutral effect on the LDL level.

The American Heart Association recommends that men should restrict themselves to 300 mg. of cholesterol a day and women to 275 mg. It also prescribes that fat should not make up more than 30 per cent of the diet and not more than one third of this should be saturated. The Association, however, urges a somewhat strict regimen for those who already have elevated levels of cholesterol.

The amount of fibre in the diet also influences the cholesterol levels and LDL cholesterol can be lowered by taking diets rich in fibres. The most significant sources of dietary fibre are unprocessed wheat bran, whole cereals such as wheat, rice, barley, rye; legumes such as potato, carrot, beet and turnips; fruits like mango and guava and green vegetables such as cabbage, lady's finger, lettuce and celery. Oat bran is especially beneficial in lowering LDL cholesterol.

Lecithin, also a fatty food substance and the most abundant of the phospholipids, is highly beneficial in case of increase in cholesterol level. It has the ability to break up cholesterol into small particles which can be easily handled by the system. With sufficient intake of lecithin, cholesterol cannot build up against the walls of the arteries and veins. It also increases the production of bile acids made from cholesterol, thereby reducing its amount in the blood. Egg yolk, vegetable oils, whole grain cereals, soyabeans and unpasteurised milk are rich sources of lecithin. The cells of the body are also capable of synthesizing it as needed, if several of the B vitamins are present.

Diets high in vitamin B_6, cholin and inositol supplied by wheat germ, yeast, or B vitamins extracted from bran have been particularly effective in reducing blood cholesterol. Sometimes vitamin E elevates blood lecithin and reduces cholesterol presumably by preventing the essential fatty acids from being destroyed by oxygen.

Persons with high blood cholesterol level should drink at least eight to 10 glasses of water every day as regular drinking of water stimulates the excretory activity of the skin and kidneys. This in turn facilitates elimination of excessive cholesterol from the system. Regular drinking of coriander (*dhania*) water also helps lower blood cholesterol as it is a good diuretic and stimulates the kidneys. It is prepared by boiling dry seeds of coriander and straining the decoction after cooling.

Regular exercise also plays an important role in lowering LDL cholesterol and in raising the level of protective HDL. It also promotes circulation and helps maintain the blood flow to every part of the body. Jogging or brisk walking, swimming, bicycling and playing badminton are excellent forms of exercise.

Yogasanas are highly beneficial as they help increase perspiratory activity and stimulate sebaceous glands to effectively secrete accumulated or excess cholesterol from the muscular tissue. Asanas like ardhamatsyendrasana, shalabhasana, padmasana and vajrasana are useful in lowering blood cholesterol by increasing systemic activity.

Hydrotherapy can be successfully employed in reducing excess cholesterol. Cold hip baths for 10 minutes taken twice every day have proved beneficial. Steam baths are also helpful except in patients suffering from hypertension and other circulatory disorders. Mud packs, applied over the abdomen improve digestion and assimilation. They improve the functioning of the liver and other digestive organs and activate kidneys and the intestines to promote better excretion.

CHAPTER 84

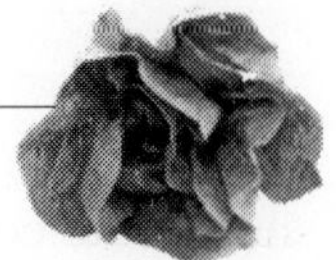

High Blood Pressure

High blood pressure or hypertension—to give it the correct medical term—is regarded as the silent killer. It is a disease of the modern age. The fast pace of life and the mental and physical pressures caused by the industrial and metropolitan environments give rise to psychological tensions. Worry and mental tension increase the adrenaline in the blood stream and this, in turn, causes the pressure of the blood to rise.

The blood which circulates through the arteries within the body supplies every cell with nourishment and oxygen. The force exerted by the heart as it pumps the blood into the large arteries creates a pressure within them and this is called blood pressure. A certain level of blood pressure is thus essential to keep the blood circulating in the body. But when the pressure becomes too high, it results in hypertension which is caused by spasm or narrowing of the small blood vessels, known as capillaries, throughout the body. This narrowing puts more stress on the heart to pump blood through the blood vessels. Hence, the pressure of the blood to get through rises in proportion to the pressure on the heart.

The blood pressure is measured with an instrument called sphygmomanometer in millimetres of mercury. The highest pressure reached during each heart beat is called systolic pressure and the lowest between two beats is known as diastolic pressure. The first gives the pressure of the contraction of the heart as it pushes the blood on its journey through the body and indicates the activity of the heart. The second represents the pressure present in the artery when the heart is relaxed and shows the condition of the blood vessels. The blood pressure level considered normal is 120/70, but may go up to 140/90 and still be normal. Within this range, the lower the reading, the better. Blood pressure between 140/90 and 160/95 is considered border line area. From 160/96 to 180/114, it is classed as moderate hypertension, while 180/115 and upward is considered severe. A raised diastolic pressure is considered more serious than the raised systolic pressure as it has a serious long-term effect. The higher the pressure the greater the danger it causes to the wall.

Symptoms

Mild and moderate hypertension may not produce any symptoms for years. The first symptoms may appear in the form of pain toward the back of the head and neck on waking in the morning, which soon disappears. Some of the other usual symptoms of hypertension are dizziness, aches and pains in the arms, shoulder region, leg, back, etc., palpitations, pain in the heart region, frequent urination, nervous tension and fatigue, crossness, emotional upset, tiredness and wakefulness.

A person suffering from high blood pressure cannot do any serious work, feels tired and out of sorts all the time. He may experience difficulty in breathing and suffer from dyspepsia. Hypertension, if not eliminated, may cause heart attacks or strokes and other disability conditions such as detachment of the retina.

Causes

The most important causes of hypertension are stress and a faulty style of living. People who are usually tense suffer from high blood pressure, especially when under stress. If the stress continues for a long period, the pressure may become permanently raised and may not become even after removal of the stress. An irregular life style, smoking and an excessive intake of intoxicants, tea, coffee, cola drinks, refined foods, destroy the natural pace of life. The expulsion of waste and poisonous matter from the body is prevented and the arteries and the veins become slack. Hardening of the arteries, obesity, diabetes and severe constipation also lead to hypertension. Other causes of high blood pressure are excessive intake of pain killers, common table salt, food allergies and eating a high fat, low fibre diet, processed foods deficient in essential nutrients.

The kidneys play an important role in controlling blood pressure through secretion of renin, a natural chemical. If increased renin is secreted by the kidneys, more salts are retained in the body, which leads to an increase in the volume of circulating blood and consequently to an increase in the blood pressure. Repeated infections and inflammation in the kidneys can also give rise to hypertension.

The Cure

The modern medical treatment of high blood pressure is highly unscientific as it brings down the pressure by drugs without making any effort to remove the underlying causes. Drugs may temporarily reduce blood pressure, but they do not cure the condition and are harmful in the ultimate analysis. All drugs against hypertension without exception, are toxic and have distressing side-effects. The safest way to cure hypertension is to remove the real cause. The natural way of dealing with it is to eliminate the poisons from the system which cause it. Persons with high blood pressure should always follow a well-balanced routine of proper diet, exercise and rest. Diet is of primary importance. Meat and eggs cause the blood pressure to rise more than any other food. The pressure is lowered and blood clotting diminished by partaking of a higher fruit content, lower protein and non-flesh diet. A natural diet consisting of fresh fruits and vegetables, instead of a traditional diet, is helpful in getting rid of the poisons from the body. A hypertension patient should start the process of healing by living on an exclusive fruit-diet for at least a week, and take fruits at five-hourly intervals thrice in the day. Oranges, apples, pears, mangoes, guava, pineapples, raspberry, water-melon are the best diet in such cases. Bananas and jack-fruit should not be taken. Milk may be taken after a week of 'fruits only' diet. The milk should be fresh and should be boiled only once. The patient can be permitted cereals in his food after two weeks.

Vegetables are also good for a patient of hypertension. They should preferably be taken raw. If they are cooked, it should be ensured that their natural juices are not burnt in the process of cooking. Vegetables like cucumber, carrot, tomatoes, onion, radishes, cabbage and spinach are best taken in their raw form. They may be cut into small pieces and sprinkled with a little salt and the juice of a lemon added to them so as to make them more palatable.

Garlic is regarded as one of the most effective remedies to lower blood pressure. The pressure and tension are reduced because it has the power to ease the spasm of the small arteries. Garlic also slows the pulse and modifies the heart rhythm besides relieving the symptoms of dizziness, numbness, shortness of breath and the formation of gas within the digestive tract. The average dosage should be two to three capsules a day to make a dent in the blood pressure.

Indian gooseberry (*amla*) is another effective food remedy

for high blood pressure. A tablespoonful each of fresh amla juice and honey mixed together should be taken every morning in this condition. Lemon is also regarded as a valuable food to control high blood pressure. It is a rich source of vitamin P which is found both in the juice and peel of the fruit. This vitamin is essential for preventing capillary fragility.

Watermelon is another valuable safeguard against high blood pressure. It was proved in recent experiments that a substance extracted from watermelon seeds has a definite action in dilating the blood vessels, which results in lowering the blood pressure.

Recent studies have revealed an important link between dietary calcium and potassium and hypertension. Researchers have found that people who take potassium-rich diets have a low incidence of hypertension even if they do not control their salt-intake. They have also found that people with hypertension do not seem to get much calcium in the form of dairy products. The two essential nutrients seem to help the body throw off excess sodium and are involved in important functions which control the working of the vascular system. Potassium is found in abundance in fruits and vegetables and calcium in dairy products.

Exercise plays an important role in curing hypertension. Walking is an excellent form of exercise. It helps to relieve tension, builds up the muscles and aids in the circulation of blood. As the blood pressure shows signs of abating, more exercise like bicycling, swimming, jogging should be taken. Yogic asanas such as surya namaskar, makarasana, matsyasana, vajrasana, ardhpadmasana, pavanmuktasana, shavasana and simple pranayama like anuloma-viloma and abdominal breathing are beneficial. All asanas should, however, be discontinued except shavasana if the blood pressure is above 200 millimeters.

Water Treatment

Prolonged neutral bath daily for an hour or so at 90° to 95° will be beneficial. Cold compress should be kept on the head during this bath. Other water treatments include hot foot or leg bath for 10 minutes, hot compress over the heart replacing it as bath cools down.

Persons suffering from hypertension must ensure at least eight hours of restful sleep, because proper rest is an important aspect of the treatment. Most important of all, the patient must avoid over-straining, worries, tension, anger and haste. He must try to be cheerful and develop a contented mind. The natural treatment may take some time, but it is the safest and the best way to get rid of this disease.

CHAPTER 85

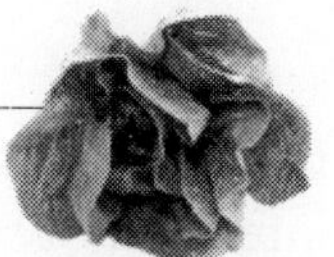

Hydrocele

Hydrocele is a common condition of men in which there is accumulation of fluid in the tunica vaginalis, the sac which surrounds the testicle. It may occur at any age, but old men are usually more prone to the condition.

The testicles are the major sex glands in the male. Each gland is composed of myriads of coiled tubes in which the sperm cells are produced. It is the function of these cells to fertilize the ovum during sexual intercourse.

Symptoms

The main symptom of hydrocele is painless, smooth and elastic enlargement of the scrotum. In some cases swelling is so much as to cause a great deal of inconvenience interfering greatly with walking. Consequently it may produce a great deal of pressure upon the testicles and the spermatic vessels causing a detrimental effect upon the generative system. The hydrocele is translucent. If a bright light is placed upon it in the dark the whole swelling lights up. If the swellings become painful, it usually denotes that it has become infected.

Causes

The apparent cause of hydrocele may be a knock or a strain but toxic condition of the system is usually at the root of the matter. This systemic toxicity results from wrong dietary habits, general wrong living and suppressive medical treatment of former diseases. Sexual excess and abuse is also an important factor in some cases, through the degeneration of the sex organism which follows. Sometimes gonorrhoel infection, obstruction of the abdominal vein, tuberculosis and dropsy may be the cause of this condition.

Hydrocele sometimes exists at birth. In this case swelling is seen when the infant is in an upright position and disappears when the infant is laid upon its back. Hydrocele usually disappears by itself in infants.

Treatment

Tapping is the method usually resorted to for removal of the fluid in hydrocele. This, however, does not remove the cause of the trouble, but only its effects. The correct way in which the condition can be really dealt with successfully is through constitutional treatment. Such a treatment should aim at removing the underlying toxicity of the system, which is at the root of the trouble.

The sufferer from hydrocele should begin with an exclusive fresh fruit diet for seven to ten days. In this regimen, he should have three meals a day of fresh, juicy fruits, such as apples, pears, grapes, grape-fruit, oranges, pineapple, peaches, melon or any other juicy fruit in season, but no bananas or dried, stewed, or tinned fruit, and no other foodstuff whatever. For drinks, lemon water unsweetened or water either hot or cold may be taken.

During this period the bowels should be cleansed daily with a warm-water enema. If constipation is habitual, all steps should be taken for its eradication. After an all-fruit diet, the patient may adopt the following regimen:

Breakfast: Fresh fruit as obtainable, or grated raw carrot or other raw salad-stuff, prunes or other dried fruits, if desired, and a cup of milk.

Lunch: Steamed vegetables, as obtainable, with either a poached or scrambled egg or a vegetarian savoury. Stewed fruit or a baked apple may be taken for dessert.

Dinner: A good-sized raw salad, of any suitable vegetables as obtainable; with wholewheat bread and butter, and prunes or other dried fruit as dessert.

Further short periods on the all-fruit diet should be undertaken at monthly intervals as required, for two or three consecutive days each time. The diet is most important and fruits and salads must form the main basis of the future dietary. Alcohol, strong tea, or coffee condiments, pickles and sauces should be avoided. Smoking, where habitual, should be given up.

Water Treatment

Treatment through water is extremely beneficial in curing hydrocele. Cold hip baths twice daily in the morning and the evening, for 10 minutes each time, are specially valuable. For a cold hip bath, an ordinary bath tub may be used. It should be filled with cold water. The patient should sit in the tub, keeping the legs outside.

A hot Epsom-salts bath is also very useful in the treatment of hydrocele and should be taken once or twice weekly, where possible. This bath is prepared as outlined in chapter 3 on Therapeutic Baths.

Every effort should be made to build up the general health-level to the highest degree. Fresh air and outdoor exercise are essential to the success of this treatment. Sun and air bathing, where possible, should be undertaken. All habits, and practices tending to lower the tone of the body should be avoided; strain should be avoided as far as possible. The wearing of a suspensory bandage is often useful.

Unless the condition persists for a long time, the foregoing treatment should soon begin to show its beneficial effects, and the whole general health-level of the sufferer will be greatly enhanced at the same time.

CHAPTER 86

Hypoglycemia

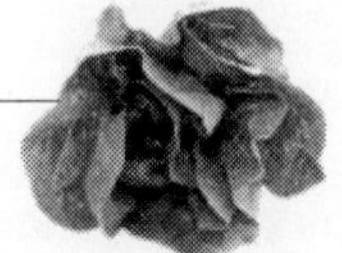

Hypoglycemia or low blood sugar is a disorder of blood sugar metabolism which may result in diabetes in later life. It is a condition in which the pancreas produces too much insulin, causing the blood sugar to drop.

Hypoglycemia sometimes occurs in healthy people some hours after a meal rich in carbohydrates, especially following muscular exertion. It is frequently found in the first few days of life, especially among premature infants.

Hypoglycemia is a serious disorder as the brain cannot function properly when the blood sugar level is too low. Like all other organs of the body, the brain receives its fuel from the diet. But it can use only the sugar produced by the body from carbohydrates. Unlike many of the body tissues, it cannot store its fuel. Therefore, it must get a constant supply of sugar through the bloodstream. Mental disturbances caused by sub-normal blood sugar levels can seriously affect a person's life.

Symptoms

A craving for sweets and starches in excessive amounts between meals is the first sign of a low blood sugar level. When the blood sugar level falls much below normal, symptoms such as nervousness, irritability, fatigue, depression, disturbed vision and headache appear. Other symptoms are sweating, trembling, numbness, absent-mindedness, dizziness, palpitation of the heart and some sexual disturbances. Most hypoglycemia patients feel hungry and eat frequently to get over the feeling of weakness and emotional irritability. They feel tense if they have to go without food for several hours.

Causes

Hypoglycemia is usually caused by an excessive intake of refined carbohydrates and sugar foods. These substances cause the pancreas, the adrenal glands and the liver to lose their ability to handle the sugar properly. Other causes of low blood sugar are a tumour, disturbed functioning of the liver, pituitary gland or adrenal glands. Stress intensifies this condition as it weakens the adrenal gland and starts a faulty pattern of glucose intolerance.

The Cure

The high animal protein diet generally prescribed for hypoglycemia is not suitable for this disorder. It may help control the condition temporarily, but it is harmful in many other respects and may result in other diseases like heart trouble, arthritis, kidney problems and cancer.

The ideal diet for hypoglycemia should be based on three basic food groups, namely grains, seeds and nuts, vegetable and fruits, supplemented by milk, milk products and vegetable oils. Seeds, nuts and grains should be the main constituents of the diet. Seeds and nuts should be taken in their raw form. Grains, in the form of cereals, should be cooked. Cooked grains are digested slowly and release sugar into the blood gradually six to eight hours after meals. This will keep the blood sugar level normal and constant for a long period.

Persons suffering from low blood sugar should take six to eight small meals a day instead of two or three large ones. Eating raw nuts and seeds such as pumpkin or sunflower seeds or drinking milk, buttermilk or fruit juices between meals will be highly beneficial. All refined and processed foods, white sugar, white flour and their by-products should be completely eliminated from the diet. Coffee, alcohol and soft drinks should also be avoided. The consumption of salt should be reduced as an excessive intake of salt causes loss of blood potassium, which causes blood sugar to drop. The following is the menu suggested for hypoglycemia.

On rising: Fresh fruits such as apples, peaches, melons, berries, avocado or a glass of fresh fruit juice.

Breakfast: Nuts, seeds, fruit, cottage cheese and buttermilk.

Mid-morning: Fruit, fruit juice or tomato juice.

Lunch: Cooked cereals and milk.

Mid-afternoon: A glass of fruit or vegetable juice or a snack consisting of nuts.

Dinner: Vegetable salad with a cooked vegetable from among those allowed, one or two slices of whole wheat bread, cottage cheese and buttermilk.

On retiring: A glass of milk or buttermilk.

Vegetables which can be taken in hypoglycemia are asparagus, beets, carrots, cucumbers, egg-plants, peas, radishes, tomatoes, spinach, kale, lettuce, beans, baked potatoes. Fruits which can be taken are apples, apricots, berries, peaches, and pineapples. Consumption of citrus fruits should be limited.

Foods rich in vitamin C, E and B-complex are highly beneficial in the treatment of low blood sugar. Vitamins C and B increase tolerance to sugar and carbohydrates and help normalise sugar metabolism. Pantothenic acid, and vitamin B_6 help to build up adrenals which are generally exhausted in persons with hypoglycemia. Vitamin E improves glycogen storage in the muscles and tissues. The patient should take vitamin C in large doses from 2,000 to 5,000 mg; B_6 50 mg, and vitamin E upto 1,600 IU daily.

Proper rest is essential for those suffering from low blood sugar. A tranquil mind is of utmost importance in this condition. Nervous strain and anxiety should be relieved by simple methods of meditation and relaxation. Yogasanas like vakrasana, bhujangasana, halasana, sarbangasana, shavasana and pranayama like kapalbhati and anuloma-viloma will be beneficial. A prolonged neutral immersion bath is also helpful in relieving mental tension.

CHAPTER 87

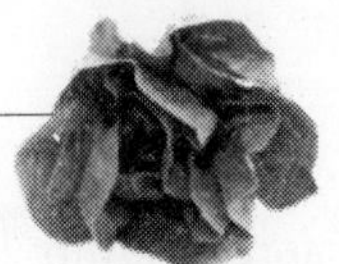

Impetigo

Impetigo is an extremely contagious skin infection. This is essentially a disease of childhood, though it may also occur frequently in adults. The infection can spread rapidly from one person to another by close contact. The disease is more common in the areas with unhygienic conditions.

Symptoms

At first, impetigo appears as a small fluid-filled vesicle usually around the nose or lips. The infection can spread to other parts of the face and occasionally other parts of the body by the patient's irresistible urge to scratch and due to presence of bacteria in large numbers on this weeping surfaces. The vesicle rapidly crusts over, forming a yellowish scab which can be easily knocked-off, leaving a raw, weeping surface.

Causes

Impetigo is caused by staphylococci and occasionally by streptococci germs. The organism can spread quickly, particularly between persons, causing an outbreak of the disease. Impetigo may also occur as a secondary phenomenon in atopic eczema, scabies and head-louse infestation.

The real cause of the disease, however, is constitutional, resulting from malnutrition due to wrong feeding and unhygienic habits of living. It is easily passed from the affected person to other persons, who are in a similar state of toxicity and impaired vitality, by contact from fingers or towels.

Treatment

Early and adequate treatment of the first small patch of impetigo can prevent the spread of the disease. The patient should be kept isolated until the condition is cleared up, so as to prevent the spread of infection. He should be prevented from scratching the scabs. He should have his own sponge and towel. No other member of the family should use these articles. They should be changed frequently and washed separately. The use of harsh detergent should be avoided for this and they should be thoroughly rinsed.

The treatment of impetigo is essentially constitutional and it should consist of proper diet, correct hygiene and fresh air. The best way to commence the treatment is to place the patient on an all-fruit diet for two or three days. In this regimen, he should be given fresh juicy fruits such as orange, apple, pineapple, peach, pear and papaya. In serious cases, however, it would be advisable to commence the treatment by a short fast on orange juice and water for about three days. This may be followed by an all-fruit diet for further three days.

After the all-fruit diet, the patient may embark upon a well-balanced diet consisting of milk, seeds, nuts, grains, vegetables and fruits. The emphasis should be on fresh fruits, raw salads, fresh milk and whole meal bread. The use of these foods is of utmost importance in the future dietary. The patient should avoid tea, coffee, condiments and highly flavoured dishes as well as sugar, white flour products, denatured cereals and tinned or bottled foods.

It will be desirable to administer warm-water enema daily during the first few days of the treatment to cleanse the bowels. If constipation is habitual, all natural methods should be adopted for its eradication.

Certain home remedies have been found beneficial in the treatment of impetigo. The use of turnip (*salgum*) is one such remedy. A few chopped turnip pieces after thorough cleaning should be immersed in cooked rice water (*kanji*) or any natural vinegar for about six hours. They should then be eaten by the patient.

Garlic is useful in relieving constant itching caused by this disease. This vegetable should be crushed and spread over irritated areas. One or two cloves of garlic should also be chewed for better results.

Other helpful measures for treating this disease are sun and air baths, a daily dry friction, breathing and other light exercise. Daily dry friction bath can be taken with a rough dry towel or with a moderately soft bristle brush. If a brush is used, the procedure should be as follows: Take the brush in one hand and begin with the face, neck and chest. Then brush one arm, beginning at the wrist and brushing towards the shoulders. Now stoop down and brush one foot, then the ankle and leg. Then do the other foot and leg, and next the hips and central portion of the body. Continue brushing each part until the skin is pink. Use the brush quickly back and forward on every part of the body. The whole process does not take very long—about a minute or so. If a towel is used, it should be fairly rough, and the same above mentioned process should be followed.

CHAPTER 88

Indigestion

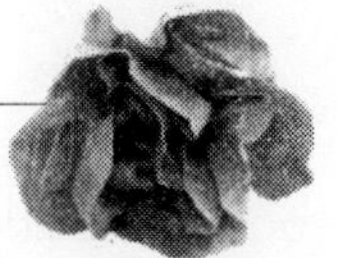

Indigestion or dyspepsia is one of the most common ailments today and is caused by dietetic errors. It is a condition of the stomach in which digestive juices are incorrectly secreted, resulting in discomfort.

The alimentary canal and the process of digestion begin at the mouth. The stomach, which is the most abused organ of the body, looks like a pear-shaped pouch. It forms part of the digestive tract which is a tube coiled in loops nearly 28 feet in length. It varies in size and position depending on how much food it contains. An overloaded stomach tends to prevent the diaphragm from functioning properly. It may also press on the heart.

Symptoms

Abdominal pain, a feeling of undue fullness after eating, heartburn, loss of appetite, nausea or vomiting and excessive wind or gas are the usual symptoms of indigestion. Other symptoms include a bad taste in the mouth, coated tongue, foul breath and pain in the upper abdomen.

Causes

The feelings of discomfort and distress in the abdomen are often caused by overeating, eating too rapidly or not chewing properly. Overeating or eating frequently produces a feverish state in the system and overtaxes the digestive organs. It produces excessive acid and causes the gastric mucus membrane to become congested. Hyperacidity is usually the result.

Overeating makes the work of the stomach, liver, kidneys and bowels harder. When this food putrifies, its poisons are absorbed back into the blood and consequently, the whole system is poisoned.

Many people gulp their food due to stress or hurry. When food is swallowed in large chunks, the stomach has to work harder and more hydrochloride is secreted. Eating too fast also causes one to swallow air. These bad habits force some of the digestive fluids into the oesophagus, causing burning, a stinging sensation or a sour taste, giving an illusion of stomach acid.

Certain foods, especially if they are not properly cooked,

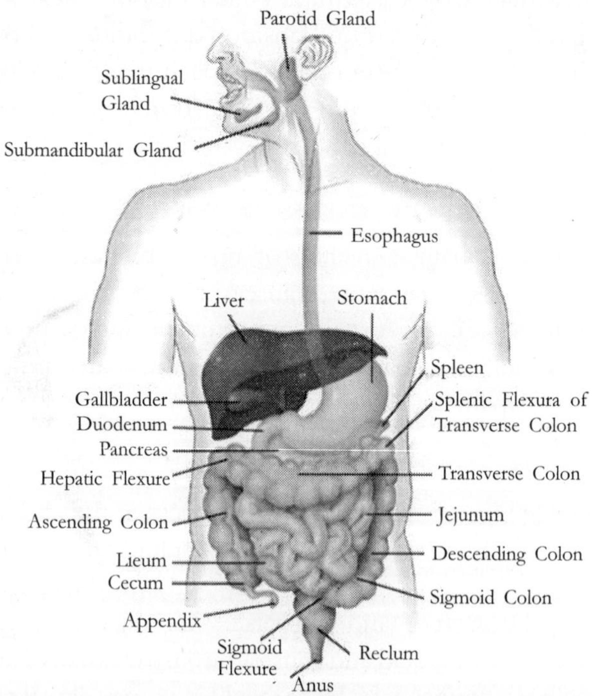

The alimentary canal and the process of digestion begin at the mouth.

cause indigestion. Some people react unfavourably to certain foods like beans, cabbage, onions, cucumber, radishes and seafood. Fried foods as well as rich and spicy foods often cause abdominal discomfort and gas, and aggravate the existing condition. Excessive smoking and intake of alcohol can also cause stomach upsets. Constipation may interfere with the normal flow of ingested matter through the gastro-intestinal tract, resulting in gas and abdominal pain. Drinking too much water with meals, insomnia, emotions such as jealousy, fear and anger and lack of exercise are among the other causes of indigestion.

The Cure

The only effective treatment for indigestion is a thorough cleansing of the digestive tract; adoption of a sensible diet and a change in the style of living. The best way to commence the treatment is to adopt an all-fruit diet for about five days. After the all-fruit diet, the patient may take to a restricted diet of easily digestible foods, consisting of lightly cooked vegetables, juicy fruits and buttermilk for about 10 days. He may thereafter gradually embark upon a well-balanced diet.

The use of fruits in general is beneficial in the treatment of indigestion. They flush out the undigested food residue and accumulated faeces and re-establish health to perfect order. Being rich in water, they clean body mechanisms thoroughly. The best among the fruits in dyspepsia is lemon. Its juice reaches the stomach and attacks the bacteria, inhabiting the formation of acids. Lemon juice removes indigestion by dislodging this acid and other harmful substances from the stomach, thereby strengthening and prompting a healthy appetite.

The orange is another effective food remedy in chronic

indigestion. It gives rest to the digestive organs and supplies nutrition in a most easily assimilable form. It also stimulates the flow of digestive juices thereby improving digestion and increasing appetite. It creates suitable conditions for the development of friendly bacteria in the intestines.

Another fruit useful in indigestion is grapes. They are a light food which removes indigestion and irritation of the stomach in a short time and relieves heat. Pineapple is also valuable. It acts as a tonic in dyspepsia and relieves much of the digestive disorders of dyspeptics. Half a glass of pineapple juice should be taken after a meal in this condition.

The sufferer from indigestion must always follow the under-mentioned rules regarding eating:

(i) Never eat and drink together. Water or other liquids should be taken half an hour before and one hour after a meal. Milk, buttermilk and vegetables soups are, however, foods and can be taken with meals.

(ii) Never hurry through a meal. Eat very slowly and chew your food as thoroughly as possible.

(iii) Never eat to a full stomach. Always leave the table with a feeling that you could eat more.

(iv) Never sit down to a meal, feeling worried, tired, excited or in a bad temper as such feelings temporarily paralyse the manufacture of digestive juices including hydrochloride.

(v) Do not eat if appetite is lacking. Miss a meal or two, if necessary, until real appetite returns.

(vi) Never boil vegetables, always steam them.

(vii) Do not mix too many foods at the same meal. Never eat raw vegetables and raw fruits together as they require a different set of enzymes. Take protein and starchy foods separate as far as possible.

Yogic asanas such as ardhmatsyasana, sarvangasana, uttanpadasana, pavanmuktasana, vajrasana, yogamudra, bhujangasana, shalabhasana and shavasana, kriyas like jalneti kunjal and pranayamas like kapalbhati, anuloma-viloma ujjai are highly beneficial in the treatment of indigestion. Light exercises such as walking, golf and swimming also help digestion.

Water Treatment

A daily enema should be administered to cleanse toxic bowel waste. Other beneficial water treatments include wet girdle pack applied at night, application of ice bag over the stomach half an hour after meals, a daily cold friction bath and alternate hot and cold hip baths at night. Massaging of the abdomen also helps.

CHAPTER 89

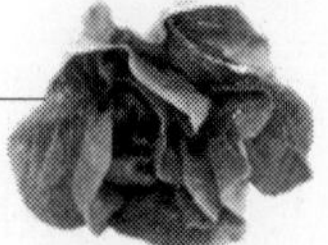

Influenza

Influenza, also known as flu, is the clinical condition that results from infection with influenza viruses. The main effects of the influenza viruses are on the upper respiratory tract, the nose and throat, with possible spread and involvement of the lungs and bronchi.

The disease is highly contagious and it has potential to cause widespread epidemics affecting sizeable portion of a population at any time. Although it is more common during winter it may strike at any time. It affects people of all ages.

Symptoms

Influenza strikes suddenly. It usually begins with a chill, fever, headache and severe muscular pains. The patient feels miserable and weak. There is an inflammation in the nose and throat, which may spread down the windpipe to the lungs, resulting in a sore throat, cough, running of the nose and eyes.

In milder cases of influenza, the temperature rises to 102°F and lasts for two or three days. In severe cases, it may go upto 104° F and last for four or five days. The consequent weakness and fatigue may continue for several weeks. This may be followed by a deep chest cough due to irritation in the windpipe.

Causes

Influenza is what is known as germ disease. It is, however, not caused primarily by the action of the germs as is generally believed, but develops due to a toxic and run-down condition of the system of the affected person. This condition is brought about by dietetic errors and a faulty style of living such as worry, over work, lack of proper exercise, living in stuffy rooms and keeping late hours. No disease germs can find lodgement and become active in the system of a person who is perfectly healthy in the true sense of the term. Influenza is passed on with ease from one affected person to an other especially to those who are also in an equally low vital state. That is how an epidemic starts.

Treatment

Influenza, like all other acute diseases, is a natural attempt at self-cleansing and if rightly treated in a natural way, immense good can ensue so far as the future health of the patient is concerned. In the acute stage of influenza, the patient should abstain from all solid foods and only drink fruit and vegetable juices diluted with water, 50—50 for first three to five days, depending on the severity of the disease. The juice fast should be continued till the temperature comes down to normal. The warm water enema should be taken daily during this period to cleanse the bowels.

After fever subsides the patient may adopt an all-fruit diet for two or three days. In this regimen, the patient should take three meals a day of fresh juicy fruits such as apples, pears, grapes, oranges, pineapple, peaches and melons at five-hourly intervals. Bananas or dried, stewed or tinned fruits however, should not be taken. No other foodstuff should be added to the fruit meals, otherwise the value of the treatment will be lost. This may be followed by a further two or three days on fruits and milk diet. Thereafter, the patient may adopt a well-balanced diet of three basic food groups, namely, (i) seeds, nuts and grains, (ii) vegetables, and (iii) fruits.

Spices and condiments, and pickles, which make food more palatable and lead to overeating, must be avoided. Lemon juice may be used in salad dressing. Alcohol, tobacco, strong tea and coffee, highly seasoned meats, over-boiled milk, pulses, potato, rice, cheese, refined, processed, stale and tinned foods should all be avoided.

Certain remedies have been found highly beneficial in the treatment of influenza. The most important of these is the use of long pepper. Half a teaspoonful of the powder of long pepper with two teaspoonfuls of honey and half a teaspoonful of juice of ginger should be taken thrice a day. This will help greatly if taken in the initial stages of the disease. It is especially useful in avoiding complications which follow the onset of the disease, namely, the involvement of the larynx and the bronchial tube.

Another excellent remedy for influenza is the green leaves of basil or *tulsi* plant. About one gram of these leaves should be boiled along with some ginger in half a litre of water till about half the water is left. This decoction should be taken as tea. It gives immediate relief.

Garlic and turmeric are other effective food medicines for influenza. Garlic is useful as a general antiseptic and should be given as much as the patient can bear. Garlic juice may also be sucked up the nose. A teaspoonful of turmeric powder should be mixed in a cup of warm milk and taken three times in the day. It will prevent complications arising from influenza and also activate the liver which becomes sluggish during the attack.

CHAPTER 90

Insomnia

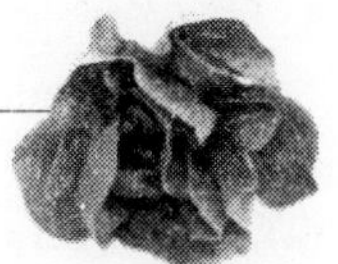

Insomnia or sleeplessness has assumed alarming proportions in present times, especially among the upper classes in urban areas. This is evident from the wide range of medication for this condition prescribed by physicians and sold by chemists. Instances of persons taking an overdose of sleeping pills with fatal results are quite frequent. Insomnia deprives a person of mental rest and thereby interferes with his activities in the daytime. It constitutes a severe health hazard when it becomes a habit.

Sleep is a periodic state of rest for the body which is absolutely essential for its efficient functioning. Sleep gives relief from tension, rests the brain and body and a person wakes up in the morning fresh and relaxed after sleep. The amount of sleep, however, varies within very wide limits from individual to individual. Normally, seven to eight hours of sleep every night is adequate for most people. Some, however, do well with four to five hours because their sleep is deeper and more refreshing.

Insomnia is common among the elderly for a variety of reasons. The sleep of the elderly is often punctuated by brief periods of wakefulness during the night. In such cases it is the quality rather than the quantity which is most affected. With age, there is a gradual reduction of periods of deep sleep. The older person, therefore, gets roused easier. Sleep requirements also diminish with ageing. From nine hours of sleep per night at the age of 12 the average sleep needs decrease to eight hours at the age of 20, seven hours at 40, six and a half hours at 60 and six hours at 80.

Symptoms

The signs of pathological insomnia are dramatic changes in the duration and quality of sleep, persistent changes in sleep patterns, lapses of memory and lack of concentration during the day. Other symptoms are emotional instability, loss of co-ordination, confusion and a lingering feeling of indifference.

Causes

The most common cause of sleeplessness is mental tension brought about by anxiety, worries, overwork and overexcitement. Suppressed feelings of resentment, anger and bitterness may also cause insomnia. Constipation, dyspepsia, over-eating at night, excessive intake of tea or coffee and going to bed hungry are among the other causes. Smoking is another unsuspected cause of insomnia as it irritates the nervous system, especially the nerves of the digestive system. Often, worrying about falling asleep is enough to keep one awake.

The Cure

Sleeping pills are no remedy for sleeplessness. They are habit forming and become less effective when taken continuously. They lower the I.Q., dull the brain and can prove fatal if taken in excess or before or after alcohol. The side-effects of sleeping pills include indigestion, skin rashes, lowered resistance to infection, circulatory and respiratory problems, poor appetite, high blood pressure, kidney and liver problems and mental confusion.

To overcome the problem, one should adhere to a regular sleeping schedule, going to bed at a fixed time each night and getting up at a fixed time each morning. Early to bed and early to rise is a good rule. Two hours of sleep before midnight are more beneficial than four after. It is sheer folly for students, at examination times, to keep awake till long after midnight, drinking one cup of tea after another, as that is only apt to cause blankness and inability to concentrate in the examination hall.

Research has shown that people with chronic insomnia almost invariably have marked deficiencies of such key nutrients as B-complex vitamins, and vitamin C and D as also calcium, magnesium, manganese, potassium, and zinc. The sleep mechanism is unable to function efficiently unless each of these nutrients is present in adequate amounts in the diet.

A balanced diet with simple modifications in eating pattern will go a long way in the treatment and cure of insomnia. Such a diet should exclude white flour products, sugar and its products, tea, coffee, chocolate, cola drinks, alcohol, fatty foods, fried foods, foods containing additives, that is chemicals for preserving, colouring and flavouring, excessive use of salt and strong condiments.

In the modified eating pattern, breakfast should consist of fresh and dried fruits, whole cereals, seeds and yogurt. Of the two main meals, one should consist of a large mixed salad and the other should be protein-based. A cup of milk sweetened with honey at bedtime is helpful as the amino-acid tryptophan contained in milk induces sleep.

Sleep is often elusive. Any attempt to force it only drives it further away. It is better to divert the mind with soft music or light reading. While going to bed, visualise a blank black wall occupying the entire field of vision. Turn your thoughts to light and cheerful matters. Use light bed clothes and relax. Do not lie on your back, but on your side with one or both knees brought well up and the head and shoulders slightly forward. During the night, the position of the arms and legs should be changed frequently and a healthy sleeper usually shifts from one side to the other several times in the course of the night.

Controlled breathing is also a great help in inducing sleep. The method is to lie on your side in bed, and then take three deep breaths expanding the abdomen completely. Then hold your breath as long as you can. Next, take three more breaths and repeat the breath-holding. While you hold your breath, carbon dioxide accumulates in the body and induces natural sleep.

Regular, active exercising during the day and mild exercise at bedtime enhances the quantity and the quality of sleep. Exercise stimulates the elimination of lactic acid from the body which correlates with stress and muscular tension. Regular exercise also produces hormonal changes which are beneficial to the body and to the sleep pattern. Walking, jogging, skipping, swimming are all ideal exercises. Vigorous exercise should, however, be avoided at night as this can be over-stimulating.

Yogasanas

Yoga helps a majority of cases of insomnia in two ways. Firstly, yoga treatment helps tone up the glandular, respiratory and nervous system. Secondly, yoga also gives physical and mental relaxation as a safety valve for one's disturbing problems. The traditional yogasanas which are effective for insomnia patients are shirsasana, sarvangasana, paschimottanasana, uttanasana, viparitakarni and shavasana.

Hydrotherapy is also effective in treatment of insomnia. Application of hot packs to the spine before retiring, hot fomentation to the spine, hot foot bath or an alternate hot and cold foot bath at bedtime are all time-tested methods. The cold hip bath with the feet in hot water and the prolonged neutral immersion bath (92° to 96°F) at bed time, when one's nerves are usually irritable, are also effective measures.

Along with the various measures for the treatment of insomnia, all efforts should be made to eliminate as many stress factors as possible. The steps in this direction should include regular practice of any relaxation method or meditation technique, cultivating the art of doing things slowly (particularly activities like eating, walking and talking) limiting the working day to nine to ten hours and five and a half days weekly, cultivating a creative hobby and spending some time daily on this, avoiding working against unrealistic targets and completing one task before starting another.

CHAPTER 91

Intestinal Worms

Worms and other intestinal parasites which infest human beings are found in all countries of the world. However they are more common in tropical and subtropical areas and are widely prevalent during the rainy seasons. Children are more infested with these worms than adults. There are several types of intestinal worms. The most common of these are roundworms, pinworms, threadworms, hookworms, tapeworms and giardia.

Symptoms

The usual symptoms of intestinal worms are diarrhoea, foul breath, dark circles under the eyes, constant desire for food, restlessness at night with bad dreams, anaemia and headache. Roundworms may give rise to inflammation of the intestine and lungs, nausea, vomiting, loss of weight, fever, nervousness and irritability. Pinworms and threadworms may bring intense itching in the area around the rectum.

Threadworms may cause periodic bouts of diarrhoea alternating with constipation, loss of weight, cough and fever. Hookworms may give rise to anaemia and nutritional disorders. The presence of giardia may result in pain in the calves and weakness in the legs.

Causes

The eggs of these parasites are introduced into the human system through the medium of food or water, especially undercooked meat. Roundworms may result from dirty fingers

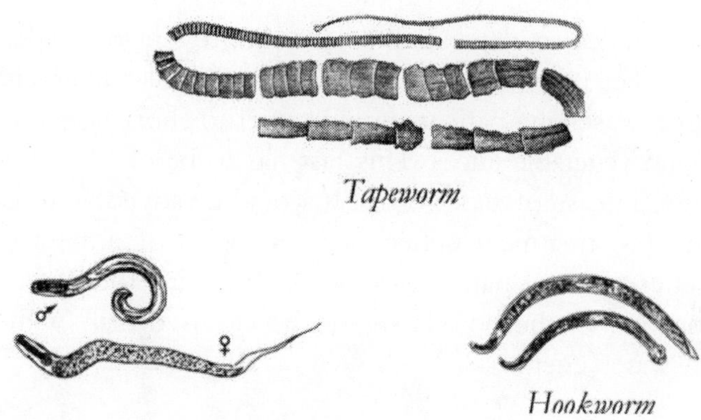

Varieities of intestinal Worms

and food. Hookworms enter the human body through the skin from infected water. The tapeworms are transmitted into the body through undercooked flesh foods or foods contaminated by dogs.

The real cause of intestinal worms, however, is wrong feeding. The eggs of these worms, taken into the human body through food and water, can breed in the intestines only if they find there a suitable medium for their propagation. This medium is an intestinal tract clogged with morbid matter and systemic refuse due to wrong feeding habits.

Treatment

The treatment for intestinal worms should begin with diet. The patient should be kept on an exclusive diet of fresh fruits for five to seven days. Thereafter he may adopt a well-balanced light diet consisting mainly of fruits, vegetables, milk and wholegrain bread. The diet should exclude fatty foods such as butter, cream, oil, refined foods and all flesh foods. This dietary should be continued till the parasites are completely eliminated.

In some cases, depending on the progress being made, the all-fruit diet may have to be repeated at regular intervals. In obstinate cases the patient should resort to short fasts on raw fruit and vegetable juices. This fast has to be of a fairly long duration in case of tapeworms. It would be advisable to carry on this fast treatment under the supervision of a naturopath or, better still, in a nature cure hospital. During the all-fruit or fasting period, the bowels should be cleansed daily with the warm water enema.

Home Remedies

Among the numerous home remedies found beneficial in the treatment of intestinal worms, the use of coconut is most effective. It is an ancient remedy for expelling all kinds of intestinal worms. A tablespoon of the freshly ground coconut should be taken at breakfast followed by a dose of Castor oil after three hours. The process may be repeated till the cure is complete.

Garlic has been used for expelling intestinal worms from ancient times by the Chinese, Greeks, Romans, Hindus and Babylonians. It is also used by modern biological practitioners for this purpose. Both fresh garlic and its oil are effective. An ancient method of its medication was to place a couple of cloves of fresh garlic in each shoe. As the person walks, it is crushed and the worm-killing garlic oil is absorbed by the skin and carried by blood into the intestines as it possesses a powerful penetrative force. This method is worth a trial by those who do not like the taste of garlic and cannot eat it.

The carrot (*gajar*) is valuable in the elimination of threadworms children as it is offensive to all parasites. A small cup of grated carrot taken every morning, with no other food added to the meal, can clear these worms quickly.

The digestive enzyme papain in the milky juice of the unripe papaya (*papita*) is a powerful anthelmintic for destroying round-worms. A tablespoon of the fresh juice and equal quantity of honey should be mixed with three to four tablespoons of hot water and taken as a dose by an adult. This should be followed two hours later by a dose of 30 to 60 ml. of castor oil mixed in 250-375 ml. of lukewarm milk. This treatment should be repeated for two days, if necessary. For children of 7 to 10 years, half the above doses should be given. For children under three years, a tablespoon is sufficient.

Papaya seeds are also useful for this purpose. They are rich in a substance called caricin which is a very effective medicine for expelling roundworms. The alkaloid Carpaine found in the leaves has also the power to destroy or expel intestinal worms. They are given with honey.

The bark, both of the root and the stems of pomegranate (*anar*) tree, is well known for its anthelmintic properties of destroying parasitic worms. The root-bark is, however, preferred as it contains greater quantity of the alkaloid punicine than the stem-bark. This alkaloid is highly toxic to tapeworms. Ninety to 180 ml. of the cold decoction of bark, preferably fresh bark, should be given three times at intervals of one hour to an adult. A purgative should be given after the last dose. The dose for children is 30 to 60 ml. The decoction is also used for expelling tape-worms.

The seeds of the ripe pumpkin (*kumra*) are useful in intestinal worms, especially tapeworms. An infusion, prepared from the seeds after they are peeled and crushed, will kill parasites and help in expelling the tapeworm. It will be necessary to fast for a day and empty the intestines by taking the juice of boiled dry prunes. The next day, three or four tumblers of this pumpkin seed infusion should be taken.

CHAPTER 92

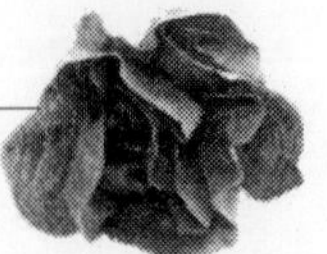

Jaundice

Jaundice is the most common of all liver disorders resulting from an obstruction in the bile duct, or the loss of function of the bile-producing liver cells. There are several forms of jaundice but all of them are marked by yellow discoloration of the skin and the whites of the eyes.

The liver, located under the diaphragm just above the stomach, is a vast chemical laboratory which performs many important functions. It inactivates hormones no longer needed, synthesizes many amino acids used in building tissues, and breaks proteins into sugar and fat when required for energy. It produces lacithin, cholesterol, bile and blood albumin, vital for the removal of tissue wastes. It also stores vitamins and minerals.

Bile is a vital digestive fluid which is essential for proper nutrition. It exercises a most favourable influence on the general processes of digestion. It also prevents decaying changes in food. If the bile is prevented from entering the intestines there is an increase in gases and other products. Normally the production of bile and its flow is constant.

Symptoms

The symptoms of jaundice are extreme weakness, headache, fever, loss of appetite, undue fatigue, severe constipation, nausea and yellow coloration of the eyes, tongue, skin and urine. The patient may also feel a dull pain in the liver region.

Causes

Jaundice is indicative of the malfunctioning of the liver. It may be caused by an obstruction of the bile ducts which discharge bile salts and pigment into the intestine. The bile then gets mixed with blood and this gives a yellow pigmentation to the skin. The obstruction of the bile ducts could be due to gall stones or inflammation of the liver, known as hepatitis, caused by a virus. In the latter case, the virus spreads and may lead to epidemics owing to over-crowding, dirty surroundings, insanitary conditions and contamination of food and water. Other causes of jaundice are pernicious anaemia and certain diseases affecting the liver such as typhoid, malaria, yellow fever and tuberculosis.

The Cure

The simple form of jaundice can be cured rapidly by diet therapy and exercises. Recovery will, however, be slow in serious cases which have been caused by obstruction or pressure in the bile ducts. The patient should rest until the acute symptoms of the disease subside.

The patient should be put on a fruit juice fast for a week. The juice of lemon, grapes, pear, carrot, beet and sugarcane can be taken. A hot water enema should be taken daily during the fast to ensure regular bowel elimination, thereby preventing the absorption of decomposed, poisonous material into the blood stream. The fruit juice fast may be discontinued after the severity of the disease is over and a simple diet may be resumed on the following lines:

On rising: A glass of warm water mixed with two teaspoons of lime juice.

Breakfast: One fresh juicy fruit such as apple, papaya, grapes berries and mango. One cup wheat dalia or one slice of whole wheat bread with a little butter.

Mid-morning: Orange juice.

Lunch: Two small chappatis of whole wheat flour, a cup of strained vegetable soup, a steamed leafy vegetable such as spinach, fenugreek or carrot and a glass of buttermilk.

Mid-afternoon: Orange juice or coconut water.

Dinner: Two whole wheat chappatis with a little ghee or butter, baked. Baked potato and one other leafy vegetable like spinach and fenugreek, a glass of hot milk with honey if desired.

All fats like ghee, butter, cream and oils must be avoided for at least two weeks, and after that their consumption should be kept down to the minimum. Digestive disturbances must be avoided. No food with a tendency to ferment or putrefy in the lower intestines like pulses, legumes, etc. should be included in diet.

The juice of bitter luffa (*karvi torai*) is regarded as an effective (home) remedy for jaundice. It is obtained by pounding and squeezing through cloth. The juice should be placed on the palm of the hand and drawn up through the nostrils. This will cause a profuse outflow of the yellow coloured fluid through the nostrils. The toxic matter having been evacuated in a considerable quantity, the patient will feel relieved. It is, however, a strong medicine and may cause in the patients with delicate nature, side effects like giddiness, migraine and at times high fever for a short duration. Its use should, therefore, be avoided by such patients.

If the green juice of bitter luffa is not available, it can best be substituted by two to three drops of the fluid obtained by soaking its dry crusts overnight in water. This produces an identical effect. Seeds of bitter luffa which are easily available can also be used for the same purpose after rubbing in water.

Another valuable food remedy for jaundice is the green leaves of radish. The leaves should be pounded and their juices extracted through cloth. One pound of this juice daily is sufficient for an adult patient. It should be strained through a clean piece of muslin cloth before use. It provides immediate relief. It induces a healthy appetite and proper evacuation of bowels, and this results in gradual decrease of the trouble. In most cases a complete cure can be ensured within eight or ten days.

Water Treatment

Drinking a lot of water with lemon juice will protect the damaged liver cells. Alternate hot and cold compresses should be applied to the abdomen. Maintain the hot compress for one minute at 120°F. Alternate with a cold compress at 60°F for few minutes. The treatment may be continued for an hour or 10 repetitions. The procedure should be repeated at five-hourly intervals. A hot immersion bath at 104°F for 10 minutes daily will be helpful in relieving the itching which sometimes accompanies jaundice and in the elimination of the bile pigment from the system through the skin and kidneys. Cold friction twice a day will be beneficial for general tone-up. Certain asanas such as uthanpadasana, bhujangasana, viparitakarani and shavasana, and anuloma-viloma, pranayama will be helpful in the treatment of jaundice.

The jaundice patient can overcome the condition quite easily and build up his sick liver until it again functions normally with the above regime. With reasonable care in the diet and life style, and regular, moderate exercise and frequent exposure to sunshine and fresh air, a recurrence of liver trouble can be prevented.

CHAPTER 93

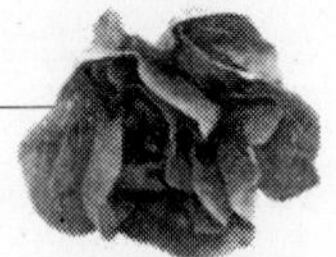

Kidney Stones

The formation of stones in the kidneys or urinary tract is a fairly common disorder. The stones are formed from the chemicals usually found in the urine such as uric acid, phosphorus, calcium and oxalic acid. They may vary in consistency from grit, sand and gravel-like obstructions to the size of bird's eggs.

Stones may form and grow because the concentration of a particular substance in the urine exceeds its solubility. This disorder occurs more frequently in middle age, with men being afflicted more often than women.

The kidneys are two bean-shaped organs, lying below the waist on either side of the spinal column on the back wall of the abdomen. They are soft, reddish brown in colour, and, on an average, measures 10 cm. in length, 6 cm. in width and is 2.5 cm. thick at its centre. They are the filtering plant for purifying the blood, removing water and salts from it which are passed into the bladder as urine.

Symptoms

Kidney stones usually cause severe pain in their attempt to pass down the ureter on their way to the bladder. The pain is first felt in the side and thereafter in the groin and thighs. Other symptoms of kidney stones are a desire to urinate frequently, painful urination, scanty urination, nausea, vomiting, sweating, chills and shock. The patient may also pass blood with the urine. Sometimes, large stones may remain in the kidneys without causing any trouble and these are known as 'silent' stones.

Causes

The formation of stones in the kidneys is the result of defects in the general metabolism. They usually occur when the urine becomes highly concentrated due to heavy perspiration or insufficient intake of fluids. They are aggravated by a sedentary lifestyle. The other causes are wrong diet, excess intake of acid-forming foods, white flour and sugar products, meat, tea, coffee, condiments and spices, rich foods and overeating. Lack of vitamin A and an excessive intake of vitamin D may also lead to formation of stones.

Types of Stones

Chemically, urinary stones are of two categories, namely, primary stones and secondary stones. Primary stones are

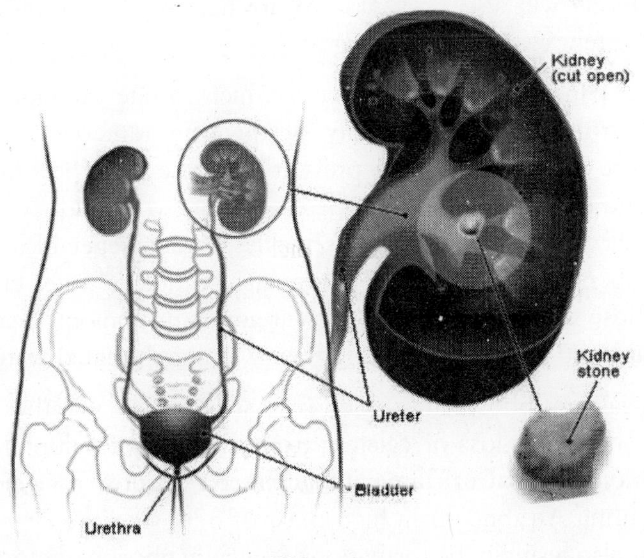

Kidney stone

ordinarily not due to infection and are formed in acidic urine. They usually result from alcoholism, sedentary life, constipation and excessive intake of nitrogenous or purine-rich foods. Secondary stones are due to local infection and are formed in alkaline urine.

Most kidney stones are composed either of calcium oxalate or phosphate, the latter being most common in the presence of infection. About 90 per cent of all stones contain calcium as the chief constituent. More than half of these are mixtures of calcium, ammonium and magnesium, phosphates and carbonates, while the remainder contain oxalate. Uric acid and cystine stones represent about four per cent and one per cent respectively of the total incidence of stones.

Treatment

A majority of patients suffering from kidney stones can be treated successfully by proper dietary regulations. These regulations will also prevent a recurrence of the symptoms. Only a few cases require surgery.

The patient should avoid foods which irritate the kidneys, to control acidity or alkalinity of the urine and to ensure adequate intake of fluids to prevent the urine from becoming concentrated. The foods considered irritants to the kidneys are alcoholic beverages, condiments, pickles, certain vegetables like cucumbers, radishes, tomatoes, spinach, rhubarb, water-cress and those with strong aroma such as asparagus, onions, beans, cabbage and cauliflower, meat, gravies and carbonated waters.

In calcium phosphate stones, over-secretion of parathyroid hormone causes loss of calcium from the bones resulting in a high blood level of calcium with increased excretion of calcium in the urine. An abnormally high intake of milk, alkalis or vitamin D may also result in the formation of calcium phosphate stones.

For controlling the formation of calcium phosphate stones, a moderately low calcium and phosphorus diet should be taken. The intake of calcium and phosphates should be restricted to minimal levels consistent with maintaining nutritional adequacy. The maintenance level of calcium is 680 mg. and of phosphorus 1000 mg. In this diet, milk should constitute the main source of calcium and curd or cottage cheese, lentils and groundnuts should form the main sources of phosphorus. Foods which should be avoided are whole wheat flour, Bengal gram, peas, soyabeans, beets, spinach, cauliflower, turnips, carrots, almonds and coconuts.

When stones are composed of calcium and magnesium phosphates and carbonates, the diet should be so regulated as to maintain an acidic urine. In such a diet, only half a litre of milk, two servings of fruits and two servings of vegetables (200 grams) should be taken. The vegetables may consist of asparagus, fresh green peas, squash, pumpkins, turnips, cauliflower, cabbage and tomatoes. For fruits, watermelon, grapes, peaches, pears, pineapple, papayas and guavas may be taken.

On the other hand, the urine should be kept alkaline if oxalate and uric acid stones are being formed. In this diet, fruits and vegetables should be liberally used and acid-forming foods should be kept to the minimum necessary for satisfactory nutrition. When the stones contain oxalate, foods with high oxalic acid content should be avoided. These foods include almonds, beetroots, brinjal, brown bread, cabbage, cherry, chocolate, French beans, potatoes, radish, spinach and soyabeans.

Uric stones occur in patients who have an increased uric acid in the blood and increased uric acid exertion in the urine. Since uric acid is an end product of purine metabolism, foods with a high purine content such as sweet bread, liver and kidney should be avoided.

Kidney beans, also known as French beans or common beans, are regarded as a very effective remedy for kidney problems, including kidney stones. It was Dr. Ramm of Germany, who first discovered the value of kidney beans as a medicine for kidney and bladder troubles. The method prescribed by him to prepare the medicine is to remove the beans inside the pods, then slice the pods and put about 60 mg. in four litres of hot water, boiling slowly for four hours. This liquid should be strained through fine muslin and then allowed to cool for about eight hours. Thereafter, the fluid should be poured through another piece of muslin without stirring.

According to Dr. Ramm, a glassful of this decoction should be given to the patient every two hours through the day for one day, and thereafter, it may be taken several times a week. Dr. Ramm also says that this decoction will not work if it is more than 24 hours old. The pods can be kept for longer periods but once they are boiled, the therapeutic factor disappears after one day.

The basil, known as *tulsi* in the vernacular, has a strengthening effect on the kidneys. In case of kidney stones, basil juice and honey should be taken for six months. It has been found that stones can be expelled from the urinary tract with this treatment. The celery is also a valuable food for those who are prone to stone formation in the kidneys or the gall bladder. Its regular use prevents future stone formation.

Research has shown the remarkable therapeutic success of vitamin B_6 or pyridoxine in the treatment of kidney stones. This treatment has to be continued for several months for obtaining a permanent cure.

The patient should take a low-protein diet, restricting protein to one gram per kg of food. A liberal intake of fluid upto 3,000 ml. or more daily is essential to prevent the production of urine at the concentration level where the salts precipitate out.

The patient should be given a large hot enema, followed by a hot bath with a temperature of 100°F, gradually increased to 112°F. The head should be kept cold with cold application. Hot fomentation applied across the back in the region of the kidneys will relieve the pain. Certain yogasanas such as pavanmuktasana, uttanpadasana, bhujangasana, dhannurasana and halasana are also highly beneficial as they stimulate the kidneys.

CHAPTER 94

Leucoderma

Leucoderma, also known as vitiligo, is a distressing skin condition. The word literally means 'white skin'. There is a gradual loss of pigment melanin from the skin layers which results in white patches. These patches look ugly, especially in persons with dark complexions.

The condition does not cause any organic harm. It, however, brings about great psychological tension to the patient who is more embarrassed than the victim of any pain or discomfort. The condition thus, besides being a medical problem, also becomes a social stigma.

Leucoderma is a fairly common disorder and it affects one per cent or more of the world's population. The incidence is a little higher in India. The disorder can occur at any age in either sex in normal skin. It is, however, more common in women than men. The most affected areas are the hands the neck the back and the wrist in that order.

Symptoms

The problem usually starts with a small white spot and later on it develops into patches. These patches are pale in the beginning but become whiter and whiter as time passes due to loss of pigment. As spots enlarge, they merge into each other and in course of time form a very broad patch. In some cases, most of the skin of the body may be covered with white patches.

Causes

Many wrong beliefs are prevalent about the causes of leucoderma. It is not caused by eating fish and drinking milk at the same time, as is generally believed because even vegetarians suffer from this disorder. Other food combinations such as pumpkin and milk, onion and milk as possible causes of leucoderma also have no basis.

Leucoderma is not caused by any germs; nor is it due to bad blood. It is neither infectious nor contagious. It cannot be transmitted from one person to another by physical contact.

The main causes of leucoderma are excessive mental worry, chronic or acute gastric disorder, impaired hepatic function such as jaundice, worms or other parasites in the alimentary canal, ailments like typhoid which affect the gastrointestinal tract, defective perspirative mechanism and burn injuries. Often the hormone secreting glands are involved in this disorder. Heredity is also a causative factor and about 30 per cent of patients have a family history of the disorder.

Treatment

In nature cure, the treatment of leucoderma consists of adoption of constitutional measures to cleanse the system of accumulated toxins. This enables the healing power within the body to assert itself, and produce normalcy. To begin with, the patient should undertake a fast on juices for about a week. In this regimen, he or she should take fruit or vegetable juices, diluted with water on 50 : 50 basis every two or three hours from 8.00 a.m. to 8.00 p.m. The bowels should be cleansed daily with warm water enema during this period.

After the juice fast, the patient may adopt a restricted diet consisting of fresh fruits, raw or steamed vegetables and whole meal bread or chappaties. Curd and milk may be added to this diet after a few days. The patient may thereafter gradually embark upon a well-balanced diet of seeds, nuts and grains, vegetables and fruits. The large proportion of the diet should consist of raw foods. Seeds and beans such as alfalfa, mung and soyabeans can be sprouted. This diet may be supplemented with cold-pressed vegetable oils, honey and yeast. Juice fasting may be repeated at intervals of two months.

The patient should avoid tea, coffee, alcoholic beverages and all condiments and highly flavoured dishes. He or she should also avoid sugar, white flour products, denatured cereals like polished rice and pearled barley and tinned or bottled foods.

Home Remedies

Certain home remedies have been found useful in the treatment of leucoderma. The best known of such remedies is the use of seeds of psoralea, known as *babchi* in Hindi. Seeds should be steeped in the juice of ginger or cow's urine for three days. The fluids should be renewed every day. The seeds should then be rubbed with hands to remove their husks, dried in the shade and powdered. One gram of this powder should be taken every day with fresh milk for 40 days continuously. The ground seeds should also be applied to the white spots.

Babchi seeds, combined with tamarind seeds, are also useful. Equal quantity of both the seeds should be steeped in water for three to four days. They should then be shelled and dried in the shade. They should be ground into paste and applied to the white patches for a week. If the application of this paste causes itching or the white spots become red and a fluid begins to ooze out, it should be discontinued. If there is no itching or reddening, babchi seeds should be taken also for 40 days.

Another useful remedy for leucoderma is red clay found by the river side or on hill slopes. The clay should be mixed in ginger juice and applied over the white spots once a day. The copper contained in the clay seems to bring back skin pigmentation and ginger juice serves as a milk stimulant, facilitating increased blood flow to the spots. Drinking water kept overnight in a copper vessel also helps.

A paste made from the seeds of the radish is valuable in treating leucoderma. About 35 grams of these seeds should be powdered in vinegar and applied on the white patches. For better results, seeds should be finely pounded, mixed with a little white arsenic and soaked in vinegar at night. After two hours, when leaves appear, it should be rubbed on the leucoderma patches.

The use of turmeric and mustard oil is also considered beneficial in the treatment of leucoderma. About 500 gms. of turmeric should be pounded and soaked in eight kgs. of water at night. It should be heated in the morning till only one kg. of water is left. It should then be strained and mixed with 500 gms. of mustard oil. This mixture should be heated till only the oil is left. It should be applied on white patches every morning and evening for a few months.

CHAPTER 95

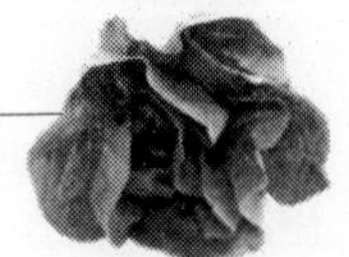

Low Blood Pressure

Low blood pressure or hypotension, to give it a proper medical term, refers to the fall in blood pressure below the normal. It is a condition in which the action of the heart in forcing the blood through the arteries is weak. This is a direct outcome of a weakened and devitalised system.

Symptoms

The patient with chronic low blood pressure may complain of lethargy, weakness, fatigue and dizziness. The patient may faint especially if arterial pressure is lowered further when he assumes an erect position. These symptoms are presumably due to a decrease in perfusion of the brain, heart, skeletal muscle and other organs.

Causes

The most important cause of low blood pressure is faulty nutrition. It makes the tissues forming the walls of the blood vessels to become over relaxed and flabby or stretched. This results in less supply of oxygen and nutrients to the tissues. Malnutrition can result from diet deficient in calories, proteins vitamin C or almost any one of the B vitamins.

Sometimes, the blood pressure falls rapidly because of haemmorrhage or loss of blood. Low blood pressure may develop gradually because of slow bleeding in the gastrointestinal tract, or through the kidneys or bladder. Emotional problems are a far more frequent cause of low blood pressure. To a lesser degree, prolonged disappointment and frustration may result in a subnormal blood pressure.

Treatment

The treatment for low blood pressure should aim at regeneration of the whole system. To begin with, the patient should adopt an exclusive fresh fruit diet for about five days, taking three meals a day of fresh juicy fruits such as orange, apple, pineapple, grapes, pear, peach and papaya at five-hourly intervals. Thereafter, he may adopt fruit and milk diet for two or three weeks. After a fruit and milk diet, the patient may gradually embark upon a well-balanced diet consisting of seeds, nuts and grains, with emphasis on fresh fruits and raw vegetables. Further periods on an all-fruit left, followed by milk and fruit diet may be necessary at two or three-monthly intervals in some cases, depending on the progress being made.

The warm-water enema should be used daily to cleanse the bowels during the first few days of the treatment, and afterwards, if necessary. Those who are habitually constipated should take all possible steps for its eradication.

Certain home remedies have been found beneficial in the treatment of low blood pressures. The juice of raw beet (chukandar) is one of the most effective of these remedies. The patient should drink a cup of this juice twice daily for treating this condition. Considerable improvement will be noticeable within a week.

The herb Indian spikenard (jatamansi) is another effective home remedy for low blood pressure. It should be taken in doses of 30 to 40 grains with the addition of a little camphor and cinnamon (dalchini). It can also be taken as an infusion in doses of 30 to 60 grams, thrice a day.

Protein, Vitamin C and all vitamins of B group have been found beneficial in the prevention and treatment of low blood pressure. Of these, pantothenic acid is of particular importance. Liberal use of this vitamin often helps in raising the blood pressure. A diet which contains adequate quantities of complete proteins, the B-Vitamins and particularly the nutrients that stimulate adrenal production quickly normalizes low blood pressure.

The use of salt is valuable in low blood pressure. Until the blood pressure reaches normal levels through proper dietary and other remedies, it is essential that the patient should take salty foods and half a teaspoon of salt in water daily.

Daily dry friction and sponge should be undertaken by those suffering from low blood pressure. They should also undertake breathing and other light exercises like walking, swimming and bicycling. The patient should take sun and air bath and spend as much time as possible in open air.

The hot Eposm-salt bath is one of the simplest remedy for low blood pressure. This bath is prepared by dissolving one to one and half kg. of commercial Epsom-salts in an ordinary bath of hot water. The patient should remain immersed in the bath from 10 to 20 minutes. This bath should be taken just before retiring to bed, and care should be exercised not to get chilled afterwards.

All habits of living tending to set up enervation of the system, such as overwork, excess of all kinds, needless worry, wrong thinking, must be eliminated.

CHAPTER 96

Malaria

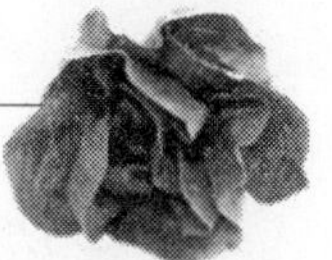

Malaria is a serious infectious disease. It is one of the intermittent fevers which have a tendency to return again and again to haunt the sufferer. The word malaria comes from the Italian *mala aria,* meaning bad air as it was once supposed to be caused by bad air. It is one of the most widespread diseases in the world, especially in tropical and subtropical regions.

Symptoms

There are three main types of malaria, depending upon the parasite which causes it. These are *vivax, falciparum* and *malariae,* commonly called tertian fever, quarten fever and the malignant tertian malaria. The most common symptom of all types of malaria is high fever, which may come every day, on alternate days or every fourth day. The fever is accompanied by chill, headache, shivering and pain in the limbs. The temperature comes down after some time with profuse sweating. One of the main effects of malaria is anaemia. Other complications of the disease are kidney failure and dysentry.

Causes

Malaria is caused by a tiny parasite called *Plasmodium.* The parasites grow in the liver of a person for a few days and then enter the bloodstream where they invade the red blood cells. The disease is spread from a sick person to a healthy one by the female anopheles mosquito. She draws a small quantity of blood containing the parasites, when she bites a person who has malaria. These parasites then pass through several stages of development within the mosquito's body and finally find their way to its salivary glands. There they lie in wait for an opportunity to enter the bloodstream of the next person the mosquito bites. The malaria-carrying mosquito breeds in stagnant water.

The real cause of malaria, however, as in case of other infectious diseases, is wrong feeding habits and faulty style of living, resulting in the system being clogged with accumulated systemic refuse and morbid matter. It is on this soil that the malaria germs breed. The liberal use of denatured foods of today such as white sugar, white flour and products made from them, as well as tinned foods, strong tea, coffee and alcoholic beverages, lower the vitality of the system and paves the way for the development of malaria.

Treatment

Diet is of utmost importance in the treatment of malaria.

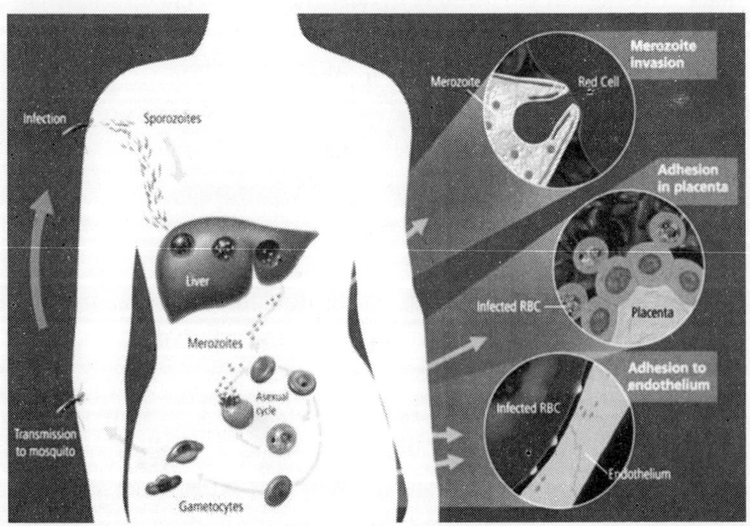

The malarial cycle in man.

To begin with, the patient should fast on orange juice and water for 7 to 15 days depending on the severity of the fever. The warm-water enema should be administered daily during this period to cleanse the bowels. After the fever has subsided, the patient should be placed on an exclusive fresh fruit diet for further three days. In this regimen, he should take three meals a day, at five-hourly intervals, of fresh, juicy fruits like oranges, grapes, grape-fruit, apple, pineapple, mango and papaya. Milk may be added to the fruit-diet after this period and this diet may be continued for a further few days. Thereafter, the patient may gradually embark upon a well-balanced diet of natural foods consisting of seeds, nuts and grains, vegetables and fruits, with emphasis on fresh fruits and raw vegetables.

The patient should avoid strong tea, coffee, refined and processed foods, fried foods, condiments, sauces, pickles, white sugar, white flour, and all products made from them. He should also avoid all meats, alcoholic drinks and smoking.

The best way to reduce temperature naturally, during the course of the fever, is by means of cold pack, which can be applied to the whole body. This pack is made by wringing out a sheet or other large square piece of linen material in cold water, wrapping it tight around the body and legs of the patient, (twice round would be best) and then covering completely with a small blanket or similar warm material. This pack should be applied every three hours during the day while temperature is high and kept on for an hour or so. Hot-water bottles may be applied to the feet and also against the sides of the body.

Home Remedies

Certain home remedies have been found beneficial in the treatment of malaria. One such remedy is the use of grapefruit (*chakotra*). This substance can be extracted from the fruits by boiling a quarter of the grapefruit and straining its pulp.

Lime and lemon are beneficial in the treatment of quartan type of malarial fever. About three grams of lime should be dissolved in about 60 ml. of water and juice of one lemon added to it. This water should be taken before the onset of the fever.

Cinnamon (*dalchini*) is regarded as an effective cure for all types of colds, including malaria. It should be coarsely powdered and boiled in a glass of water with a pinch of pepper powder and honey. This can be used beneficially as a medicine in malaria.

Alum (*phitkari*) is also useful in malaria. It should be roasted over a hot plate and powdered. It should be taken about four hours before the expected attack and every two hours after it. This will give relief.

Preventive Measures

The preventive aspect in malaria is as important as the curative one. The best way to protect against malaria is to adopt all measures necessary for preventing mosquito bites. For this purpose, it is essential to maintain cleanliness of surroundings, environmental hygiene and to eradicate stretches of stagnant water. As the mosquito generally perches itself on the walls of the house, after biting a person, it would be advisable to spray the walls with insecticides.

The leaves of the holy basil (*tulsi*) are considered beneficial in the prevention of malaria. An infusion of some leaves can be taken daily for this purpose. The juice of about 11 grams of tulsi leaves mixed with three grams of black pepper, powder, can be taken beneficially in the cold stage of the malarial fever. This will check the severity of the disease.

CHAPTER 97

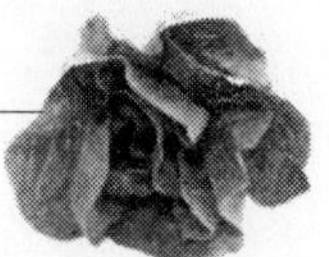

Measles

Measles, a highly infectious disease, is very common in childhood. It is so common at this stage of life that nearly all children everywhere in the world go through this brief period of red spots. The disease appears in epidemic form, often in the winter season.

Symptoms

The first symptoms which appear during 7 to 14 days after exposure to the virus are feverishness, cold, watering of the eyes and dry cough. Rashes appear on the skin in three to five days after the onset of these symptoms. These rashes, which consist of small rounded spots with reddened skin in between, initially appear on the sides of the face and the neck and then gradually spread all over the body, appearing last on the extremities. Initially pink in colour, these rashes grow darker as time passes.

Measles is usually accompanied with slight fever and diarrhoea. In rare cases of great severity, high fever and delirium may occur. Complication which can arise from this disease include pneumonia, bronchitis, and ear abscess. One serious but rare complication is the inflammation of the brain.

Causes

Measles is one of the most contagious diseases, caused by a virus. The measles virus is so infectious that in cities, children catch this disease before they reach the age of five years. Mothers generally pass their antibodies to their children which immunize them passively. This protection, however, does not last beyond the sixth month. Measles is easily transmitted in the early stages through the invisible droplets of moisture which are discharged from a patient's nose or mouth when he coughs or sneezes.

The real cause of this disease, like other diseases of childhood, is, however, wrong feeding and unhygienic living conditions. Measles is thus a natural healing crisis aimed at cleansing the infant organism of the toxins and deleterious products resulting from the assimilation of the excesses of starchy and sugary foods consumed by young children today.

The Cure

In the beginning of the treatment, the patient should be given juices of fresh fruits like orange and lemon frequently. This is sufficient as the child suffers from lack of appetite during this period. He should be kept in a well-ventilated room. As light has a detrimental effect upon the eyes during measles, because of the weakened condition of the external eye tissues, the child should have his eyes shaded or the room should have subdued light.

The treatment should aim at bringing down the temperature and eliminating the toxins from the system. This can be achieved by administration of warm water enema every morning, application of mud packs on the abdomen twice a day in the morning and evening and repeated application of chest packs. Lukewarm water bath can be given every day to ease itching. Addition of extracts of neem leaves to this water will prove beneficial.

As the condition improves, the child can be placed on an all fruit diet for a further few days. Thereafter he may be allowed to gradually embark upon a well-balanced diet.

Home Remedies

Certain home remedies have been found beneficial in the treatment of measles. The most valuable among these is the use of orange. When the digestive power of the body is seriously hampered, the patient suffers from intense toxaemia and the lack of saliva coats his tongue and often destroys his thirst for water as well as his desire for food. The agreeable flavour of orange juice helps greatly in overcoming these drawbacks. Orange juice is the most ideal liquid food in this disease.

The juice of lemon is another remedy. It also makes an effective thirst-quenching drink in measles. About 15 to 25 ml. of lemon juice, should be taken diluted with water for this purpose.

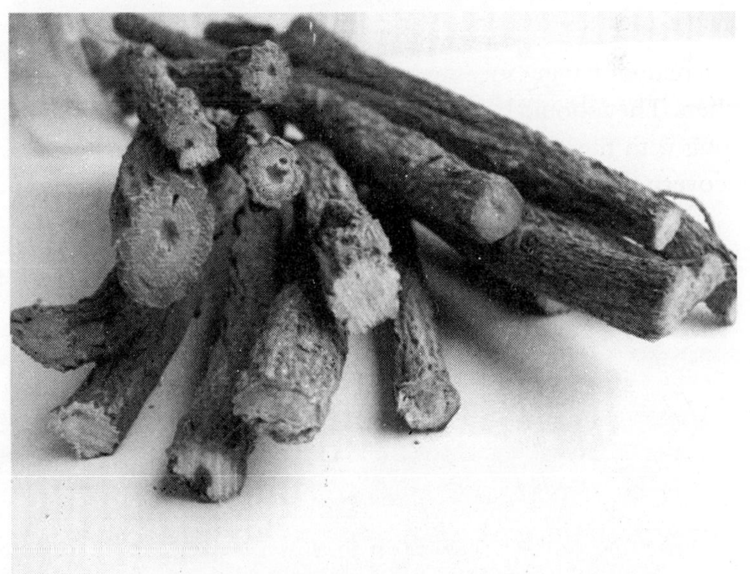

Powdered liquorice relieves cough in measles.

Turmeric (*haldi*) is beneficial in the treatment of measles. Raw roots of turmeric should be dried in the sun and ground to a fine powder. This powder, mixed with a few drops of honey and the juice of a few bitter gourd leaves, should be given to the patient suffering from measles.

Powdered liquorice (*mulethi*) has been found valuable in relieving the cough, typical of measles. The child patient should be given this powdered liquorice mixed with honey.

The use of barley (*Jau*) water has proved beneficial in case of troublesome cough in measles. This water should be taken frequently, sweetened with the newly drawn oil of sweet almonds.

The seeds of eggplant (*baingan*) are stimulant. According to Dr. Sanyal of Calcutta, intake of half a gram to one gram of these seeds daily for three days will help develop immunity against measles for one year.

Children having measles should not be allowed to mix with others. They should be given complete rest. Hygienic conditions along with the above mentioned treatment will lead to speedy recovery. Medications should be strictly avoided.

CHAPTER 98

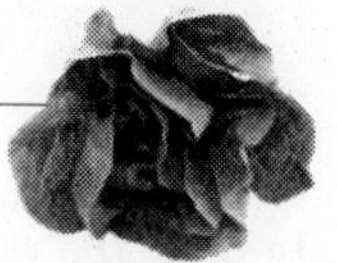

Meningitis

Meningitis is a severe inflammation of the meninges or inner lining of the brain and spinal cord. This may result from invasion of bacteria or virus into meninges. The infection usually spreads from the base of the brain up over the surface and down the spinal cord. It appears to reach the inside from the throat and nose via the blood stream. It is one of the most serious of all the acute diseases.

Epidemic meningitis sometimes occurs in densely populated areas during the cold season. It is also known as spotted fever, as spots appear upon the face and body.

Symptoms

The source of infection in most persons who develop meningitis is from throat, nose, ear or lungs. But if they are subject to damp, cold and overcrowding, the organism is liable to pass into the blood stream. The incubation period is short, ranging between one and five days, and the onset is sudden. Persons with this disease usually have a high fever and stiffness in the neck and back. The patient tends to lie in a curled position with the knees drawn up towards the chin and the eyes turned away from light. He becomes drowsy, confused and may become unconscious. There may also be a skin rash and an obstinate constipation. Vomiting is common in epidemic meningitis.

Causes

Meningitis usually follows an attack of otitis media (middle ear disease), or mastoiditis (infection of bone projecting behind the ear), or brain abcesses or even tonsillitis. Any skull fracture or penetrating head wound may also result in meningitis. Some times, tuberculosis may spread to the brain and cause the disease. In case of epidemic meningitis, the germs are apparently spread by persons who have a mild sore throat or cold.

Treatment

The patient with meningitis should be placed on complete bed rest and nursed very carefully. He should be given the juice of an orange diluted in a glass of warm water several times daily for the first few days of the treatment. This will provide energy, increase urinary output and promote body resistance against infection, thereby facilitating recovery. A warm-water enema should be administered daily to cleanse the bowels during this period. If the constipation is present, all steps should be taken to eradicate it through natural methods.

Cold compresses may be applied to the head in case the temperature rise above 103°F. If this method does not succeed, cold pack may be applied to the whole body. The procedure is to wring out a sheet or other large square piece of linen material in cold water, wrap it twice right round the body and legs of the patient and then cover completely with a small blanket or similar warm material. This pack should be applied every three hours during the day while temperature is high and kept on for an hour or so each time. Hot water bottles may be applied to the feet and also against the sides of the body.

After the temperature has come down to normal and the tongue has cleared, the patient may be given liquid foods and fresh juicy fruits like apple, pear, peach, grapes, orange, pineapple and melon, for further four or five days. For drinks, unsweetened lemon water or plain water, either hot or cold, may be given. Thereafter, he may be gradually allowed to embark upon a well-balanced diet consisting of seeds, nuts, grains, vegetables and fruits. The emphasis should be on whole grain cereals, fresh fruits and raw or lightly-cooked vegetables. Normal diet should be resorted to only after complete recovery.

The use of garlic has been found beneficial in the treatment of meningitis. The juice of three cloves of garlic should be given to the patient mixed with some fruit or vegetable juice.

The patient should take neutral immersion bath, as this bath is very useful in organic diseases of brain and spinal cord, including meningitis. This bath should be taken for 20 to 30 minutes at water temperature ranging from 26°C to 28°C (92 to 98°F) before retiring at night. A cold wet cloth should be applied to the head and forehead before entering the bath. This bath will equalize the circulation so as to reduce the amount of blood in the brain and spinal cord. Application of hot fomentation to the spine every two hours with spinal ice-bag during intervals will also be beneficial in the treatment of meningitis.

CHAPTER 99

Middle-Ear Infection

The ear is the organ of hearing and one of the most important parts of the body. It is divided into three parts, known as the external part, middle part or drum and the internal part. Ear being a very sensitive organ its inner structure is inaccessible. It is therefore necessary to deal with the disorders of this organ promptly. The most serious of these disorders is middle-ear infection, known as otitis media in medical parlance.

Symptoms

In otitis media, inflammation occurs on that portion of the ear which is directly behind the ear drum. There is discharge of pus into the outer ear. As the condition progresses, the inner ear becomes seriously affected, and hearing is considerably impaired. There is suppuration of middle-ear through a perforation of drum. In case of children, suppuration may start slowly without any reason. If the suppuration is left unattended, it may result in deafness.

Causes

Middle-ear infection generally follows the infection of upper respiratory tract. The swelling of the mucosa in the throat blocks the Eustachian tube which connects the ears with the throat and nose. This cause pus to collect in the middle ear cavity.

The real cause of middle-ear infection is, however, the outcome of previous medical treatment of childhood fevers

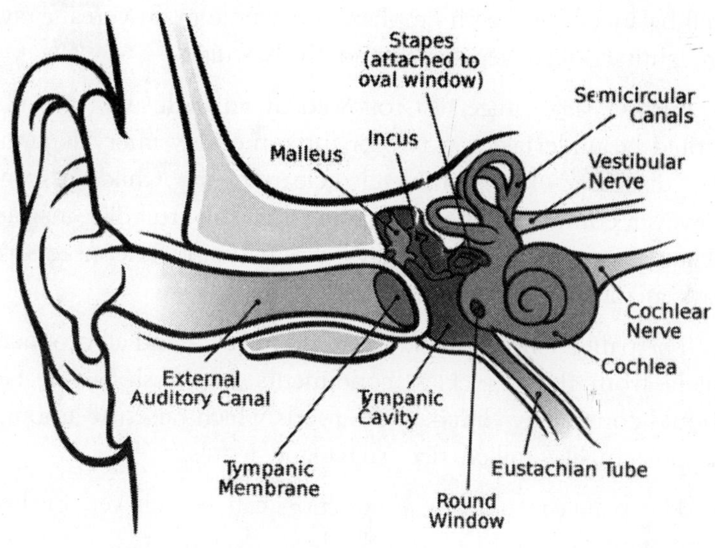

Section of ear

or due to operations for the removal of tonsils or adenoids. The disease denotes that toxins, which nature has been trying to throw off through the usual channels of elimination, have been diverted back into the system and have been lodged in the inner-ear structure. This causes the continual suppuration and discharge associated with the disease.

Treatment

A thorough internal cleansing of the system is essential to get rid of toxins, which is the root of the trouble, and clear up the infection. To begin with, the patient should be on an orange juice diluted with water for three to five days. A warm-water enema should be administered daily during this period to cleanse the bowels. After the short juice fast, the patient should adopt an exclusive diet of fresh fruits for further three to five days. Thereafter, he may gradually adopt a well-balanced diet, with emphasis on whole grain cereals, raw or lightly-cooked vegetables and fresh fruits.

Further short juice fast followed by an exclusive fruit diet should be undertaken at two or three monthly intervals, until the discharge has completely cleared up. Children can, however, commence the treatment with an all-fruit diet, instead of juice fast, for four or five days, with two or three consecutive days at monthly intervals.

The patient should avoid white flour, sugar and all products made from them, pickles, condiments and flesh foods. He should completely eliminate the foods which raise the amount of phlegm like milled rice, sugar and lentils.

The pain of middle-ear infection can be relieved by hot fomentations to the side of the head over the ear or by hot foot bath. The procedure for this bath has been explained in chapter 3 on 'Therapeutic Baths'. Irrigation of the ear with very hot water temperature (120 to 130°F) will also help relieve the pain.

Certain home remedies have been found beneficial in the treatment of earache and discharge from the ear resulting from middle-ear infection. The most important of these is the use of garlic. A few cloves should be warmed and mashed with salt. This mixture should be wrapped in a piece of woolen cloth and placed on the painful ear. Simultaneously, two or three cloves of garlic should be chewed daily for few days. It will give relief.

Garlic oil is also a popular remedy for earache. If garlic oil is not available, a few peeled cloves of garlic can be put in a tablespoon of any sweet oil, except groundnut oil. This oil should be heated, till the oil becomes brown with charred garlic pieces. The oil should then be filtered and cooled and a few drops should be put in the affected ear. This will give immediate relief.

The use of margosa (*neem*) oil has been found effective in infection and inflammation of the ear. One or two drops of this oil can be instilled into the ear with beneficial results.

The use of breast milk is a popular remedy for the inflammatory condition of the ear. Few drops of this milk put in the affected ear will give relief. Mother's milk would be preferable, but if it is not available, the milk of any healthy lactating women can be used.

Onion (*piyaaz*) is beneficial in the treatment of pus in the ear. The juice extracted from an onion should be slightly warmed and put in the ear two or three times daily. It will bring good results.

The patient should undertake regular exercises and outdoor games. Fresh air and sun bathing are of vital importance. The patient should sit in the sun so that sunlight penetrates the inner part of his ear for 15 minutes, it will help stop the discharge of pus from the ear.

CHAPTER 100

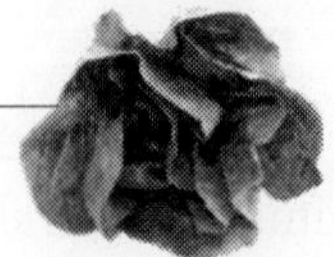

Multiple Sclerosis

Multiple sclerosis is a disease of the central nervous system. It is a chronic, progressive and demyelinating disease. It destroys the covering or insulating material around the nervous fibres, known as myeline.

The central nervous system is the nerve centre of the body. It is usually defined as the brain and spinal cord. It is linked with most nerve systems in the body, and some nerve from it continue on into parts of the body outside the brain and spinal cord. It is a wonderfully efficient system. With the help of other nerve systems, it is constantly at work, transmitting message into and out of the brain and spinal cord to and from all parts of the body 24 hours a day, even during sleep. Even the simplest action may involve scores of messages to different muscle fibres. In multiple sclerosis, these messages do not travel through the central nervous system properly and are slowed, distorted or, in some cases, blocked completely due to damage to the nerve tissue.

The disease is called multiple because many parts of the brain and spinal cord are affected. It is called sclerosis because the disease involves 'sclerosed' or hardened tissue in damaged areas of the brain and spinal cord. The disease usually affects people between the ages of 20 and 40 years, but can also occur before 20 or after 50 years. Women are slightly more affected by this disease than men.

Symptoms

Symptoms of multiple sclerosis vary greatly from person to person. Typical pattern is short period of acute symptoms, followed by an easing or disappearance of symptoms for weeks, months or even years. Some persons have mild attacks that never return. Common initial symptoms may include extreme fatigue, loss of balance and co-ordination, numbness and weakness of limbs, eye trouble, speech difficulties, and loss of bladder control. The patient may experience one, several or all of these symptoms, depending on the location and extent of damage to the nerve tissue.

Causes

Multiple sclerosis is a mystery in many ways. Medical science has not as yet been able to identify the cause of multiple sclerosis. Scientists have ascribed three probable causes for the onset of this disease. The most important of these is the viral attack. When viruses enter the body, they multiply rapidly inside the body cells. Most viruses cause symptoms quickly. Certain slow-acting viruses reappear later, causing new symptoms. Other slow-acting viruses stay inside the body for months or years before triggering illness.

The second probable cause is related to immune reaction. Our bodies have a built-in defense system which destroys viruses and bacteria. The defense system can backfire and start attacking the body's own cells. This is called an auto-immune reaction. Multiple sclerosis might involve an auto-immune reaction in which the body attacks its own tissues.

The third possible cause of multiple sclerosis is the combination of both viruses and immune reaction. When viruses invade the body, they take over body cells. The body defense system might become confused because some viruses take over parts of cells, and it might attack both host cells and virus.

The most important factors which might precipitate multiple sclerosis are exposure to cold, mental distress, over-exertion, some acute disease, an actual lesion of the central nervous system of traumatic or other nature and some specific febrile disease. There is evidence to suggest that multiple sclerosis patients tend to have experienced, on average, up to three times the unwanted stressful events in their lives within two years prior to the onset of their first symptoms compared with average number of patients with other disease.

Treatment

Diet plays an important role in the treatment of multiple sclerosis. To begin with, the patient should restore to a short juice fast for five days. In this regimen, he should take a glass of fresh fruit or vegetable juice, diluted with water on 50 : 50 basis, every two hours from 8 a.m. to 8 p.m. All available fresh, raw vegetables and fruits in season may be used for juices. A warm water enema should be used daily to cleanse the bowels during the period.

After the short juice fast, the patient should adopt a well-balanced lacto-vegetarian diet. The emphasis should be on organically grown, poison-free, whole, unprocessed raw foods, raw fruits and raw vegetables, especially root vegetables, raw milk, raw sprouted seeds and grains, particularly sprouted wheat and rye and raw nuts. Other foods beneficial in the treatment of multiple sclerosis are raw unpasturized home-made cottage cheese and home-made soured milk, raw fresh unsalted fresh butter, crude cereal germ oils, unsaturated fatty acids. Raw unfiltered honey is the only sweetener allowed.

The patient should avoid coffee, tea, chocolate, salt, spices, sugar, all refined foods, especially refined carbohydrates, processed, canned and frozen foods. All fruit and berries are beneficial. Best vegetables for multiple sclerosis are carrot, cabbage, radish, cucumber, red beet and tomato. Liquid whey contains erotic acid which has been shown to be of special value in the treatment of multiple sclerosis. When raw cottage cheese is made at home, liquid whey should not be thrown away but used for drinks.

Vitamin supplementation is vital in the treatment of multiple sclerosis. Large doses of thiamine or B1, niacin or B3 and pyridoxine or B6 can be used with success. Vitamin F and Vitamin E are also specific. Cortisone products may give temporary relief, but may not affect the general course of the disease.

The patient should avoid overwork and fatigue. Weakened muscles should be given a massage, and all the joints should be put through their normal range of motion every day. This will also help spastic muscles. Other useful measures are exercises, swimming, cold showers morning and evening, hot baths, and hot mineral baths. The patient should continue with his normal occupation as long as possible. Most patients with multiple sclerosis will have less trouble in a warmer climate.

CHAPTER 101

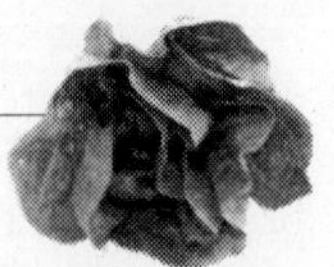

Mumps

Mumps or the epidemic Parotitis refer to a virus infection of the salivary glands, gonads, and occasionally other parts of the body. It is a contagious disease that occurs most frequently in children and young persons between the ages of five and fifteen years. The disease spreads from children to children in school. Babies are immune to this disease. Most persons have mumps only once in their lives, but one person in ten may have a second attack.

Symptoms

The first sign of mumps is swelling and pain. The pain is first felt under one ear with stiffness of the neck and jaw. There is a slight fever which subsides in three or four days. The swelling appears first under one jaw and then extends under the other jaw. The gland becomes tender on pressure. Mastication and swallowing becomes difficult due to the pressure of the swelling.

If the disease occurs after puberty, the testicles may be affected. The ovary may be infected in females, in males, the gonads are usually swollen. If the disease spreads to the testicles, the swelling and pain are very considerable, there is high fever, and the patient may become depressed and even a little confused. Mumps can also lead to meningitis (inflammation of the soft membranes of the brain) and encephalitis (inflammation of the brain) with delirium, severe headache and other signs of irritation of the meninges, or it may spread to the pancreas, when the symptoms include pain in the abdomen and loss of appetite. The patient may vomit.

Causes

Mumps are caused by a virus which attacks the salivary glands of the mouth, particularly the parotid glands located on each side of the face just below and in front of the ear. The infecting organism is a paramyxovirus. After a person is exposed to a case of mumps, it takes about two weeks for the disease to appear. Dietetic errors are at the root of the trouble.

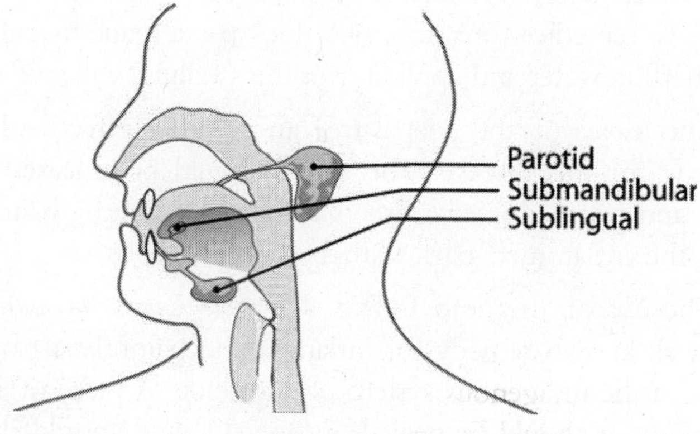

The Salivary Glands

Treatment

The patient should be put in bed for several days until the temperature returns to normal. He should be kept on a diet of orange juice diluted with warm water on a 50 : 50 basis for a few days. If the orange juice does not suit, the juices of other fruits such as mossambi, apple, pineapple, grapes or vegetables like carrot should be given. The warm water enema should be used daily during this period. Hot and cold fomentations should be applied every two hours during the day for about 10 minutes, and should consist of two or three hot applications, followed by a cold one. The mouth should be cleaned with an antiseptic wash.

When the child can swallow food comfortably and the swelling has subsided, an all-fruit diet should be adopted for a day or two. Thereafter, he may be allowed to gradually embark upon a well-balanced diet of natural foods, with emphasis on fresh fruits and raw vegetables.

Home Remedies

Chebulic myroblen (*harad or haritaki*) is one of the most effective remedies for mumps. A thick paste made by rubbing this herb in water and applied over the swelling, will give relief.

The leaves of the peepal tree are another effective home remedy for this disease. The leaves should be smeared with ghee and warmed over a fire. They should then be bandaged over the inflammed part, with beneficial results.

The use of the herb Indian aloe (*ghee kunwar or musabbar*) is a well known remedy for inflamed and painful part of the body, in the indigenous system of medicine. A piece of a leaf of this herb should be peeled on one side and sprinkled with a little turmeric (haldi) and extract of Indian barberry (*rasaut*) should be bandaged over the swelling after warming.

The seeds of asparagus (*halon*) are valuable in mumps. These seeds combined with fenugreek seeds (*methi*) should be ground together to the consistency of a paste. This paste can be applied beneficially over the swelling.

Dry ginger (*adrak*) is considered beneficial in the treatment of mumps. It should be made into a paste and applied over the swollen parts. As the paste dries, the swelling will be reduced and the pain will also subside.

The leaves of margosa (*neem*) are also useful in the treatment of mumps. The leaves of this tree and turmeric (*haldi*) should be made into a paste and applied externally over the affected parts. It will bring good results.

CHAPTER 102

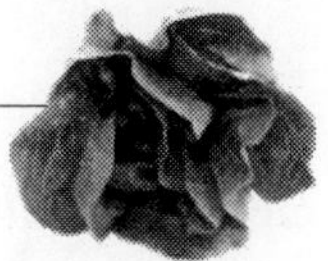

Muscle Cramps

Muscle cramps refer to painful spasmodic contraction of muscles in the limbs. They may occur in any of the muscles in the body. They are, however, more common in the calf of legs and feet, as in these parts of the leg, the muscles are more easily strained. It is estimated that 50 per cent of the people between the ages 15 and 80 years suffer from cramps or abnormal sensation in the legs at some stage or the other in their lives.

Leg cramps are especially prevalent in old age. They most often occur or are aggravated at night and are quite disabling. Occasionally, they are very disturbing leading to depression in older patients.

Causes

Muscle cramps are usually caused by dietary deficiencies of vitamins and minerals, particularly of calcium, potassium, magnesium, vitamins D and B_6, or the body's inability to assimilate these nutrients from the diet. They may also result from oxygen deficiency in the tissues. Other causes of muscle cramps are mental stress, nervous irritability and other psychic factors. Muscle cramps are sometimes associated with menstrual cycle and menopausal disorders due to the influence of sex hormones on calcium metabolism.

The contributory underlying causes of muscle cramps associated with old age, where there has been adequate dietary calcium supply, are the lack of sufficient hydrochloric acid in the stomach, lack of dietary magnesium or Vitamin D, without which calcium cannot be properly utilized. Other causes include uraemia, peripheral vascular disease and neurological disability.

Treatment

Muscle cramps caused by nutritional deficiencies can be treated successfully through diet. The patient should take a diet

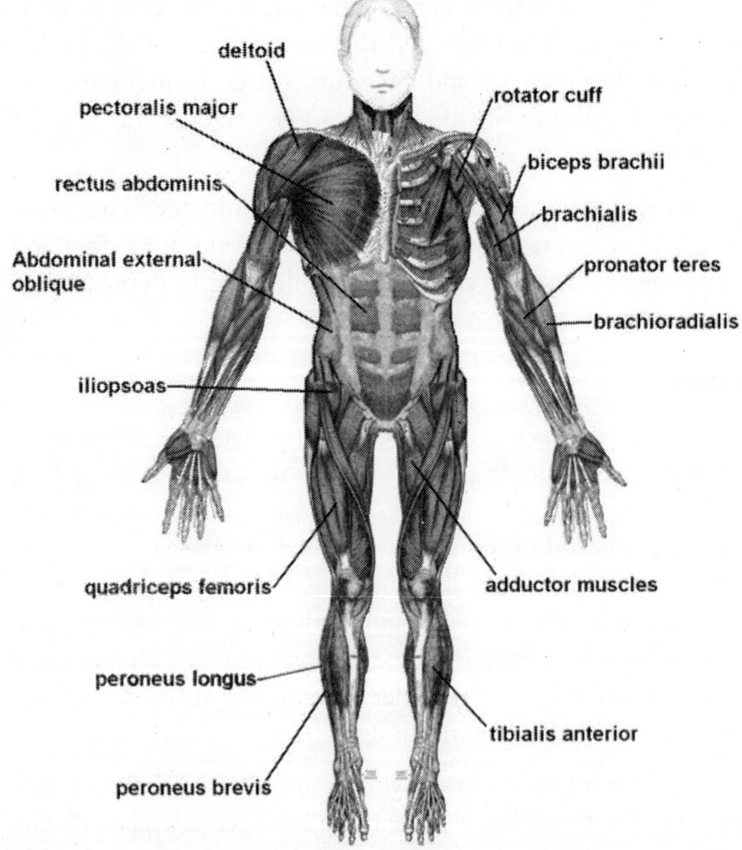

Types of muscles in human body—Front

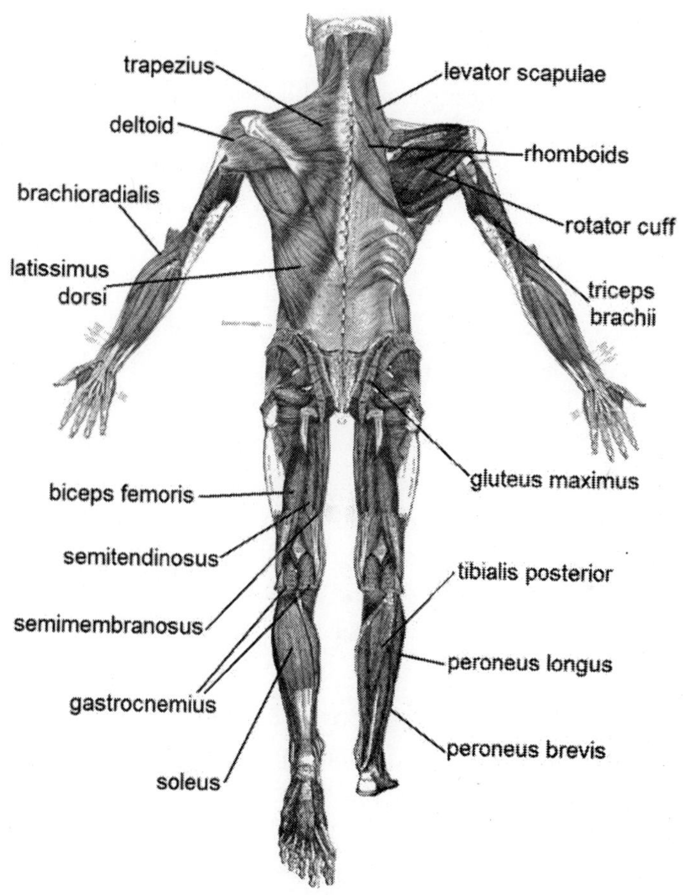

Types of muscles in human body—Back

which contains liberal quantities of all the essential nutrients. This diet may consist of seeds, nuts and whole grain, cereals, vegetables and fruits. The emphasis should be on calcium and magnesium-rich foods, such as green leafy vegetables, fresh fruits, particularly apricots, and soured milk products. The best sources of calcium are most vegetables, cereals like millet, oats, rice, sesame seeds, beans, milk and homemade cottage cheese.

The patient should avoid excess of citrus fruits, especially their juices, meats and excess of grains especially wheat, as all of them are deficient in calcium. Millets are the best cereals for relieving muscle cramps and they should be consumed liberally by the patient. Other foods which are valuable in this disease are sesame seeds and almond, especially in the form of milk.

The use of vitamin C and E in large doses has been found beneficial in the treatment of muscle cramps caused by Oxygen deficiency in the tissue. Vitamin C has been found to be valuable in the assimilation of calcium in the body and preventing it from piling in the joints. Vitamin E helps circulation in the legs. Leg cramps in some cases have responded to adding vegetable oils, which is a rich source of Vitamin E, to the diet. Organic minerals, especially potassium, can be helpful in cases, where the disease is caused by mental tension and nervous disorders. Elimination of contributory psychic causes are however, also essential in such cases.

Foot cramp may sometimes be caused by deficiency of vitamin B. Many strong persons also suffer from foot cramps because of lack of this vitamin. In such cases, it is essential to take Vitamin B_6 on a regular basis. This vitamin can be taken upto 50 mg. daily for months together without any ill effects. It is however, essential that while taking vitamin B_6, the whole family of vitamin B complex should be taken simultaneously, as too much of one of the B vitamins may cause imbalance of the other vitamin of B group.

Cramps associated with menstrual cycle and menopause can be treated successfully by large doses of vitamin E, B_6 and B_{12}. Certain herbs like Indian Sarsaparilla (*Magarbu or anantmue*) and liquorice (*mulethi*) can also be used beneficially in treating such cases. Leg cramps during pregnancy can often be relieved by vitamin B_6 and calcium.

In case of cramps associated with old age due to lack of hydrochloric acid, the addition of magnesium, vitamin D and two tablets of betaine hydrochloride after each meal can be helpful.

A useful method for relieving muscle cramps is to apply heating pad over the cramping area. Massaging the area will also be helpful. Persons suffering from leg cramps at night should keep their bed covers loose, or use a foot cradle at night to keep the weight of the covers off the feet, Those sleeping on their stomach may extend their feet over the edge of the mattress to maintain a neutral foot position.

Certain exercise have been found beneficial in the treatment of muscle cramps. One such exercise is to lean forward, bracing against the wall with hands and arms. Keeping the heels on the floor, tilt forward to the wall until a moderate pulling sensation develops in the calf muscles. Hold the stretching position for ten seconds, stand up straight for a five second rest, and repeat the exercise for a total of three stretches. This exercise should be carried out three times daily.

Another exercise useful in muscle cramps is to lie flat on the back in a bed with the feet elevated for two minutes or until they become balanced. Sit on the edge of the bed with the legs dangling over for three minutes, or until the legs become pink. Move the feet up and down, flex the ankles in and out, massage and manipulate the toes, feet and lower legs. Lie back on the bed, cover with blankets to keep the legs warm, and rest for two minutes. This exercise should be carried out six times each, four times a day.

Lower back and leg exercises assist in improving circulation to the extremities. Sit on the floor with the legs straight out in front of you, with your feet against the wall. Slowly reach for your toes with your fingers, then sit back slowly. Reach for the left foot with the right hand, then the right foot with the left hand. With hands locked behind the head, twist slowly to the right to touch the left leg with the right elbow. Return to the starting position and twist, to the left.

For relief from cramps at night, turn over in bed on your back. Point your toes toward the ceiling. This position will probably break the clutch of the cramp so that you can get back to sleep. If not, get up and walk around. If that does not help, get into a tub of hot water until the cramp subsides.

CHAPTER 103

Neurasthenia

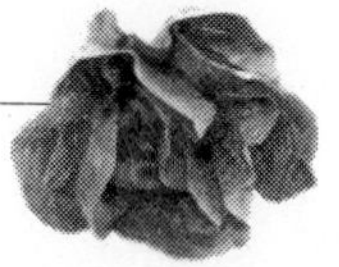

Neurasthenia is a chronic debility of the nerve cells. It is a condition in which the whole nervous system has lost tone and become exhausted. This disease is commonly known under such names as nervous prostration, nervous weakness and nervous exhaustion. It is essentially the disease of civilisation and the direct outcome of modern ways of living and thinking.

Symptoms

There are many and varied symptoms of neurasthenia. Some of these symptoms are weakness of the mental faculties, coldness of the hands and feet, sleeplessness, digestive disturbances, sexual disorders, an apprehension of sexual impotence in the male, painful menstruation in the female, restlessness, fear, muscular weakness and a host of symptoms accompanying general nervousness.

Causes

The main causes of neurasthenia are mental exertion, overwork and sexual excesses. Other causes of this disease include use of tobacco, sedentary habits, neurotic temperament and various chronic diseases.

The real causes of neurasthenia are, faulty diet, wrong style of living and wrong thinking. The present-day dietary consisting of refined, tinned, processed and preserved foods, all have adverse effects upon the health of the system in general and upon the nerves in particular. Foods 'denatured' in this way are deprived to a very great extent of their invaluable mineral salts and vitamins. The lack of these nutrients cause nerve starvation and nervous disorders like neurasthenia. The present-day high pressure standards and artificial ways of living also contribute greatly to this disease.

Treatment

There cannot be a hope for lasting cure for this disease, unless the whole life style of the patient is changed. Adequate rest is of utmost importance for those who have been overworked nervously and physically and for those who need a rapid gain of fat and blood. Muscular exercises and diversion are important factors for those who are mentally and nervously tired.

In the beginning of the treatment, the patient should adopt an exclusive diet of fresh fruits for about five days. During this period, he should take three meals a day of fresh juicy fruits such as orange, apple, pineapple, pear, peach, grapes and papaya at four-hourly intervals. While on the all-fruit diet, a warm-water enema should be administered daily to cleanse the bowels. Thereafter, the patient may spend further five to ten days on fruit and milk diet. In this regimen, the meals are exactly the same as the exclusive fresh fruit diet, but with milk added to each fruit meal. The patient should begin with one litre of milk, the first day and increase by 250 ml. daily upto two litres or more a day, according to how the milk agrees. The milk should be fresh and unboiled, but may be slightly warmed, if desired. It should be sipped very slowly.

After the fruit and milk diet, the patient may gradually adopt a well balanced diet consisting of seeds, nuts and grains, with emphasis on fresh fruits, raw vegetables and fruit and vegetable juices. This diet should be supplemented with vegetable oil, honey and milk, preferably in soured form like curd and butter-milk.

Further periods on the all-fruit diet followed by the fruit and milk diet may be necessary in some cases, depending on the progress being made. The patient should avoid all highly flavoured dishes, cakes, pastries, heavy puddings, pies and similar rich foods which over-tax digestion. He should also avoid white bread, sugar, refined cereals, condiments, tea, coffee and alcohol. He should drink liberal quantities of water. Smoking, if habitual, should be given up completely.

A regime of general health-building measures should be followed to improve the nervous and muscular systems. Mental exertion, sexual excess, worry and anxiety must be avoided. All steps should be taken to increase vitality and the nervous energy. These include the morning dry friction and sponge, as well as neutral immersion bath daily for one hour before retiring. The procedure for taking this bath has been explained in Chapter 3 on 'Therapeutic Baths'.

A hot epsom salt bath will also be beneficial and should be taken by the patient once or twice every week. This bath is prepared by dissolving one kg. of commercial epsom-salt in an ordinary bath of hot water. The patient should remain immersed in the bath from 10 to 20 minutes. Care should be taken not to get chilled afterwards. No soap should be used with the epsom-salt bath, as this interferes with its beneficial effects.

Fresh air, physical and breathing exercises and yogasanas should all form part of the treatment. The patient should take adequate rest, relax both mentally and physically. He should sleep in a well-ventilated room. He should avoid late hours and pay special attention to personal hygiene.

CHAPTER 104

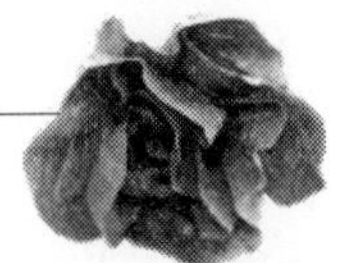

Neuritis

Neuritis is one of the serious nervous disorders. It refers to an inflammation of the nerves, involving a single nerve or a series of nerves. At times, several different groups of nerves in various parts of the body may be involved. This condition is known as polyneuritis. It is also known as polyneuropathy, for strictly speaking, the condition is not an inflammation, but a change in the state of the nerves resulting in weakness, loss of the reflexes and changes of sensation.

Symptoms

The main symptoms of neuritis are tingling, burning, and stabbing pains in the affected nerves. In severe cases, there may be numbness and loss of sensation and paralysis of the nearby muscles. Thus a temporary paralysis of the face may result from changes in the facial nerve on the affected side. During the acute stage of this condition, the patient may not be able to close the eyes due to loss of normal tone and strength by the muscles on the affected side of the face. Neuritis may also be caused by pernicious anaemia, involving the nerves of the spine. The patient with this condition may find it very difficult to walk in the dark.

Causes

The chief cause of neuritis is chronic acidosis, that is, excessive acid condition of the blood and other body fluids. All the body fluids should be alkaline in their reaction, but when the acid waste matter is continuously formed in the tissues over a long period due to a faulty diet, it results in acidosis. Wrong habits of living, overwork, etc., lower the tone of the nervous system and contribute towards neuritis. This disease can also result from a variety of nutritional deficiencies and metabolic disturbances such as faulty calcium metabolism, deficiencies of several B vitamins like B_{12}, B_6, B_1, pantothenic acid and B_2 and general toxaemia.

Other causes of neuritis include a blow, a penetrating injury, a bad bruise or heavy pressure over a nerve trunk and dislocation and fractures of the bones. Any violent muscular activity or over-extension of the joint as in sprains may injure the nerves and cause neuritis. The condition may also result from certain infections such as tuberculosis, diptheria, tetanus, leprosy and diabetes mellitus, poisoning with insecticides, mercury, lead, arsenic and alcohol.

Treatment

Treatment of neuritis by painkilling drugs may give temporary relief but it does not remove the trouble effectively. The pain is relieved for the time being at the cost of the health of other parts of the body, especially the heart and kidneys, and the neuritis remains.

The best treatment for neuritis is to ensure that the patient gets optimum nutrition, well assimilated with all the vitamins and other nutrients. The emphasis should be on whole grains, particularly whole wheat, brown rice, raw and sprouted seeds, raw milk, especially in soured form, and home-made cottage cheese.

In this regimen, the breakfast may consist of fresh fruits, a handful of raw nuts or a couple of tablespoons of sunflower and pumpkin seeds. Steamed vegetables, whole wheat chappatis and a glass of butter-milk may be taken for lunch. The dinner may comprise a large bowl of fresh, green, vegetable salad, fresh home-made cottage cheese, fresh butter and a glass of butter-milk.

In severe cases, the patient should be put on a short juice fast for four or five days before being given the optimum diet. Carrot, beet, citrus fruits, apple and pineapple may be used for juices.

All vitamins of the B group have proved highly beneficial in the prevention and treatment of neuritis. The disorder has been helped when vitamins B_1, B_2, B_6, B_{12} and pantothenic acid have been given together, and extreme pain, weakness and numbness in some cases have been relieved within an hour.

The patient should avoid white bread, white sugar, refined cereals, meat, fish, tinned foods, tea, coffee and condiments which are at the root of the trouble, by continuously flooding the tissues with acid impurities.

Certain remedies have been found highly beneficial in the treatment of neuritis. One such remedy is soyabean milk. A cupful of soyabean milk mixed with a teaspoonful of honey should be taken every night in this condition. It tones up the nervous system due to its rich concentration of lecithin, vitamin B_1 and glutanic acid. Soyabean milk is prepared by soaking the beans in water for about 12 hours. The skin of the beans is then removed and after a thorough wash, they are turned into a fine paste in a grinding machine. The paste is mixed with water, three times its quantity. The milk should then be boiled on a slow fire, stirring it frequently. After it becomes little cooler, it should be strained through a cheese cloth and sugar added.

Barley brew is another effective remedy for neuritis. It is prepared by boiling one-quarter cup of all natural pearled barley in two quarters of water. When the water has boiled down to about one quarter, it should be strained carefully. For better results, it should be mixed with butter-milk and lime juice.

Raw carrot and spinach have proved valuable in neuritis as both these vegetables are rich in elements, the deficiency of which has led to this disease. The quickest and most effective way in which the body can obtain and assimilate these elements is by drinking daily at least half a litre of the combined raw juices of carrot and spinach.

The patient should be given two or three hot Epsom-salt baths weekly. He should remain in the bath for 25 to 30 minutes. The affected parts should also be bathed several times daily in the hot water containing Epsom salt—a tablespoon of salt to a cupful of hot water. The patient should undertake walking and other moderate exercises.

CHAPTER 105

Nepthritis

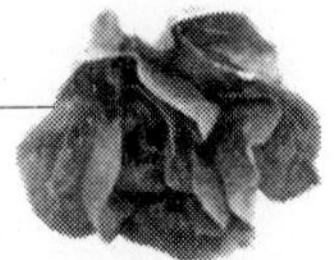

Nepthritis refers to an inflammation of the kidneys. It is a serious condition and may be either acute or chronic. A synonym for nepthritis is 'Bright's disease,' for Bright (1789-1858) described examples of many different diseases which can be included under the term.

This disease, most often strikes during childhood or adolescence. It can become progressively worse and result in death, if not treated properly in the initial stages. In the alternative, it may subside into a chronic stage where the patient gets better but not too well.

Symptoms

The main symptoms of acute nepthritis are pain in the kidneys extending down to the ureters, fever, dull pain in the back and scanty and highly coloured urine. Often the urine may contain blood, albumin and casts consisting of clumps of red and white cells which come from the damaged kidneys. The patient suffers from puffiness in the face and swelling of the feet and ankles.

In the chronic stage of nepthritis, which may drag on for many years, the patient passes large amounts of albumin in the urine. Later there may be rise in blood pressure and the patient may develop uraemia. There may be frequent urination, especially during night.

Causes

Nepthritis usually follows some streptococcus infection of the throat or an attack of scarlet fever or rheumatic fever. The underlying causes of nepthritis are however, the same as for diseases of the kidneys in general, namely wrong dietary habits, excessive drinking, the suppressive medical treatment of former diseases, the habitual use of chemical agents of all kinds for the treatment of indigestion and other stomach disorders and frequent use of aspirin and other painkillers.

Nutritional deficiencies can also lead to nepthritis. The disease has been produced in many species of animals by diets deficient in the B vitamin, choline. Animals lacking essential fatty acids and magnesium also develop nepthritis. When vitamin B_6 and magnesium are undersupplied, the kidneys are further damaged by sharp crystals of oxalic acid combined with calcium. Nepthritis also occurs if vitamin E is deficient.

Treatment

The safest treatment for acute nepthritis is fasting. By means of the fast, the toxins and systemic impurities responsible for setting up of the inflammatory kidney conditions are removed rapidly. The patient should resort to juice fasting for seven to 10 days till the acute symptoms subside. Mostly vegetable juices such as carrot, celery and cucumber should be used during this period. A warm water enema should be taken each day while fasting, to cleanse the bowels of the toxic matter being thrown off by the self-cleansing process resulting from the fast.

After the juice fast, the patient may adopt an all-fruit diet for four or five days. Juicy fruits such as apples, grapes, oranges, pears, peaches and pineapples should be taken during this period at five-hourly intervals. After the all-fruit diet, the patient may adopt fruits and milk diet. In this regimen, milk, preferably raw goat's milk, may be added to the fruit diet for further seven days. The patient may thereafter gradually embark upon a well-balanced low-protein vegetarian diet, with emphasis on fresh fruits and raw and cooked vegetables.

In case of chronic nepthritis a short juice fast for three days may be undertaken. Thereafter, a week or 10 days may be spent on a restricted diet. In this regimen, oranges or orange juice may be taken for breakfast. Lunch may consist of a salad of raw vegetables which are in season, and dinner may consist of one or two vegetables, steamed in their own juices and a few nuts. Thereafter, the patient may gradually adopt a well-balanced low-protein vegetarian diet.

Further short juice fasts followed by a week on the restricted diet should be undertaken at intervals of two or three months until such time as the kidney condition has shown signs of normalisation.

The patient should avoid vegetables containing large quantities of oxalic acid such as spinach and rhubarb. Chocolate and cocoa also contain oxalic acid and must not be used. Garlic, asparagus, parsley, watercress, cucumber and celery are excellent vegetables. The best fruits are papaya and bananas. Both have a healing effect on kidneys. A small amount of soured milk and home-made cottage cheese can be included in the diet. All salt should be eliminated from the diet. Five or six small meals should be taken in preference to a few large ones.

A glassful of carrot juice mixed with a tablespoonful of honey and a teaspoonful of fresh lime juice is a very effective home remedy for nepthritis. It should be taken every day early in the morning before breakfast.

Bananas are also valuable in nepthritis because of their low protein and salt content and high carbohydrates content. In this condition, a diet of bananas only should be taken for three or four days, consuming eight to nine bananas a day.

Smoking and drinking, where habitual, must be completely given up. Studies have shown that smoking impairs kidney function. The patient should avoid white bread, sugar, cakes, pastries, puddings, refined cereals, greasy, heavy or fried foods. He should also avoid tea, coffee, all flesh foods, condiments, pickles and sauces.

All measures should be adopted to relieve the kidneys of work by increasing elimination through other channels. Hot Epsom salt bath should be taken every alternate day to induce elimination through the skin as much as possible.

Fresh air and outdoor exercises will be of great benefit in all cases of nepthritis and where possible, the patient should have a walk for at least three kilometres once or twice daily. The sufferer from chronic nepthritis should never exert himself when doing anything. He should avoid all hurry and excite-ment. He should also avoid late hours.

If the above treatment is faithfully carried out, the patient of acute nepthritis should soon be on the way to recovery. Even in advanced cases of chronic nepthritis, the sufferer's condition should improve with this treatment.

CHAPTER 106

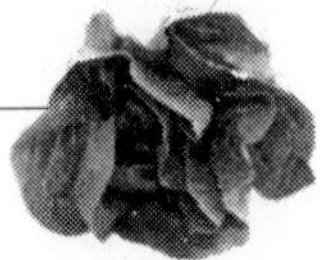

Obesity

Obesity may be described as a bodily condition characterised by excessive deposition or storage of fat in adipose tissue. It usually results from consumption of food in excess of physiological needs. Obesity is common among people in Western countries and among the higher income groups in India and other developing countries.

Obesity can occur at any age in either sex. Its incidence is higher in persons who consume more food and lead sedentary lives. Among women, obesity is liable to occur after pregnancy and at menopause. A woman usually gains about 12 kg. weight during pregnancy. Part of this is an increase in the adipose tissue which serves as a store against the demands of lactation. Many women gain more and retain part of this weight. They become progressively obese with each succeeding child.

Obesity is a serious health hazard as the extra fat puts a strain on the heart, kidneys and liver as well as the large weight-bearing joints such as the hips, knees and ankles, which ultimately shortens the life span. It has been truly said, 'the longer the belt, the shorter the life'. Overweight persons are susceptible to several diseases like coronary thrombosis, heart failure, high blood pressure, diabetes, arthritis, gout and liver and gall-bladder disorders.

Causes

The chief cause of obesity, most often, is overeating—that is, the intake of calories beyond the body's energy requirement.

Some people are habituated to eating too much while others may be in the habit of consuming high-calorie foods. These people gain weight continuously as they fail to adjust their appetite to reduce energy requirements. There has, in recent times, been an increasing awareness of psychological aspects of obesity. Persons who are generally bored, unhappy, lonely or unloved, those who are discontented with their families, or social or financial standing usually tend to overeat as eating is a pleasure and solace to them.

Obesity is sometimes also the result of disturbances of the thyroid or pituitary glands. But glandular disorders account for only about two per cent of the total incidence of obesity. In such persons the basal metabolism rate is low and they keep gaining weight unless they take a low-calorie diet.

Treatment

A suitably planned course of dietetic treatment, in conjunction with suitable exercise and other measures for promoting elimination is the only scientific way of dealing with obesity. The chief consideration in this treatment should be the balanced selection of foods which provide the maximum essential nutrients with the least number of calories.

To begin with, the patient should undertake a juice fast for seven to 10 days. Juices of lemon, grapefruit, orange, pineapple, cabbage, celery may be taken during this period. Long juice fast upto 40 days can also be undertaken, but only under expert guidance and supervision. In the alternative, short juice fasts should be repeated at regular intervals of two months or so till the desired reduction in weight is achieved.

After the juice fast, the patient should spend a further four or five days on an all-fruit diet, taking three meals of fresh juicy fruits such as oranges, grapefruit, pineapple and papaya.

Thereafter, he may gradually embark upon a low-calorie well-balanced diet of three basic food groups, namely (i) seeds, nuts and grains, (ii) vegetables and (iii) fruits, with emphasis on raw fruits, vegetables and fresh juices.

The foods which should be drastically curtailed or altogether avoided are high-fat foods such as butter, cheese, chocolate, cream, ice cream, fat meats, fried foods and gravies; high carbohydrated foods like bread, candy, cake, cookies, cereal products, legumes, potatoes, honey, sugar, syrup and rich puddings; beverages such as all-fountain drinks and alcoholic drinks.

One sure method of reducing weight is by practising what is known as "Fletcherism". It was discovered in 1898 by Horace Fletcher of the U.S.A. Fletcher, at 40, considered himself an old man. He was 50 pounds overweight, contracted flu every six months and constantly complained of indigestion and a tired feeling. After a deep study, he made some important discoveries and prescribed the rules for "Fletcherism" which are as follows:

1. Chew your food to a pulp or milky liquid until it practically swallows itself.
2. Never eat until hungry.
3. Enjoy every bite or morsel, savouring the flavour until it is swallowed.
4. Do not eat when tired, angry, worried, and at meal-time refuse to think or talk about unpleasant subjects.

Horace Fletcher followed these rules for five months. As a result he lost more than 60 pounds and felt better than he had for 20 years. A weight reducing programme built on Fletcherism works wonders and is worth a trial.

Ingestion of honey is an excellent home remedy for obesity.

It mobilises the extra deposited fat in the body and puts it into circulation which is utilised as energy for normal functions. One should start with small quantity of about 10 grams to be taken with hot water. The dose can be gradually increased.

Fasting on honey-lime juice water is highly beneficial in the treatment of obesity without the loss of energy and appetite. In this mode of treatment, one spoon of fresh honey should be mixed with a juice of half a lime in a glass of lukewarm water and taken at regular intervals.

Another effective remedy for obesity is an exclusive lemon juice diet. On the first day the patient should be given nothing but plenty of water. On the second day juice of three lemons mixed with equal amount of water should be given. One lemon should be subsequently increased each day until the juice of 12 lemons is consumed per day. Then the number of lemons should be decreased in the same order until three lemons are taken in a day. The patient may feel weak and hungry on the first two days, but afterwards the condition will be stabilised by itself.

Cabbage is considered to be an effective home remedy for obesity. Recent research has discovered in this vegetable a valuable content called tartroric acid which inhibits the conversion of sugar and other carbohydrates into fat. Hence, it is of great value in weight reduction. A helping of cabbage salad would be the simplest way to stay slim, a painless way of dieting.

A hundred grams of cabbage yields only 27 kilo calories of energy while the same quantity of wheat bread will yield about 240 calories. Cabbage is found to possess the maximum biological value with minimum calorific value. Moreover, it gives a lasting feeling of fullness in the stomach and is easily digestible.

Along with dietetic treatment, the patient should adopt all other natural methods of reducing weight. Exercise is an important part of weight reduction plan. It helps to use up calories stored in body fat and relieves tension, besides toning up the muscles of the body. Walking is the best exercise to begin with and may be followed by running, swimming, rowing and other outdoor sports.

Certain yogic asanas ate highly beneficial. Not only do they break up or re-distribute fatty deposits and help slimming, but they also strengthen the flabby areas. Sarvangasana, halasana, bhujangasana, shalabhasana, dhanurasana, chakrasana, naukasana, ardh-matsyendrasana, paschimottanasana, vajrasana, yogamudra and trikonasana are recommended. These asanas work on the glands, improve circulation, strengthen many weak areas and induce deep breathing which helps to melt off excess fat gradually. Yogic kriyas like kunjal and jalaneti and pranayamas such as kapalabhati and bhastrika are also helpful in normalising body weight.

The patient should also adopt measures which bring on excessive perspiration such as sauna baths, steam bath and heavy massage. They help to reduce weight. Above all, obese persons should make every effort to avoid negative emotions such as anxiety, fear, hostility, insecurity and develop a positive outlook on life.

CHAPTER 107

Osteoporosis

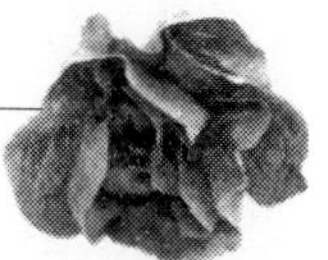

Osteoporosis, commonly known as soft or brittle bones, refers to increased porousness of bones. The word literally means porous or honeycombed bones. In this disorder, the bones of the skeleton become fragile due to excessive loss of bone tissues. It may cause the bones to fracture more easily than they should. If the disease affects the spine, it may lead to collapse of the vertebral bodies and consequent deformity.

Normal bone consists of a series of thin, intersecting plates, called 'trabeculae'. These plates are surrounded by a dense shell. These plates form, what is called the Bone mass. In osteoporosis, they become filled with holes or may even totally disappear. This causes a diminution of bone mass. With loss of bone mass, the shell also becomes thin. All these changes make the bones extremely fragile and it can crack with the most trivial injury.

Osteoporosis is often found in old age, although it may occur at any age. Bone mass increases rapidly upto adolescence and continues to increase at a reduced rate until the early 30s. In women, at menopause, there is a particularly rapid loss of bone for several years, followed by a slower decline throughout the rest of life. In men, bone mass declines steadily from the age of 45 onwards. There is wide individual variation. The bones commonly affected are wrist bones, spine and hip bones.

Symptoms

Osteoporosis is usually accompanied by severe pain. In

elderly patients, the disease is accompanied by an actual loss of height and by bending causing a humpback, deformity that crowds lungs and digestive organs. Other symptoms of osteoporosis are backache and spasms of the back muscles, aching of the long bones and, thinning of the pelvic bones, loss in twisting and bending strength and frequent occurrence of spontaneous fractures.

Causes

Abnormal porosity of bones in older people usually results from nutritional deficiencies and the body's inability to absorb and utilise nutrients. Prolonged deficiency of calcium and vitamin D in particular leads the skeleton to become demineralised and shrunken. The disease is far more prevalent in women than in men, because of calcium loss during pregnancies and menstruation. A broken hip bone is usually considered to be the result of a fall. But in reality, the collapse of the bone is the cause of a fall, which first draws attention to osteoporosis.

Other causes of this disease are over consumption of meat, heavy smoking of chronic alcoholism post-menopausal hormonal imbalances and diminished physical activity with age. Prolonged cortisone treatment, by blocking the bone-building activity and decreasing the intestinal absorption of calcium, may also cause osteoporosis.

Treatment

Diet plays an important role in the treatment of osteoporosis. To begin with, the patient should adopt a raw-juice diet for about five days. In this regimen, he should take juices of fresh fruits and vegetables, diluted with water on 50 : 50 basis, every two hours during the day. Fruits and vegetables which can be used for juices are orange, lemon, pineapple, papaya, green leafy vegetables, red beet and carrot. A warm water enema should be taken daily during this period to cleanse the bowels.

After the raw juice diet, the patient may gradually embark upon a well-balanced diet consisting of seeds, nuts, grains, vegetables and fruits. The emphasis should be on mineral-rich foods such as whole grains, seeds, nuts, cooked and raw vegetables and fruits, milk and milk products such as homemade cottage cheese.

Foods rich in Calcium, magnesium, potassium and silicon will be specially beneficial in the treatment of this disorder. These four are green vegetables, cabbage, carrots, fruits and berries of all kinds. Strawberries, raspberries, blueberries, sesame seeds and sunflower seeds are excellent foods for use in this disease.

The patient should also take liberal quantities of foods rich in lactic acid, sour milk products, oats, barley, millet and rice.

The diet should be supplemented with a good all-inclusive mineral and trace mineral supplement and Betaine Hydrochloride tablets with each meal to ensure proper assimilation.

The patient should avoid large meals and overeating. He should eat slowly and chew his food extremely well. He should avoid tea, coffee, flesh food, white sugar and white flour products, processed, refined and denatured foods, smoking and alcoholic beverages are completely forbidden.

Latest studies indicate that trace mineral boron can exercise great influence on osteoporosis. This mineral is found in fruits and nuts. A deficiency of baron can hamper calcium metabolism, and thereby make the bones brittle. New research shows that boron dramatically boosts blood levels of the hormone oestrogen and other compounds that prevent calcium loss and bone demineralization. Boron can thus serve as a mild 'oestrogen replacement therapy.'

The liberal use of pineapple is considered beneficial in the prevention and treatment of osteoporosis and bone fractures. This is attributable to high content of manganese in the fruit. In a study Dr. Freeland-Graves, professor of nutrition at the university of Texas at Austin, discovered that women with osteoporosis had about one-third less manganese in their blood than healthy women. Further, when given manganese the diseased woman absorbed twice as much, showing that their bodies needed it.

The patient should undertake regular physical exercise for the prevention and treatment of osteoporosis. Exercises which put stress on long bones such as walking, jogging and cycling will be specially beneficial.

CHAPTER 108

Parkinson's Disease

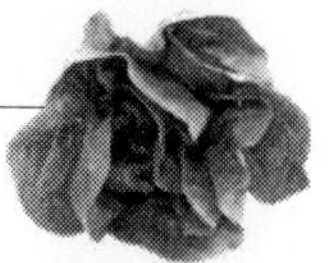

Parkinson's disease, also known as Paralysis agitans or shaking palsy, is serious chronic disease of the nervous system. It is characterised by stiffness of muscles and a continuous tremor or shake. It is a disease of the extra-pyramidal system.

Symptoms

The description of the disease originally given by Dr. James Parkinson of Shoreditch in 1817 is as follows: 'involuntary tremulous motion, which lessened muscular power, in parts not in action and even when supported, with a propensity to bend the trunk forwards, and to pass from a walking to a running pace, the senses and intellect being uninjured'. The patient shows a combination of tremor of the limbs and muscular stiffness. These tremors are more noticeable when the patient is at rest, and tend to disappear when he attempts to move or when he is asleep. The tremors are more pronounced, when he is excited or fatigued.

Older patients occasionally exhibit involuntary rapid jerking movements of their arms and legs. In a less extreme form the condition presents as purposeless mastication and lip smacking movements. The condition is embarrassing both to the patient and his relatives, but; is not associated with mental impairment and rarely causes severe incapacity.

Later, there may be impairment of speech, and the patient may complain of cramping pains in the back because of muscle spasm. His mind usually remains clear, and his other sensations are normal. In many cases, the patient may have only a mild form of Parkinson's disease and continue this way for many years before any serious symptoms develop. In severe and advanced cases, however, the patient is not able to move, and presents a distressing spectacle, for his mind may be uninjured while he cannot speak or write.

Causes

The brain changes that lead to parkinsonism are not fully understood. It, however, appears that they involve the nerve cells containing melanin, the pigment that gives skin its colour. These cells, called substantia nigra, are concentrated in the part of the brain called the basal ganglia. As the cells deteriorate, production of dopamine-a chemical that carries messages within the brain-falls, and the result is the characteristic symptoms.

Parkinsons' disease may follow severe attacks of encephalitis or some type of poisoning, such as carbon monoxide. In older patients, this type of palsy may be due to hardening of the arteries in certain vessels leading to the brain. In most cases, however, the disease begins to show itself in later middle age, and is considered to be a consequence of 'degeneration', particularly in the basal ganglia.

Parkinson's disease may also result from deficiency of antioxidant Vitamin E earlier in life. According to Dr Lawrence Golbe, M.D., a neurologist at the University of Medicine and Dentistry of New Jersey, too little Vitamin E foods earlier in life may somehow leave the brain vulnerable to the onset of Parkinson's years later. In most cases the cause of Parkinson's disease, is unknown.

Treatment

Diet plays an important role in the treatment of Parkinson's disease. To begin with, the patient should resort to a short juice fast for five days. In this regime, he should take a glass of fresh fruit or vegetable juice, diluted with water on 50 : 50 basis, every two hours from 8 a.m. to 8 p.m. Fruits and vegetables which may be used for juices are apple, pineapple, grapes, orange, tomato, carrot, cabbage and spinach. A warm water enema should be used daily to cleanse the bowels during the period of fasting.

After the short juice fast, the patient may adopt an all fruit diet for further 5 days. During this period, he should take three meals a day of fresh juicy fruits, such as apple, pear, peach, papaya, grapes, orange and pineapple, at five-hourly intervals. Thereafter, he may gradually adopt a well-balanced lacto-vegetarian diet. The emphasis should be on raw seeds, nuts and grains, plenty of sprouts, raw milk, preferably goat's milk, and raw fruits and vegetables. Green leafy vegetables and yellow turnips are especially beneficial. Sesame seeds and sesame seed butter can be taken with beneficial results. In general, a low-protein diet of raw, organically grown foods is best for the patient with Parkinsons' disease.

The patient should avoid tea, coffee, chocolate, salt, spices, condiments, pickles, flesh foods, white flour and white sugar and all products made from them. He should also avoid all processed, tinned, canned and frozen foods. The short juice fast followed by an all fruit diet should be repeated at monthly intervals till condition improves.

The patient should always follow certain rules regarding eating. These include taking of water or other liquids half an hour before and one hour after a meal and not with meals, eating very slowly and chewing your food as thoroughly as possible and never eat to full stomach.

Use of vitamin E in high doses is considered beneficial in the treatment of Parkinsons' disease. There is preliminary evidence to suggest that massive doses of Vitamin E may slow down the progress of the disease. Extensive studies about the efficacy of vitamin E therapy for Parkinsons' disease are, however still being carried out.

Stress can lead to Parkinsonism, Meditation and relaxation methods, especially Shavasana can help reduce it. Combining meditation with yoga may also improve muscle tone and control. Meditation can also be helpful in inducing sleep, if insomnia is a problem.

Everything possible should be done to help the patient to maintain a cheerful mental outlook. He should remain as active as possible and lead a quite life. Hot moist packs may be applied to the stiffened muscles which should also be gently massaged. The daily warm bath are useful. Fresh air and light exercise, especially walking, are essential to the treatment of Parkinson's disease.

CHAPTER 109

Peptic Ulcer

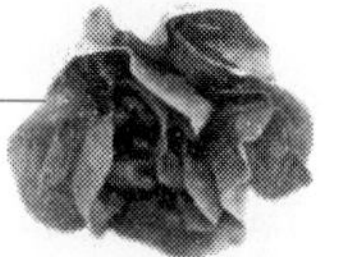

Peptic ulcer refers to an eroded lesion in the gastric intestinal mucosa. An ulcer may form in any part of the digestive tract which is exposed to acid gastric juice, but is usually found in the stomach and the duodenum. The ulcer located in the stomach is known as gastric ulcer and that located in the duodenum is called a duodenal ulcer. Usually both are grouped together and termed peptic ulcer.

Symptoms

The most common symptoms of peptic ulcer are sharp and severe pain and discomfort in the upper central abdomen. The pain is commonly described as burning or gnawing in character. Gastric ulcer pain usually occurs an hour after meals, but rarely at night. Duodenal ulcer pain usually occurs between meals when the stomach is empty and is relieved by food, especially milk. It is often described as hunger pain and gets the sufferer out of bed between 2 and 4 a.m. As the disease progresses there is distension of the stomach due to excessive flatulence, besides mental tension, insomnia and a gradual weakening of the body. It may also cause constipation with occasional blood in the stools. If an ulcer bleeds slowly, there is anaemia.

Causes

Peptic ulcers result from hyperacidity which is a condition caused by an increase in hydrochloric acid in the stomach. This strong acid, secreted by the cells lining the stomach, affects much of the breakdown of food. It can be potentially dangerous and, under certain circumstances, it may eat its way through the lining of the stomach or duodenum producing, first, irritation of the stomach wall and eventually an ulcer.

Dietetic indiscretion, like overeating, taking of heavy meals or highly spiced foods, coffee, alcohol and smoking are the main factors contributing to this condition. The ingestion of certain drugs, particularly aspirin, food poisoning, infections like influenza and septicaemia and gout may also cause ulcers. Emotional stress or nervous tension also plays a major role in the formation of ulcers.

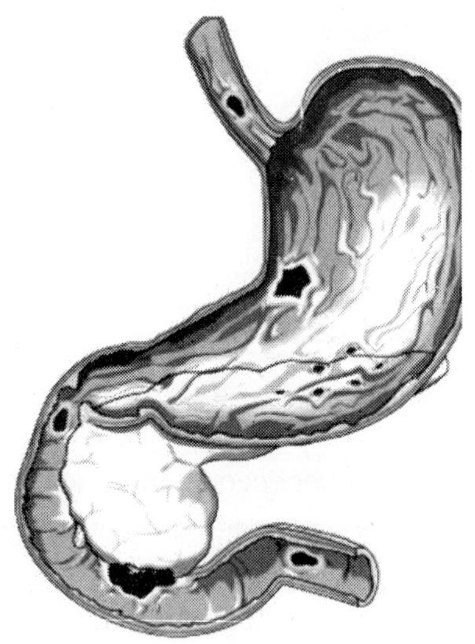

Peptic ulcer

Treatment

Diet is of utmost importance in the treatment of ulcer. The diet should be so arranged as to provide adequate nutrition to afford rest to the disturbed organs, to maintain continuous neutralisation of the gastric acid, to inhibit the production of acid and to reduce mechanical and chemical irritation. Milk, cream, butter, fruits and fresh, raw and boiled vegetables, natural foods and natural vitamin supplements are the best diet for an ulcer patient.

The most effective remedy for peptic ulcers is bananas. They are said to contain an unidentified compound called, perhaps jokingly, vitamin U (against ulcers). Banana neutralises the overacidity of the gastric juices and reduces the irritation of the ulcer by coating the lining of the stomach. Banana and milk are considered an ideal diet for the patients who are in an advanced state of the disease.

Almond milk made from blanched almonds in a blender is very beneficial as it binds the excess of acid in the stomach and supplies high quality protein. Raw goat's milk is also highly beneficial. It actually helps to heal peptic ulcer.

Cabbage is regarded as another useful home remedy for peptic ulcers. Cabbage is boiled in water. This water is allowed to cool and taken twice daily. The leaves of kalyana murangal tree, which is a variety of drumstick found in South India, have also proved helpful in the healing of ulcers. The leaves of this tree are ground into a paste and taken mixed with yogurt daily.

Raw vegetable juices, particularly carrot and cabbage juices are beneficial in the treatment of peptic ulcers. Carrot juice may be taken either alone or in combination with spinach or beet and cucumber. The formula proportions in case of the first combination are 300 ml. of carrots and 200 ml. of spinach, and in case of the second combination, 300 ml. of carrots and three ounces each of beets and cucumbers to make half a litre of juice.

The observance of certain rules by an ulcer patient with regard to eating habits are essential. He should never eat when tired or emotionally upset, nor when he is not hungry even if it is meal time, nor when his mouth is dry. He should chew every morsel thoroughly. He should eat only natural foods and take food in as dry a form as possible. Meals must be small and frequent. All foods and drinks which are either too hot or too cold should be avoided.

The ulcer patient should drink eight to 10 glasses of water every day. However, he should not drink water during or with meals, but only half an hour before or one hour after he has eaten. He should bathe, preferably in cold water, twice daily. Alternate hot and cold hip baths for 10 to 15 minutes and a mud pack applied over the lower abdomen for half an hour daily will help the ulcers to heal. The hip bath or the mud pack should be taken on an empty stomach and should be followed by a walk. In case of haemorrhage in the stomach, a rectal enema should be administered four times daily with water temperature at 110 to 115°F. In case of abdominal or stomach pain, hot packs should be placed on the abdomen with water temperature at 120°F. A hot pack should also be placed between the shoulder blades.

Daily massages and deep breathing exercises also help. Above all, the patient must try to rid himself of worries and stay cheerful. He should also cultivate regularity in his habit— be it work, exercise or rest. Asanas which are beneficial in the treatment of hyperacidity and ulcers are vajrasana, uttanpadasana, pavanamuktasana, bhujangasana, paschimottanasana. Yogic kriyas like jalneti and pranayamas like anuloma-viloma, shitali and sitkari are also beneficial.

Hyperacidity does not appear suddenly; it develops gradually and its cure is also a gradual process. The patient should not lose patience but must continue the regimen suggested; this will help him get relief from his ailment.

CHAPTER 110

Piles

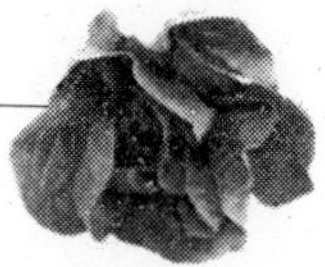

Piles or haemorrhoids are among the most common ailments today, especially in the Western world. They are a varicose and often inflamed condition of the veins inside or just outside the rectum. In external piles there is a lot of pain, but not much bleeding. In case of internal piles there is discharge of dark blood. In some cases the veins burst and this results in what is known as bleeding piles.

Symptoms

Pain at passing stools, slight bleeding in the case of internal trouble, and a feeling of soreness and irritation after passing a stool are the usual symptoms of piles. The patient cannot sit comfortably due to itching, discomfort and pain in the rectal region.

Causes

The primary cause of piles is chronic constipation and other bowel disorders. The pressure applied to pass a stool to evacuate constipated bowels and the congestion caused by constipation ultimately lead to piles. The use of purgatives to relieve constipation, by their irritating and weakening effect on the lining of the rectum, also result in enlargement and inflammation of veins and bleeding of the mucus lining. Piles are more common during pregnancy and in conditions affecting the liver and upper bowel, Prolonged periods of standing or sitting, strenuous work, obesity and general weakness of the tissues of the body are the other contributory causes of piles.

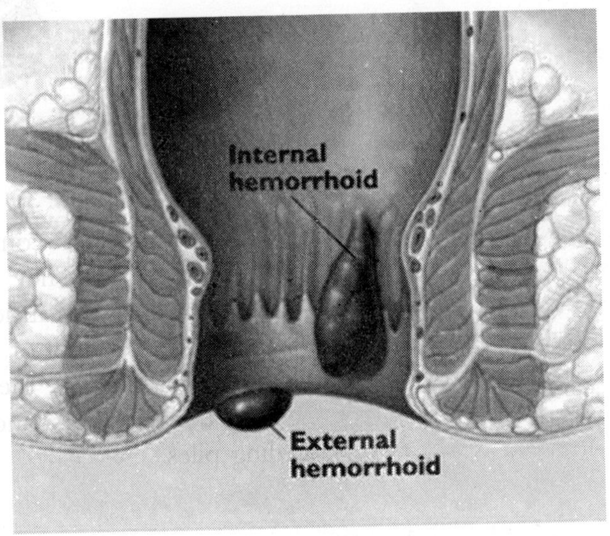

Internal Haemorrhoid and External Haemorrhoids

Mental tension is also one of the main causes of haemorrhoids. Persons who are always in a hurry often strain while passing stools. They rush through defecation instead of making it a relaxed affair. The pressure thus exerted by the anal muscles affect the surrounding tissues. The extra rectal pressure and the resultant congestion of veins ultimately leads to haemorrhoids. There is probably a hereditary factor also involved in the development of piles.

Treatment

The treatment of the basic cause, namely, chronic constipation, is the only way to get rid of the trouble. To begin with, the whole digestive tract must be given a complete rest for a few days and the intestines thoroughly cleansed. For this purpose the patient should adopt an all-fruit diet for at least seven days. After the all-fruit diet, the patient may adopt a diet of natural foods aimed at securing soft stools.

The most important food remedy for piles is dry figs. Three or four figs should be soaked overnight in water after cleansing them thoroughly in hot water. They should be taken the first thing in the morning along with the water in which they were soaked. They should also be taken in the evening in a similar manner. This treatment should be continued for three or four weeks. The tiny seeds of the fruit possess an excellent quality of stimulating peristaltic movements of intestines. This facilitates easy evacuation of faeces and keeps the alimentary canal clean. The pressure on the anus having thus been relieved, the haemorrhoids also get contracted.

Mango seeds are regarded as an effective remedy for bleeding piles. The seeds should be collected during the mango season, dried in the shade and powdered and kept stored for use as medicine. It should be given in doses of about one and a half gram to two grams with or without honey.

The jambul fruit is another effective food remedy for bleeding piles. The fruit should be taken with salt every morning for two or three months in its season. The use of the fruit in this manner in every season will effect a radical cure and save the user from bleeding piles during his/her entire life.

White radish is considered highly valuable in the treatment of piles. Grated radish mixed with honey may be taken in this condition. This vegetable can also be taken in the form of juice mixed with a pinch of salt. It should be given in doses of 60 to 90 ml. in the morning and evening. White radish well ground into a paste in milk can also be beneficially applied over inflamed pile masses to relieve pain and swelling.

The patient should drink at least six to eight glasses of water a day. He should avoid straining to pass a stool. Cold water treatment helps the veins to shrink and tones up their walls. The treatment is done by sitting in a tub filled with cold water for two minutes with knees drawn up to your chin. The water level should cover the hips. This should be done twice a day. Other water treatments beneficial in curing piles include cold perineal douche and cold compress applied to the rectal area for an hour before bedtime.

A patient with piles must make an all-out effort to tone up the entire system. Exercise plays an important corrective role in this condition. Movements which exercise the abdominal muscles will improve circulation in the rectal region and relieve congestion. Outdoor exercises such as walking and swimming are excellent methods of building up general health. Yogic kriyas like jalneti and vamandhouti and asanas such as sarvangasana, vipritakarani, halasana and gomukhasana are also useful. Sarvangasana is especially beneficial as it drains stagnant blood from the anus.

CHAPTER 111

Pleurisy

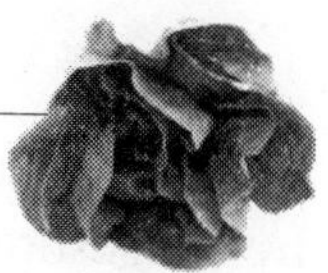

Pleurisy is an inflammation of the pleura, a serous membrane which envelopes the lungs and also lines the inside of the chest. It may be acute or chronic, and mild or severe. The disease may be limited to one side of the chest or it may include both the sides.

This disease can attack people of all ages, from children to the very elderly. Like any other viral infection, pleurisy can occur in small epidemics.

The membranes that cover the lungs are called pleura. The outer membrane, known as parital pleura, is applied to the inner wall of the thorax, and the inner membrane, known as the visceral pleura, covers the substance of the lungs. There is a capillary space between the two membranes, which is filled with fluid. This fluid enables the lungs to move freely in the chest. The parietal membrane is reflected from the chest wall to cover the upper surface of the diaphragm, and in the midline, it covers the mediastinum, the partition which separates the two sides of the chest and contains the heart, great vessels and other structures which run through the thorax.

Symptoms

The onset of pleurisy is generally marked by a sharp and stabbing pain, which may be felt in any part of the chest wall or over the diaphragm. Deep breathing or coughing increases the pain. In many cases, the disease begins with a chill, followed by congestion of the pleura and later by fever. The degree of the fever determines the severity of the disease. The inflammation destroys the tissues and chokes the circulation within the tissues. Breathing becomes difficult due to clogging of the circulation, and pain and swelling within the chest. Later a liquid effusion escapes from the pleura, filling the open spaces in the chest cavity till the effect of the distension becomes oppressive. After absorption takes place or after a drainage of the effusion, the pressure is lowered, the pain is reduced and the patient feels relieved. It is sometimes dry pleurisy, a form where there is little or no effusion, or the

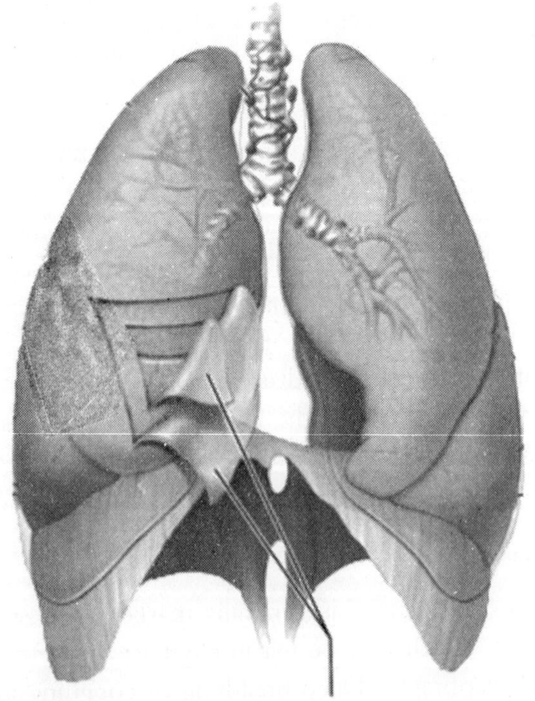

Two layers of Pleura

effusion may be circumscribed. The effusion may become gangrenous, or become mixed with blood, or be of a dirty brown colour with an offensive odour, leading to much suffering.

Causes

The most common among the immediate causes of pleurisy is that of 'catching cold' followed by congestion and swelling of the pleural membrane. It is a disease that is not caused by germs. There will be germs of putrefaction later in the ooze of serum from the tissue. The disease may be a complication of pneumonia, or pneumonia may be a complication of pleurisy. In a few cases, the diseases may also occur in rheumatic fever, uraemia and other conditions.

Treatment

At the first sign of pleurisy, the patient should observe a complete fast, abstaining from all liquid and solid foods. Nothing should be taken except plain water, hot or cold, as desired. Water may have bad taste, but at least three or four glasses should be taken daily for the first few days. The quantity of water should be gradually increased to five or six or more glasses each day. It would be helpful if during this period of fasting, a full hot enema is also taken once daily.

A hot chest pack should be applied two or three times a day, allowing it to remain for an hour or so each time. If the fever becomes high, the packs may be changed to cold ones. If, however the reaction is not prompt and complete, it would be advisable to use the hot packs.

Heat is always helpful for relieving the sharp pain associated with pleurisy. This should be applied for half an hour twice daily. The patient should practise deep breathing during this treatment. Adequate rest and abundant fresh air are essential.

In cases of dry pleurisy, further relief from the pain can be obtained by strapping the chest. Heat is not used when the taping is employed. A neutral immersion bath at 100°F for one hour daily has also been found beneficial in the treatment of pleurisy.

After the acute symptoms have subsided, the patient may adopt a milk diet. In this regimen, he should take 250 ml, of milk every two hours on the first day, every 1½ hour on the second day, every hour on the third day and every three-quarters of an hour on the fourth day and onwards. The quantity of milk should not exceed four litres daily. The patient may also take one orange daily along with the milk diet.

As soon as the patient has slightly gained some strength, he should undertake moderate exercise as a routine, avoiding fatigue. Air bath, sun bath and dry friction bath are of particular importance. If there is any particular disease present along with the pleurisy whether as a causative or as a complicating condition the same should also be given appropriate attention.

Chronic pleurisy should be treated in the same manner as to diet and the application of heat. All efforts should be made to increase the vitality, reduce toxaemia, and restore normal freedom of chest movements. Several short fasts, at regular intervals, followed by milk diet may be necessary depending on the progress for complete recovery.

CHAPTER 112

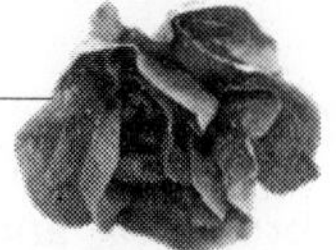

Pneumonia

Pneumonia refers to the acute inflammation of the lungs. It is one of the most serious infectious diseases. There are basically two types of pneumonia, called lobar pneumonia and broncho-pneumonia. They, however, run into each other and are treated in the same way. The disease becomes more serious if both the lungs are affected. It is called double pneumonia in common parlance.

Symptoms

Most cases of pneumonia begin with a cold in the head or

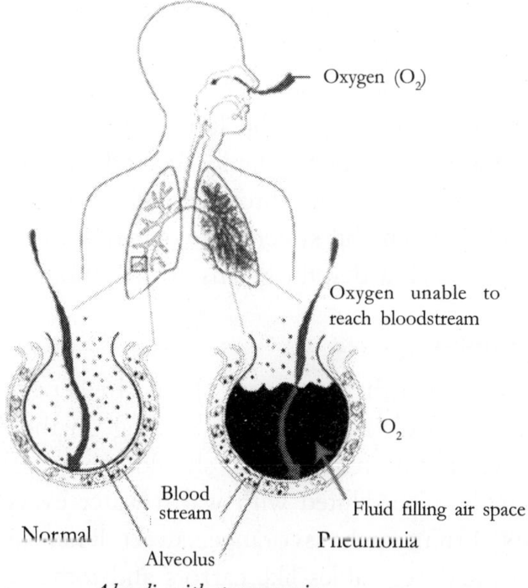

Alveoli with pneumonia

throat. The patient generally feels chill, shivering, difficulty in breathing and sharp pain in the chest. This may be followed by a cough with pinkish sputum which may later become brownish. The patient usually suffers from fever and headache. In more serious cases of pneumonia, the sputum may be of rusty colour. In young children, the disease may cause delirium and convulsions. Most patients feel very miserable and sweat profusely. The temperature may rise to 105°F and pulse may go upto 150 beats per minute. A common complication of all kinds of pneumonia is pleurisy.

Causes

Pneumonia is caused by various types of germs such as streptococcus, staphyloccus and pneumococcus varieties. At times, certain viruses are also responsible for the disease. Other causes of this disease are fungal infection, irritation by worms, inhaling foreign matter, irritant dust or noxious gases and vapours such as ammonia, nitrogen dioxide or cadmium. The real cause of pneumonia, however, is the toxic condition of the body, especially of the lungs and air passages, resulting from wrong feeding and faulty life style. Persons with healthy tissues and strong vital force are unlikely to catch pneumonia. It is only when the system is clogged with toxic matter and the vitality is low that the germs of pneumonia invade a person.

Treatment

To begin with, the patient should be kept on a diet of raw juices for five to ten days, depending on the severity of the disease. In this regimen, he should take a glass of fruit or vegetable juice diluted with warm water every two or three' hours. Fruits such as orange, sweet lime, apple, pineapple, grapes and vegetables like carrots and tomatoes may be used for juices.

After a diet of raw juices, when the fever subsides, the patient should spend three or four further days on an exclusive fresh fruit diet, taking three meals a day of juicy fruits such as apple, grapes, pineapple, mangoes, orange, lemon and papaya. Thereafter he may gradually adopt a well-balanced diet of natural foods consisting of seeds, nuts and grains, vegetables and fruits with emphasis on fresh fruits and raw vegetables. The patient should be given warm water enema daily to cleanse the bowels during the period of raw juice therapy and all fruit diet and thereafter, when necessary.

The patient should avoid strong tea, coffee, refined foods, fried foods, white sugar, white flour and all products made from them, condiments and pickles. He should also avoid all meats as well as alcoholic beverages and smoking.

To reduce temperature naturally, during the course of the fever, the procedure outlined in the chapter on malaria may be followed. Sipping of cold water has also been found beneficial in the treatment of pneumonia. The patient should sip cold water at short intervals so long as the fever continues. The cold water is cooling to the feverish blood.

Home Remedies

Certain home remedies have been found beneficial in the treatment of pneumonia. During the early acute stage of this disease, a herbal tea made from fenugreek seeds will help the body to produce perspiration, dispel toxicity and shorten the period of fever. It can be taken upto four cups daily. The quantity should be reduced as condition improves. To improve flavour, a few drops of lemon juice can be used. During this treatment, no other food or nourishment should be taken as fasting and fenugreek will allow the body to correct these respiratory problems in a few days.

According to Dr. F.W. Crosman, an eminent physician, garlic is a marvellous remedy for pneumonia, if given in sufficient quantities. This physician used garlic for many years in the treatment of pneumonia, and said that in no instance did it fail to bring down the temperature as well as the pulse and respiration within 48 hours. Garlic juice can also be applied externally to the chest with beneficial results as it is an irritant and rubefacient.

Sesame seeds (*til*) are valuable in pneumonia. An infusion of the seeds, mixed with a tablespoon of linseed, a pinch of common salt and a desertspoon of honey, should be given in the treatment of this disease. This will help remove catarrhal matter and phlegm from the bronchial-tubes.

The pain of pneumonia can be relieved by rubbing oil of turpentine over the rib cage and wrapping warmed cotton wool over it.

CHAPTER 113

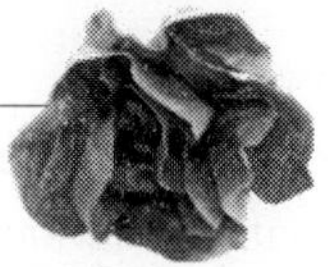

Premature Greying of Hair

The hair has a tendency to lose its natural colour with advancing age. It is therefore natural for the hair to turn grey with age. But premature greying is a morbid condition and it makes even the young look older. This causes a great deal of concern to affected persons, especially women.

The hair is an appendage of the skin. It is composed of the same kind of cells as are found in the outer layer of the skin, known as epidermis. It grows from a hair follicle which is a deep recess in the epidermis. The sebaceous glands of the scalp secrete an oily substance called sebum, which is the source of nutrition, lustre and blackness of the hair. The hair cannot be fed externally, for such nourishment as the scalp requires must come to it from the bloodstream.

Causes of Greying

A faulty diet and mental worries are the two primary causes of premature greying of hair. It is mainly due to the lack of some of the B vitamins, of iron, copper and iodine in the daily diet that this hair disorder is caused at a young age these days. Mental worries produce an extraordinary tension in the skin of the scalp which interferes with the supply of vital nutrition necessary for the health of the hair. Similarly, anxieties, fear, jealousy and failures have adverse effects on the hair. They dry out the scalpular marrow, the vital sap at the root of the hair.

Other causes of premature greying of hair are unclean condition of the scalp which weakens the roots of the hair as the pores are blocked by the collected dirt; washing the hair with hot water and drying them with electric dryers which emit a blast of hot air; the use of hair dyes in the earlier stages when the hair have just started greying; diseases like chronic cold, sinusitis, anaemia, chronic constipation; and the use of factory-made hair oils, which are generally cleaned with acids and some of the acids have a tendency to remain in the oil. Heredity is another predisposing factor which gives rise to this ailment.

Treatment

Diet is of utmost importance in the prevention and treatment of premature greying of hair and persons suffering from this disorder should take a diet rich in all essential nutrients. The vitamins considered useful in premature greying of hair are pantothenic acid, para-aminobenzoic acid or PABA and inositol. The minimum daily requirement of these vitamins appears to be 10 mg. of pantothenic acid, 100 gm. of para-aminobenzoic acid and 2000 mg. of inositol. To obtain satisfactory results, all three of these vitamins, belonging to B group, should be supplied at one time preferably in a form which gives all B vitamins, such as yeast, wheat germ and liver. The three anti-grey hair vitamins can be produced in the intestinal tract by bacteria. Thus drinking a litre of yogurt daily with a tablespoon of yeast before each meal will be an excellent remedy for the prevention and treatment of premature greying of hair. If one wishes to take tablets of calcium pantothenate and paba, they should be taken in addition to the yeast and yogurt and not as a substitute for them.

Gayelord Hauser, one of the best known world nutritionists, in his book, 'The New Diet Does it', claims that this treatment will restore the grey hair back to its natural colour. He also advises addition of iron and iodine in the form of sea food, to an otherwise adequate diet for obtaining better results. Besides fish, which is the main source of iodine, the requirement of this mineral can be met by adequate intake of carrots, bananas and similar other vegetables and fruits. Carrots are especially useful in furnishing fresh blood and maintaining the health of the hair.

Home Remedies

Certain home remedies have been found useful in the prevention and treatment of premature greying of hair. The foremost among these is the use of Indian gooseberry or *amla* which is a valuable hair tonic for enriching hair growth and hair pigmentation. The fruit, cut into pieces, should be dried, preferably in the shade. These pieces should be boiled in coconut oil till the solid matter become like charred dust. This darkish oil is very useful in preventing greying.

The water in which dried *amla* pieces are soaked overnight is also nourishing to the hair. This water should be used for

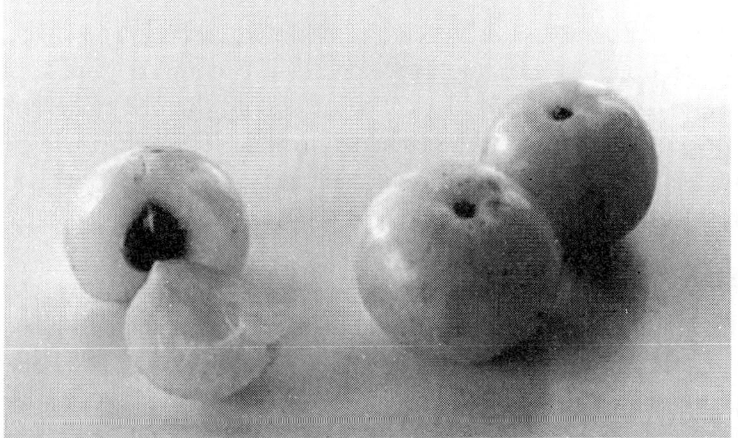

Indian gooseberry (amla) is considered highly beneficial in the treatment of premature greying of hair.

the last rinse while washing the hair. Massaging the scalp with a teaspoonful of *amla* juice mixed with a teaspoonful of almond oil or few drops of lime juice, every night has proved beneficial in the prevention and treatment of premature greying of hair.

Liberal intake of curry leaves is considered beneficial in preventing premature greying of hair. These have the property to give vitality and strength to hair roots. New hair roots that grow are healthier with normal pigment. The leaves can be used in the form of *chutney or* these may be squeezed in butter-milk or *lassi.* When the leaves are boiled in coconut oil, the oil forms an excellent hair tonic to stimulate hair growth and bring back hair pigmentation.

The butter made from cow's milk has the property to prevent premature greying of hair. A small roll may be taken internally and a little quantity may be massaged into the hair roots twice a week.

Ribbed gourd, known as *torai* in the vernacular, boiled in coconut oil is another effective remedy for premature greying of hair. Pieces of this vegetable should be dried in the shade. These dried pieces should be soaked in coconut oil and kept aside for three or four days. The oil should then be boiled till the solid is reduced to a blackened residue. This oil should be massaged into the scalp. It will help enrich the hair roots and restore pigment to the hair.

Hair Dye

The paste of henna leaves, boiled in coconut oil to get a darkish oil, can be used as a hair dye to blacken grey hair. The paste itself can be applied to the hair and washed away after a few hours to dye the grey hair. Washing the hair with concentrated tea extract twice a week is also considered useful in colouring grey hair to brown or black.

CHAPTER 114

Prostate Disorders

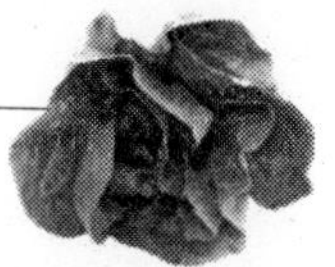

Nearly one-third of all men over 50 years suffer from prostate troubles of one form or another. The percentage rises with age and reaches 75 after the age of 80 years. Prostate and bladder disorders can lead to numerous other ailments such as arthritis, kidney disorders and uremia.

The prostate gland is a male gland, comparable in shape and size to a large chestnut. It is reddish brown in appearance. It measures approximately 3.8 cm. in width and about 2.5 cm. in length and weighs approximately 25 grams. It is situated at the base of the urinary bladder and around the commencement of the urethra, the membranous tube for the passage of the urine. It is thus vital in relation to the emptying of the bladder and bears a close relationship to the rectum. The gland plays an important role in normal sexual life and its function is to secrete a fluid which is added to semen during sexual intercourse.

Various Disorders

There are various types of prostate disorders. Of these the most important are prostatitis or inflammation in the prostate gland and hypertrophy or enlargement of the prostate gland. Prostatitis may be acute or chronic. It is a painful and distressing disorder, but can be cured with proper treatment without any adverse effects.

Enlargement of the prostate gland or hypertrophy is the most common complaint affecting the gland. This occurs

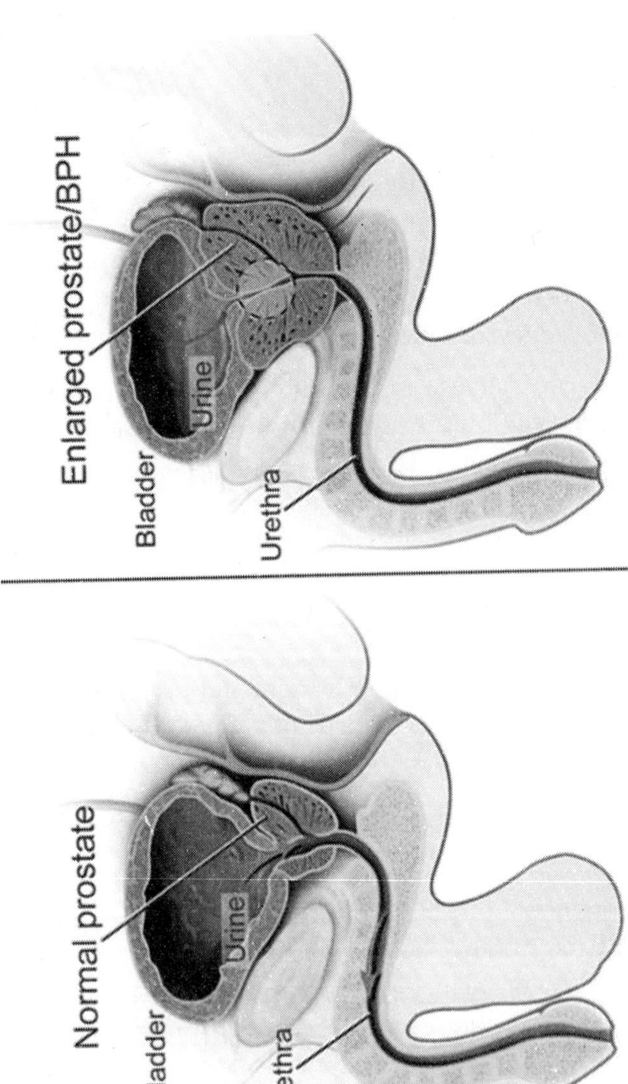

Kidney and bladder troubles

mostly in men of middle or advanced age. The enlargement develops so gradually over a long period that it often assumes serious proportions before it is detected.

Symptoms

There are two warning signals to indicate the possibility of prostate disorders. The first is the interference with the passage of urine and the second is the need to void the urine frequently during the night's sleep. Other symptoms are a dull aching pain in the lower back and pain in the hips, legs and feet. Prostate enlargement affects the glandular system as a whole. The patient experiences all the symptoms of disturbed health such as lack of energy and physical, mental and nervous disturbances.

Causes

The position of the prostate gland makes it liable to congestion and other disorders. In an erect position, pressure falls on the pelvic region just where the prostate gland is situated. With ageing, the body gets heavier and loses its flexibility which makes the pressure on the pelvis even greater and increases the vulnerability of the prostate gland. Prolonged periods of sitting down, as in certain occupations, also increases the pressure on the pelvic region resulting in congestion of the tissues in and around the prostate gland. With the passage of time, changes such as inflammation or enlargement occur in the gland. Acute prostatitis may also result from exposure to cold and chill and from an infectious disease. Chronic prostatitis is an after-effect of the acute condition. It may also result from continual irritation of the gland due to excessive sexual excitement.

Another important cause of prostate disorders is constipation. In constipation, the faeces becomes hardened and the rectum or lower bowel overloaded. This causes undue pressure on the prostate gland. It also entails a great deal of straining at stools and this adversely affects the prostate gland due to its proximity to the rectum.

Treatment

To begin with, the patient should forgo all solid foods and subsist on water only for two or three days. The intake of water should be as plentiful as possible. Nothing should be added to the water except a little lemon juice, if desired. The water may be taken cold or hot and it should be taken every hour or so when awake. This will greatly increase the flow of urine.

An enema may be taken once a day during fasting to clear the lower bowel of accumulations. After a thorough cleansing of the bowels, hot and cold applications may be used directly on the prostate gland and its surrounding parts. The heat relieves the tissues and a brief cold immersion tones them up. The patient should take alternate hot and cold hip baths. These are of great value in relieving pain and reducing congestion. The hot bath should be taken first for 10 minutes, followed by a cold bath for one minute only.

After the short fast, the patient should adopt an all-fruit diet for three days. The fruits should include apples, pears, oranges, grape-fruit, grapes, sweet limes, mangoes, melons and all other juicy fruits. This will help to clear toxins from the body and will also enable excess fat to be reduced to some extent.

The exclusive fruit diet should be followed by a diet, consisting of two meals of fruits and one of cooked vegetables for further seven days. The vegetable meal should be taken in the evening and should consist of all kinds of cooked vegetables, preferably steam cooked. Thereafter, the patient may adopt a well-balanced diet of three basic foods groups, namely (i) seeds, nuts and grains, (ii) vegetables and (iii) fruits.

The short lemon juice fast followed by an all-fruit diet and a further period on fruits and vegetables may be repeated after two or three months if necessary depending on the progress being made.

Pumpkin seeds have been found to be an effective home remedy for prostate problems and many patients have been helped by their use. These seeds are rich in unsaturated fatty acids which are essential to the health of the prostate.

Heavy starches, sweet stimulants and highly seasoned foods are entirely forbidden, as they cause direct irritation on the prostate gland and bladder. The diet should also exclude spices, condiments, salt in excess, sauces, red meats, cheese, asparagus, watercress, greasy or fried foods, alcohol, tobacco and too much tea or coffee. The patient should avoid hurried meals and must chew his food thoroughly and slowly. Water should be taken between meals and not at mealtime.

The patient should avoid sexual excess, irregularities in eating and drinking, long periods of sitting and vigorous exercise. He should guard against constipation by taking plenty of fruits, bran and nuts. All efforts should be made to tone up the general condition of the body. With a general improvement in health, the condition will be greatly relieved. Surgery should be resorted to only if the condition does not improve even after the dietary treatment and other measures outlined here.

CHAPTER 115

Psoriasis

Psoriasis is one of the most stubborn skin diseases. It is a chronic disease characterised by thick, red, silvery, scaled patches of skin. This disease affects both sexes equally and usually first appears at the age ranging from 15 to 30 years, although it may appear at any age. It is, however, rare in infancy and old age. Psoriasis is not contagious.

Symptoms

Generally, the skin of the person suffering from psoriasis appears red and irritated and may be covered with bright silvery scales. Sometimes there is also a little itching. Areas usually involved are elbows, knees, the skin behind the ears, trunk and scalp. The disease may also affect the underarm and genital areas. The lesions vary in size from minute papules only just visible, to sheets covering large parts of the body. Quite often, they are discs from 1.5 cm. to several centimetres in size. The lesions of psoriasis are always dry and rarely become infected.

Causes

The modern medical system has not been able to establish the exact cause of psoriasis. Recent studies have shown that psoriasis involves an abnormality in the mechanism in which the skin grows and replaces itself. This abnormality is related to the metabolism of amino-acids, the protein chemicals which are nature's basic building blocks for the reproduction of cell tissues. Heredity also plays a role in the development of psoriasis as it tends to occur in families. About 30 per cent of the patients have a family history of the disease.

The factors that aggravate and precipitate the outbreak of psoriasis are injury to the skin in the form of cuts, burns, minor abrasions, changes in the seasons, physical and emotional stress, infections and use of certain medicines for the treatment of other diseases.

Treatment

Since psoriasis is a metabolic disease, a cleansing juice fast for about seven days is always desirable in the beginning of treatment. Carrots, beets, cucumbers and grapes may be used for juices. Juices of citrus fruits should be avoided. The warm water enema should be used daily to cleanse the bowels during the fast. After the juice fast, the patient should adopt the diet of three basic food groups, namely (i) seeds, nuts and grains, (ii) vegetables and (iii) fruits, with emphasis on raw seeds and nuts, especially sesame seeds, pumpkin seeds, sunflower seeds and plenty of organically grown raw vegetables and fruits.

All animal fats, including milk, butter and eggs should be avoided. Refined or processed foods and foods containing hydrogenated fats or white sugar, all condiments, tea and coffee should also be avoided. After noticeable improvement, goat's milk, yogurt and home made cottage cheese may be added to the diet. Juice fast may be repeated after four weeks on diet.

Vitamin E therapy has been found effective in the treatment of psoriasis. The patient should use this vitamin in therapeutic doses from 200 to 800 I.U. a day. It will help reduce itching and scabs.

Lecithin is considered a remarkable remedy for psoriasis. The patient may take six to nine lecithin capsules a day—two or three capsules before or after each meal. In the form of granules, it may be taken four tablespoonfuls daily for two months. It may thereafter be reduced to two tablespoonfuls.

Too frequent baths should be avoided. Soap should not be used. Regular sea-water baths and application of sea water externally over the affected parts once a day are beneficial. The hot Epsom-salts bath has proved valuable in psoriasis. Three full baths should be taken weekly until the trouble begins to subside. The number of baths thereafter may be reduced to two weekly and finally to one. The affected areas should also be bathed twice in hot water containing Epsom salts. After the bath, a little olive oil may be applied. The skin should be kept absolutely clean by daily dry friction or sponge.

In many cases, psoriasis responds well to sunlight. The affected parts should be frequently exposed to the sun. The daily use of a sunlamp or ultra-violet light are also beneficial.

Cabbage leaves have been successfully used in the form of compresses in the treatment of psoriasis. The thickest and greenest outer leaves are most effective for use as compresses. They should be thoroughly washed in warm water and dried with a towel. The leaves should be made flat soft and smooth by rolling them with a rolling pin after removing the thick veins. They should be warmed and then applied smoothly to the affected part in an overlapping manner. A pad of soft woolen cloth should be put over it. The whole compress should then be secured with an elastic bandage.

The use of mud packs in the treatment of psoriasis has also been found highly beneficial. The packs are made by mixing the clay with a little water and applying to the affected areas. After the clay has dried, it is removed and fresh pack applied. Mud packs are eliminative in their action. They absorb and remove the toxins from the diseased areas.

The patient should undertake plenty of regular exercise in fresh air, especially exposing the affected parts, and deep breathing exercises. He should avoid all nervous tension and should have adequate rest.

CHAPTER 116

Pyorrhoea

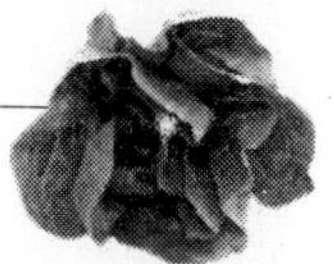

Pyorrhoea, or periodontal disease to give it a proper medical term, is a disease of the teeth socket. It is one of the most widely prevalent diseases these days. It affects the membrane surrounding the teeth-root, with loosening of the teeth, pus formation and shrinkage of the gum. This disease is the primary cause for tooth loss among adults.

Pyorrhoea affects persons of all ages. About half the adult population over the age of 18 suffer from early stages of this disease. Even children of five years or so may have signs of the disease. It progresses with increasing age. Unless treated properly, it may lead to loss of supporting bone of teeth and ultimately to tooth loss.

Symptoms

The gum becomes tender and on pressing pus oozes out along the margin of teeth. Pus from the cavities continually finds its way into the stomach. When the disease is far advanced, the gums become swollen and the stomach, being dosed with increasing quantities of pus, does not function properly. Sepsis may appear in various forms, digestion is disturbed, liver trouble sets in and the whole system is adversely affected.

Causes

Pyorrhoea is triggered by bacterial activity. A thin layer of harmful bacteria is continuously building up in our teeth. If it is not removed by tooth-cleansing, especially after meals, it forms an organised mass on the tooth surface in a short time. This is referred to as a "bacterial plaque" when accumulated, bacteria in plaque produce many toxins which irritate the gums, cause them to become inflamed, tender and bleed easily. The bacterial activity is, however, facilitated by the lowered vitality of the system caused by acidosis as a result of wrong feeding habits. The habitual use of white bread, white sugar, refined cereals and much meat, leads to swamping of the blood and tissues with acid waste matter, and to the development of disease in one form or another. Pyorrhoea is one of the many forms this swamping of the system with acid impurities takes.

Other factors contributing to the development of pyorrhoea include injury to the gums and supporting structures by physical and chemical irritants in the mouth, wrong brushing, stagnation of food particles and improper use of tooth picks. In many cases, prolonged tension and even allergy can lead to this disease. In some cases, the use of the pill and pregnancy can give rise to or aggravates the condition.

Treatment

Any treatment for pyorrhoea, to be effective, should be constitutional. It should aim at cleansing the blood and tissues of the acid impurities which are at the root of the trouble. The extraction of teeth affected with the disease will not help clear the systemic toxaemia.

The patient should begin the treatment with a short juice fast for three to five days. The juice of a fresh orange diluted with water on 50 : 50 basis, should be taken at two-hourly intervals from 8 a.m. to 8 p.m. during this period. If the orange juice does not agree, carrot juice may be taken. The bowel should be cleansed daily during this period with a warm water enema. If constipation is habitual, all steps should be taken for its eradication.

After the juice fast, the patient should spend a further three to five days on an exclusive fresh fruit diet. In this regimen, he should have three meals a day, at five-hourly intervals, of fresh juicy fruits such as apples, pears, grapes, grape-fruit, oranges, pineapple and melon. If losing much weight on the all-fruit diet, those already under weight may add a glass of milk to each fruit meal. Thereafter the patient may gradually embark upon a balanced diet, with emphasis on fresh fruits, green salads, whole meal bread, properly cooked vegetables, cheese, nuts and milk.

White bread, white sugar and all refined and tinned foods must be completely given up. Condiments, sauces, alcohol, coffee and strong tea as well as meat and other flesh foods should also be avoided. The patient should also keep away from starchy and sticky foods.

The teeth and gum, like other parts of the body require exercise. This can be achieved by eating hard and fibrous foods. Wheat is especially valuable in the prevention and treatment of pyorrhoea. It takes time to eat wheat chappaties and as it is generally taken with other foods, it compels the chewing of other foods also. This not only provides the needed exercise for the teeth and gum but also a great aid to digestion.

Chewing unripe guava is an excellent tonic for teeth and gums. It stops the bleeding from gums due to its styptic effect and richness in vitamin C. Chewing its tender leaves also helps in curing bleeding from gums and keeps the teeth healthy. A decoction of root-bark can also be beneficially used as mouth-wash for swollen gums.

Lemon and lime are also useful in pyorrhoea due to their

high vitamin C content. They strengthen the gums and teeth and are very effective for preventing and curing acute inflammations of the gum margins.

Raw spinach juice is another valuable food remedy for the prevention and treatment of pyorrhoea because of its beneficial effect on the teeth and gums. This effect is greatly enhanced if the spinach juice is taken in combination with carrot juice. A permanent aid for this affliction has been found in the use of natural raw foods and in drinking an ample quantity of carrot and spinach juice.

The daily dry friction and hip bath and the breathing and other exercises should form a part of the morning routine. A hot Epsom-salts bath taken twice weekly will also be beneficial.

As regards local treatment, the teeth should be cleansed every morning and night with a little lemon juice squeezed on the toothbrush, after it has been dipped into warm water. Afterwards mouth should be well rinsed with warm water containing lemon juice. The forefinger of the right hand should be rubbed gently over the gums for a minute or two after each brushing.

CHAPTER 117

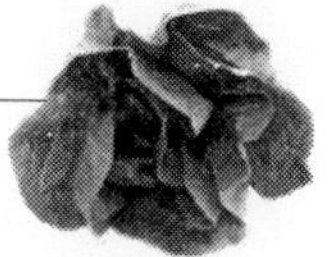

Rheumatism

The word rheumatism is derived from the Greek word "rheuma", which means a swelling. This disease is recognised as one of the most serious threats to health. It is a crippling disease which causes widespread invalidism, but seldom kills.

Rheumatism refers to an acute or chronic illness which is characterised by pain and swelling of the muscles, ligaments and tendons or of the joints. It affects men and women, both young and old. Quite often, this disorder extends to the heart and the valves and the lining of this vital organ becomes inflamed. It is the most common cause in 80 per cent of the cases of valvular organic diseases of the heart.

Rheumatism, perhaps, more than any other disease, although readily diagnosed, is never the same in any two individuals. There are too many variations in the development of this disease. Broadly speaking, however, rheumatism, which may be acute or chronic, can be roughly grouped into two classes. These are muscular rheumatism which affects the muscles and articular rheumatism which affects the joints. The muscular variety is, however, far less common than that affecting the joints. In the acute form, it is often found among children and young people, but in the chronic form, it is generally confined to the adults.

Symptoms

The onset of the acute type of rheumatism is characterised

by fever and rapid pulse with intense soreness and pain. In the acute muscular type, the tissues become so sensitive that even the weight of bed clothing aggravates the pain. The liver is found to be swollen. Acute rheumatism is extremely painful but it leaves no permanent defects, if treated properly. It may settle into a chronic state under a wrong mode of treatment.

The symptoms of chronic muscular rheumatism are pain and stiffness of the affected muscles. The pain increases when an effort is made to move these muscles. In case of chronic articular rheumatism, pain and stiffness are felt in one or more joints of the body, with swelling in most cases. It is not usually fatal but there is a danger of permanent deformity.

Causes

The chief cause of rheumatism is the poisoning of the blood with acid wastes, which results from imperfect elimination and lowered vitality. Meat, white bread, sugar and refined cereals, to which modern man is most addicted, leave a large residue of acid toxic wastes in the system. These acid wastes are not neutralised due to absence of sufficient quantities of alkaline mineral salts in the foods eaten, This upsets the acid-alkaline balance in the body and produces the conditions described as acidosis.

When there is abundant vitality, excess acids are ejected almost before they reach any appreciable concentration in one or the other of the acute cleansing efforts such as colds and fevers. When the vitality is low, the acid wastes are concentrated around the joints and bony structure, where they form the basis of rheumatism. The reason why large quantities of acid wastes piling up in the system are attracted towards body structure for storage is that lime, which is the most prominent constituent of the bony structure, and is an alkaline substance.

In certain cases, infection from the teeth, tonsils and gall bladder may produce rheumatism. The disease is aggravated by exposure to cold water.

Treatment

In the case of acute rheumatism, the patient should be put on a short fast of orange juice and water for three or four days. While fasting, the bowels should be cleansed through a warm water enema. After the juice fast, the patient should be placed on a restricted diet for 14 days. In this regimen, orange or grapefruit may be taken for breakfast, lunch may consist of a raw salad of any vegetables in season, with raisins, prunes, figs, or dates; and for dinner, one or two steamed vegetables such as spinach, cabbage, carrots, turnips, cauliflower etc., and a few nuts or some sweet fruit may be taken. No bread or potatoes or other starchy food should be taken; otherwise the effect of the diet will be lost. Thereafter, the patient may gradually commence a well balanced diet of three basic food groups, namely (i) seeds, nuts and grains (ii) vegetables and (iii) fruits.

In case of chronic rheumatism, the patient may be placed on an all-fruit diet for four or five days. In this regimen, he should have three meals a day of fresh, juicy fruits such as apples, grapes, peaches, pears, oranges, pineapples and grapefruit. He may thereafter gradually adopt a well-balanced diet.

The patient should take ripe fruits and fresh vegetables in abundance. Lots of buttermilk should be taken. The foods which should be avoided are meat, fish, white bread, sugar, refined cereals, rich, indigestible and highly seasoned foods, tea, coffee, alcohol, sauces, pickles and condiments.

Raw potato juice is regarded as an excellent food remedy for rheumatism. One or two teaspoonsful of the juice pressed out of mashed raw potato should be taken before meals. This will help eliminate an acid condition and relieve rheumatism. In some rural areas in Great Britain, it is a custom for rheumatic sufferers to carry a potato in their pockets, in the belief that the potato will absorb in itself some of the acid from the sufferer's body. The old potato is thrown away and replaced by a new one after a few days.

The skin of the potato is also an excellent food remedy for rheumatism. The skin is exceptionally rich in vital mineral salts and the water in which the peelings have been boiled is one of the best medicines for the ailments caused by excess of acid in the system. The potato peelings should be thoroughly washed and boiled for a few minutes. The decoction should then be strained and a glassful of the same should be taken three or four times daily.

Celery is another effective food remedy for rheumatism. A fluid extract of the seeds is more powerful than the raw vegetable. This also has a tonic action on the stomach and kidneys. Five to ten drops of this fluid should be taken in hot water before meals. Powdered seeds can be used as a condiment. Lemons are also valuable and the juice of two or three lemons may be taken each day.

Other helpful methods in the treatment of rheumatism are application of radiant heat and hot packs to the affected parts, a hot tub bath, cabinet steam bath, dry friction and a sponge bath. Hot Epsom-salt baths are also beneficial and should be taken twice a week for three months in case of chronic rheumatism and once weekly thereafter. The affected parts should also be bathed twice daily in hot water containing Epsom-salt after which some olive oil should be applied. Fresh air, deep breathing and light outdoor exercises are also beneficial. Dampness and cold should be avoided.

CHAPTER 118

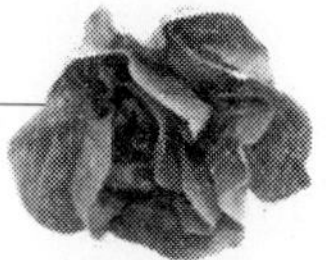

Rickets

The word ricket is derived from the Anglo-Saxon 'wrikken' which means 'to twist'. It is a deficiency disease of infancy and early childhood in which the bones are softened and deformed. The disease most likely makes its first appearance at the teething. It is known as the disease of poverty and darkness and is more prevalent in children of poor class.

The history of rickets as a deficiency disease is much older than our knowledge of preventing it. In the early 19th century, cod-liver oil was a well-known folk remedy, and later on as therapeutic agent for rickets in European countries. McColloumn, in 1922, isolated vitamin A and D from cod-liver oil and described vitamin D as an antirachitic vitamin which resists oxidation.

Symptoms

The child is restless, fretful and pale, with flabby and toneless muscles, which cause the limbs to assume unnatural postures. Excessive sweating of the head is common. The child's abdomen protrudes. He may suffer from diarrhoea and anaemia. The bones become soft and easily bent. Under the constant pull of the muscles, the joints lose their shape and are unable to function normally. In young infants, there may be a marked softening of the skull bones. The head may be flattened on one side. The chest is also deformed due to softening of ribs and is called pigeon breast. The marked weakness in the bones delays the child's ability to sit up, crawl and walk. The weight of his body may bend the bones and joints out of shape, causing such deformities as bow-legs and knock-knees.

Causes

Rickets arises as a result of deficiency of vitamin D. This vitamin is also essential for the proper absorption of calcium and phosphorus. It has been proved that poor absorption and metabolism of both these minerals, checks the formation of strong and healthy bones resulting in rickets. Sunlight prevents the disease by irritating the skin, which contains a provitamin which is changed into Vitamin D by ultra-violet light. Smoke in the cities prevents sunlight shining in the streets. In many tropical countries, where adequate sunshine is available the practice of covering the child from sunrays leads to this disease.

Another cause of rickets is relaxation of the solid parts, which may arise from being born of weak and sickly parents, or of those who have followed a wrong style of living and lived on faulty diet such as excessive intake of tea, coffee, sugar, fatty foods and white flour products, or who have had the venereal disease, which was not thoroughly cured.

Treatment

Rickets are generally curable especially in the initial stages. Proper nursing of the child, is very essential and all factors that might promote the disease must be carefully removed.

Diet is of utmost importance in the prevention and treatment of this disease. As far as possible, the child should be breast-fed for the first year of its existence. He should be given goat's or cow's milk, diluted with water, whenever breast feeding is not possible. Other foods should be introduced gradually, with emphasis on fruits, steamed vegetables, whole grain cereals and milk.

Adequate intake of Vitamin D and calcium is very essential for recovery. The child-patient should be given liberal quantities of Vitamin D-rich foods such as milk, cream and butter, eggs and fish liver oil. Vitamin D can also be given in supplement form from 1,000 to 4,000 I.U. per day for six to 12 weeks, depending on the severity of the disease. This can be followed by daily supplements of 200 to 400 I.U. which are adequate to prevent the development in otherwise normal children.

The best source of calcium is milk and a young child with rickets should drink at least 500 ml. per day. For severe cases, a supplement of calcium lactate should also be given orally. The diet after weaning may include daily an egg and butter. An adequate intake of iron and ascorbic acid is also necessary.

Besides proper diet and adequate intake of nutrients outlined above, all effects should be made to improve the hygienic environment of the child. Unnecessary clothing should be removed and if the child was previously confined indoors, he should be allowed to enjoy the sunshine and fresh air. Light massage once or twice a week will also be beneficial in the treatment of rickets.

Skeletol deformities could be corrected by maintaining a good posturs and bracing could help in ruducing deformities.

CHAPTER 119

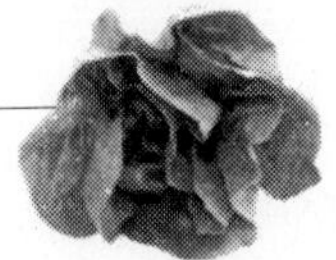

Ringworm

The word ringworm used for this disease does not correctly describe it. For the disease is not caused by any worm but by a fungus which is very minute form of vegetable plant life that grows on the skin.

The disease is more annoying than dangerous. It is serious only when the skin break up due to scratching and this leads to secondary infection.

Symptoms

Ringworm infection occurs in the scalp, the body, the feet and the nails. Ringworm of the scalp is most common in children because of the lack of protective fatty acids in their scalps. These fatty acids are produced only in adult life and make the scalp of an adult person resistant to ringworm infection. The infection is more frequent in boys than in girls because boys have shorter hair and the scalp is relatively less protected.

The disease spreads on the skin and extends deeper into the hair roots and also up along the hair. The affected hair becomes dull and breaks off near its root. This leaves bald spots on the scalp which may assume a shabby appearance on account of the raised grey scales that protrude from the infected areas. The patches of ringworm of the body are usually round or oval, with raised pink and scaly rings, which show a clean space in the centre. The itching in the infected parts helps to spread infection through the nails to other healthy parts of the body. If it is not treated for a long time, the infection becomes chronic and is, then, difficult to get rid of.

Ringworm of the body commonly affects the face and the neck. Ringworm of the feet, also known as 'athlete's foot' is more prevalent in summer. Infection is conveyed from one person to another through bath mats, bath tubs and swimming pools. The fungus, which causes the ringworm grow easily in the warm and moist parts of the body, thrives between the toes. It finds suitable place to live there on account of the perspiration in this region.

Causes

Ringworm is passed from an infected person to a healthy one by contact. It may also spread by use of articles such as towels of infected person. Sometimes, it is contracted from infected domestic animals, such as dogs and cats.

Treatment

The use of suppressive lotions or ointments for the treatment of ringworm may give temporary relief, but does not remove the cause. The best way to deal with this disease is to cleanse the blood stream and the body.

To begin with, the patient should be placed on an all-fruit diet for two or three days. He should take fresh juicy fruits, such as apple, orange, pineapple, papaya and pomegranate during this period. This will help eliminate morbid matter from the body and lead to substantial improvement. A warm-water enema may be administered during this period to cleanse the bowels, if possible.

Fruits, salt-free raw or steamed vegetables with whole wheat chappatis may be taken after the all-fruit diet. After a few days, curd and milk may be added to the diet. The patient may thereafter start with normal diet. The patient's emphasis should be on whole grain cereals, raw or lightly-cooked vegetable and fresh fruits. This diet may be supplemented with vegetable oils, honey and yeast.

The patient should avoid tea, coffee, all condiments, highly flavoured dishes, as well as sugar, white flour products, denatured cereals and tinned or bottled foods.

Certain home remedies have been found beneficial in the treatment of ringworm. One of the most effective of these is the use of mustard (*raye*) seeds. A paste made from these seeds should be applied externally over the areas affected with ringworm. The skin should be washed thoroughly with hot water, before application of this paste.

The use of raw papaya has also been proved beneficial in the treatment of ringworm. A few slices of this unripe fruit should be rubbed on the ringworm patches, twice daily. A paste made from dry seeds of papaya can also be applied beneficially on these patches.

The use of castor (*arandi*) oil, is valuable in case of ringworm on the head. This oil should be rubbed liberally on the affected parts. Noticeable improvement will be visible within two or three days.

Raw vegetable juices, especially carrot juice in combination with spinach juice, have proved beneficial in the treatment of ringworm. The formula proportions considered helpful in this combination are carrot juice 300 ml. and spinach 200 ml. to make 500 ml. of combined juice.

The patient should get as much fresh air as possible. He should drink plenty of water and bathe twice daily. The skin, with the exception of part affected with ringworm, should be vigorously rubbed with the palms of the hands before taking a bath.

Coconut oil may be applied to the portions with ringworm. It will help the skin to stay soft. Sunbathing is also beneficial and should be resorted to early in the morning, in the first light of dawn. A light mud pack applied over the sites of the ringworm is also helpful. The pack should be applied for half an hour twice daily.

CHAPTER 120

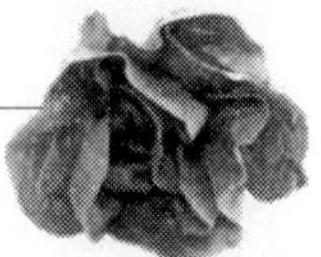

Scabies

Scabies is a skin infection, popularly known as itch. It is caused by the mite sarcoptes scabiei or itch-mite. It is a contagious disease and is more common among people who live in crowded places under unhygienic conditions. The incidence of scabies is highest in children under the age of 15 years.

Symptoms

The disease is characterised by severe itching. It tends to be more marked at night or after a hot bath. This is due to increased activity of the parasite because of the greater warmth of the body. The common sites for scabies are the genital areas, the space between the fingers, the front surface of the wrists, around the elbows, under the arm-pits, around the nipples, along the belt-line, and on the lower part of the buttocks. In infants, burrows are often present on the palms on the trunk. The burrow made by the itch-mite appears as a fine, wavy, dark line, if it can be seen at all. Often there is swelling, as well as scratch marks and local eczema over the irritated areas and this may cover up the tiny tunnels, so that they will not be seen. Infected individuals with good personal hygiene, usually have few lesions and burrows there by making it difficult to identify.

Causes

The female itch-mite, measuring 0.4 mm, burrows under the outer layer of the skin and deposits her eggs along the tunnel. Within a few days, the larvae hatch and tend to congregate around the hair follicles of the skin. The disease is transmitted from person to person by close bodily contact, particularly among family members. Those who spend nights with friends or exchange clothing with others are at increased risk. Prolonged holding of hand is also a frequent means for spreading the disease.

Treatment

As the disease is contagious, the suffering patient and all the affected members of the family should be treated simultaneously. The oldest and the most effective of treatments is the application of a paste, prepared by mixing two teaspoons of sublimed sulphur with eight tablespoons of coconut oil. The whole body should be soaked for 20 minutes in a warm-bath using plenty of soap. Particular attention should be paid to the itching areas, scrubbing them thoroughly. After the bath, a paste should be rubbed well over the entire skin surface, below the chin line, but particularly over the affected areas. This should be done for three successive nights, wearing the same under-clothing during this period. About 10 to 12 hours after the last application, a hot-soap bath should be taken and a clean under-clothing and outside clothing should be worn. All clothes next to the skin, bed sheets and pillow cases should be boiled in hot water and occasionally sun-dried.

Another effective treatment is that of Benzyl-Benzoate. After a warm soap bath, as mentioned above, a mixture of equal parts of soap, ethyl alcohol and benzyl benzoate should be brushed for five minutes, while still wet. It should be allowed to dry and again painted for five minutes. After it is dry, the same old clothes should be worn. A bath should be taken after 24 hours and clean clothing should be worn.

Benzyl-Benzoate, being an irritant, should be diluted to half the strength, if it is used for treating babies. Any of the other regimes can be used in the treatment of young children. Recently, gamuna benzene lotion is being used in place of benzyl-benzoate, as it is effective and less irritating to skin. Its burrows are present on the head and neck areas in babies, they can be treated with topical Eurax cream.

During the treatment period, the patient should be given light foods, preferably fresh juicy fruits such as orange, apple, pineapple, pear, peaches and melon. Warm water enema should be used daily during this period to ensure regular bowel movements.

Certain home remedies have been found beneficial in the treatment of scabies. The use of apricot (*khubani*) leaves is one such valuable remedy. Fresh juice of these leaves should be extracted and applied with beneficial results in scabies. Application of the juice of mint (*pudina*) leaves over the affected areas has also proved valuable in treating this disease.

The use of bitter gourd (*karela*) has proved beneficial in the treatment of this disease. Half a cup of juice of this vegetable, should be taken mixed with one teaspoon of lime juice. This juice should be sipped slowly on an empty stomach once daily for a week or so.

The flour of unroasted Bengal gram (*besan*) is a very effective cleansing agent. Washing the skin with this flour will be beneficial in treating scabies.

CHAPTER 121

Sciatica

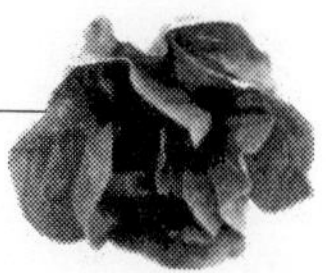

Sciatica is a serious disease of the nervous system. It is a neuritic condition of the sciatica nerve. It refers to a severe pain running down the course of the sciatic nerve, which supplies sensation to the back of the leg and foot.

The sciatica nerve is the largest nerve in the body. It has branches in the thigh muscles, the knee joints, and down into the muscles of the legs and feet. This nerve begins in the lower part of the back and passes down behind the thigh. It is more exposed to injury and inflammation than most other nerves.

Symptoms

The patient of sciatica feels severe pain in the buttock which may radiate down the posterior aspect of the thigh and calf to the outer border of the foot. In severe cases, he may feel weakness of the calf muscles or foot-drop. Sometimes the pain is so severe that the patient cannot stand and is crippled. In the case of a ruptured disc, the pain is often aggravated by coughing, sneezing, bending forward, or straining at the stool. Often the pain disappears with bed rest, only to return days or weeks later after some slight injury or extra exertion.

Causes

Sciatica may be caused by any type of injury to the spine, because of compression of the sciatica nerve at its roots. Any infection or toxic material near the area of the nerve may result in this disease. But in most cases, the trouble is due either to a ruptured disc or else osteoarthritis of the lower spine. Other

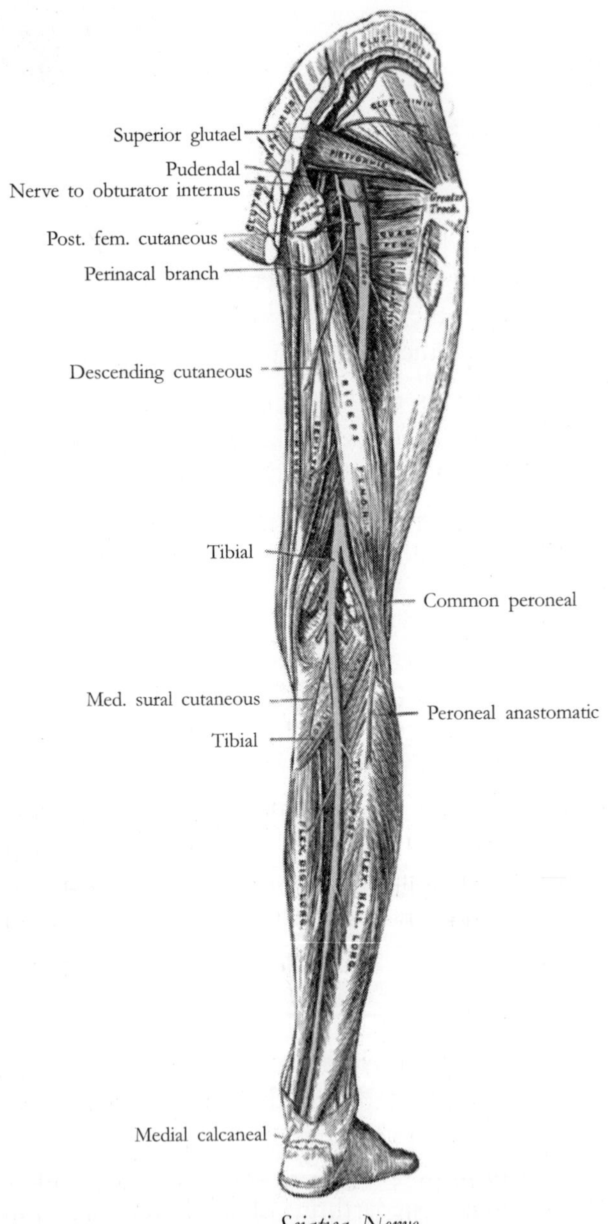

Sciatica Nerve

causes include pregnancy, tumours of the pelvis, deformities of the lower spine and exposures to cold and damp. The sciatica nerve may even be injured by walking, running, or riding a bicycle. Prolonged standing, or sitting on one side of the edge of a chair may also lead to this disease.

The real cause of sciatica, however, is the direct outcome of excess acidity of the blood and tissues and a rundown condition of the system generally. It is one of the many forms of "acidosis."

Treatment

Treatment of sciatica by painkillers drugs may give temporary relief but it does not remove the trouble effectively. The pain is relieved for the time being at the cost of the health of other parts of the body, especially the heart and kidneys, and the sciatica remains.

The best way to commence the treatment is to take complete bed rest on firm mattress supported by fracture boards for a few days. Rest must be absolute and in no case, the patient should assume sitting position. If the disease is acute, the patient should adopt a raw juice diet for atleast five days. In this regimen, he should take juices of fresh fruits or vegetables, such as orange, apple, pineapple, pear, peach, carrot and beet, every two hours from 8 a.m. to 8 p.m. Warm water enema should be used daily during this period to cleanse the bowels.

After the juice fast, the patient may embark upon a restricted diet for about seven days. In this regimen, breakfast may consist of orange, sweet lime, pineapple or grapefruit. The lunch may comprise of fresh raw vegetables salad, such as carrot, cabbage, cucumber, tomato and radish, with lime juice and olive oil dressing and soaked raisins, prunes, figs or dates.

Dinner may consist of fresh raw vegetables salad or one or two vegetables steamed in their own juices, such as spinach, cabbage, carrots, turnips and cauliflower. This may be followed by few nuts or some fruits like apple, pear, plum or cherries.

After the restricted diet, the patient may adopt a well-balanced optimum diet, well assimilated with all vitamins and other nutrients. The emphasis should be on whole grains, particularly whole wheat, brown rice, raw and sprouted seeds, milk, especially in soured form, and home-made cottage cheese.

The patient should avoid tea, coffee, sugar, white flour, all products made from white flour sugar, and all fresh foods. He should also avoid fried foods, condiments, pickles, alcoholic beverages, tobacco and smoking.

Certain home remedies have been found beneficial in the treatment of sciatica. The most important of these remedies is the use of garlic and garlic milk. This vegetable should be cut into small pieces and taken with a teaspoon of honey with each meal. Taken over a period of time, it will yield good results in relieving pain and suffering.

Garlic milk can be prepared both in cooked and uncooked states. In raw state uncooked form is more powerful. This milk is prepared by adding the pulp of the crushed garlic in uncooked buffalo milk. The proportion is four cloves to 110 ml of milk. Another method is to boil the garlic in milk.

The use of lemon is beneficial in the treatment of sciatica. It is sour in taste, but its reaction in the body is alkaline and as such it is valuable in rheumatic affections, including sciatica. A sufficient intake of lemon juice prevents the deposit of uric acid in the tissues.

Nutmeg (jaiphal) is another effective remedy for sciatica. A nutmeg should be coarsely powdered and fried in gingelly (til) oil until all the particles become brown. This oil can be applied beneficially on the affected parts as a pain reliever.

The herb chamomile (babunah or babuni-ke-phul) is valuable in sciatica. Its extracted oil, diluted in vegetable oil should be rubbed on the affected parts. A compress of chamomile flowers can also be used beneficially to treat this disease.

The herb Indian aloe (ghee kanvar or musabbar) is also beneficial in the treatment of sciatica. The pulp of a leaf of this herb should be taken daily for obtaining relief.

Certain water treatment have proved effective in sciatica. These include the cold hip-bath in the morning and the hot and cold hip-bath at night. For hip-baths, a common tub may be used. The tub should be filled with water in such a way that it covers the hips and reaches upto the navel when the patient sits in it. Generally, four to six gallons of water are required. A support may be placed under one edge to elevate it by two or three inches. The water temperature for cold and hot hip-baths should be 10°C to 18°C and 40°C to 45°C respectively.

Other helpful measures include sleeping on firm mattress, dry friction bath every morning and sun baths taken every alternate day. The patient should also undertake some exercises aimed at strengthening the back. Yoga asanas considered beneficial in the treatment of sciatica are pavanmuktasana, bhujangasana, shalabhasana, uttanpadasana and shavasana.

CHAPTER 122

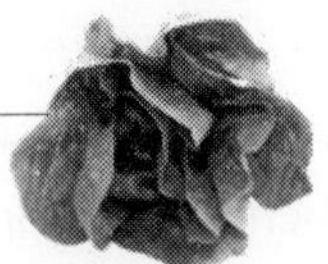

Scurvy

Scurvy is perhaps the oldest known deficiency disease. However, its specific relationship to ascorbic acid was not recognised until the 20th century. The disease is common in children and is often mistaken for rheumatism, rickets or paralysis.

Scurvy was prevalent in Europe during the 19th century and earlier. For centuries, the disease was attributed to a limited food supply. On the long voyages which followed the discovery of America, sailors were often obliged to subsist for long periods on salt, fish, meats and breadstuffs, entirely deprived of any fresh food. The outbreaks of scurvy on such voyages were frequently so severe that there was scarcely enough of the crew left to man the vessel. In 1772, however, Captain Cook commanded a voyage which lasted three years. Not one man was lost during this period because of scurvy. This fact he attributed to the use of a 'sweet wort' made from barley and sauerkraut.

In the 18th century, a British Naval Surgeon for the first time demonstrated that citrus fruit juices prevented and cured scurvy. As a result of this discovery, the two important citrus fruits, lime and lemon, were included in the supplies for sailors. It was much later discovered that the common anti-scurvy factors in all citrus fruits was vitamin C.

Symptoms

The onset of scurvy is gradual. The first signs of the disease

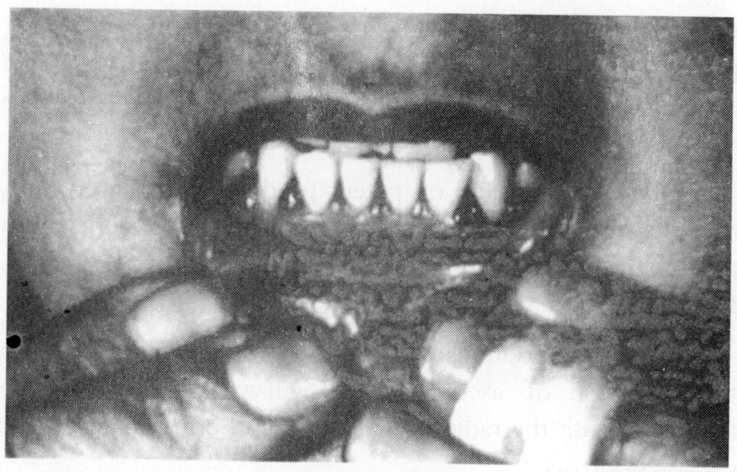

Scorbutic gums, a symptom of scurvy

are breathlessness, exhaustion and mental depression. In the later stages, there is bleeding of the gums because the lack of Vitamin C (ascorbic acid) makes the capillaries fragile and their rupture is common. This may lead to extensive haemmorrhage and fermentation of glandular patches, similar to boils, all over the body, particularly in the lower limb. The disease is characterised by pain on motion, swelling of the extremities, frequently by paralysis of one or more limbs, and black and blue spots on the body.

The blood from the gums may pass into the skin, leading to formation of large bruises. It may also pass into the vital organs. Bleeding beneath the membrane covering the bones may cause extreme tenderness of the limbs. Anaemia may also occur due to loss of blood.

Causes

Scurvy is caused by lack of vitamin C or ascorbic acid. Inadequate intake of fresh fruits and vegetables can lead to this condition. The disease is likely to attack the rich as well as the poor, because it arises in the system not from an insufficient diet but from the diet lacking in the organic mineral salts so essential to health and vitality.

Children brought up on patent foods, on condensed milk, are most prone to scurvy. These foods are almost deficient in the life-giving organic minerals found abundantly in fresh milk, fresh fruits and vegetables.

Another important cause of scurvy is stress which increases the utilisation of ascorbic acid. Scurvy in adults may be associated with the radiological changes in bone characteristic of osteoporosis.

Treatment

Diet plays an important role in the prevention and treatment of scurvy. The patient should take a well-balanced diet consisting of seeds, nuts, grains, vegetables and fruits. This diet should be supplemented with certain special foods such as milk, vegetable oils, and honey. The emphasis should be on fresh fruits, raw vegetables and whole grain cereals. Breakfast may consist of fresh fruits, a glass of fresh milk sweetened with honey and some nuts or seeds. Lunch may comprise a bowl of freshly prepared steamed vegetables, whole wheat chappatis or brown rice and a glass of buttermilk. Dinner may consist of a large salad of raw vegetables with lime juice dressing, sprouts such as alfalfa or mung, a hot course like vegetable soup, if desired, cottage cheese, or a glass of butter milk.

The patient should be given liberal quantities of vitamin C-rich foods. This vitamin is found in fresh fruits and vegetables but is largely destroyed in cooking, especially if baking soda is used. The amount of this vitamin required is between 10 and 20 mg. daily. The normal diet, however, contains much less amount than this. It can therefore, if necessary, be taken as a tablet of ascorbic acid.

One of the best remedies for scurvy is the use of Indian gooseberry (*amla*), which is the richest known source of vitamin C. A teaspoon of dry amla, mixed with equal quantity of sugar should be given thrice daily with milk. If fresh amla is available, it should be cooked as vegetable and eaten.

The use of lime and lemon is beneficial in the prevention and treatment of scurvy. As rich sources of vitamin C, they have been regarded as foods of exceptional therapeutic value. They have saved the lives of innumerable crews of ocean-going vessels from scurvy. The juice of these two fruits, diluted with water and mixed with a teaspoon of honey, should be taken for treating this condition.

Another effective remedy for scurvy is the use of amchur, a popular article of diet in Indian houses, consisting of green mangoes skinned, stonned, cut into pieces and dried in the sun. Fifteen grams of it is believed to be equivalent to 30 grams of good lime on account of its citric content.

Potato (*alu*) is regarded as an excellent food remedy in scurvy. It has been noted that scurvy in Europe has become more and more uncommon with the progress of potato cultivation and it makes its appearance only when the crop fails.

Fresh air and sunshine are essential for the treatment of scurvy and the patient should spend as much time outdoors as possible. A cold towel sponge twice daily and a gentle massage twice or thrice a week will also be beneficial in the treatment of this disease. Another helpful measure is neutral immersion bath. This bath can be taken on alternate days from half an hour to one hour.

CHAPTER 123

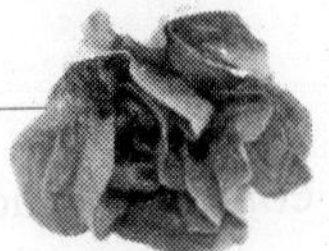

Sexual Impotence

Sex is now regarded as a basic instinct like hunger. Sexual activity, however, demands complete concentration and relaxation. It cannot be performed in haste and tension. Persons who are usually tense and over-occupied are unable to follow these norms. Many persons, therefore, suffer from sexual dysfunctions. The most common male sexual dysfunction is impotence or loss of sexual power.

Symptoms

Impotence takes three forms. There is primary impotence when the man's erectile dysfunction is there from the very beginning of sexual activity and he simply cannot have an erection. This is a rare manifestation of the problem. Secondary impotence is the commonest and this implies that the man can normally attain an erection but fails on one or more occasions in between normal activity. The third form is associated with age and is a continuous and serious form with poor prognosis.

Causes

Since erection is the result of erotic excitement, intact nervous pathways and adequate hormonal functioning, the pathological causes of impotence are numerous. It may occur as a result of psychological illness such as depression, which lowers both sexual drive and erectile function, tiredness, alcohol abuse, the therapeutic use of oestrogens, paralysis of parasympathetic nerves by drugs or permanent damage to them and diabetes. Other causes of impotence are abuse or misuse of the sexual organism over a long period and a devitalised condition of the system in general.

However, the main problem of secondary impotence is the apprehension created by failure which generates a good deal of anxiety. If in fact, intercourse is attempted again and the same failure results, then a vicious circle is established. Anxiety of failure is established as an anticipatory reflex which in turn impairs the capacity of the penis.

Treatment

Taking of drugs or so called 'remedies' in case of impotence is not only useless but dangerous. Diet is an important factor in these conditions. To begin with, the patient should adopt an exclusive fresh fruit diet from five to seven days. In this regimen, he can have three meals a day, at five hourly intervals, of fresh juicy fruits such as grapes, oranges, apples, pears, peaches, pineapple and melon. The bowels should be cleansed daily during this period with a warm-water enema.

After the all-fruit diet, the patient may gradually embark upon a balanced diet of seeds, nuts and grains, vegetables and fruits, with generous use of special rejuvenative foods such as whey, soured milks, particularly made from goat's milk, millet, garlic, honey, cold-pressed vegetable oils and brewer's yeast. The patient should avoid smoking, alcohol, tea, coffee and all processed, canned, refined and denaturated foods, especially white sugar and white flour and products made from them.

Certain foods are considered highly beneficial in the treatment of impotence. The most important of these is garlic. It is a natural and harmless aphrodisiac. According to Dr. Robinson, an eminent sexologist of America, garlic has a pronounced aphrodisiac effect. It is a tonic for loss of sexual power from any cause and for sexual debility and impotence resulting from sexual over-indulgence and nervous exhaustion.

Onion is another important aphrodisiac food. It stands second only to garlic. It increases libido and strengthens the reproductory organs. The white variety of onion, is however, more useful for this purpose.

Carrot is also considered useful in impotence. For better results, carrot should be taken with a half-boiled egg dipped in a tablespoonful of honey once daily for a month or two. This recipe increases sex stamina by releasing sex hormones and strengthens the sexual plexus. It is for this reason that carrot *halwa,* prepared according to Unani specifications is considered a very effective tonic to improve sexual strength.

The lady's finger is another great tonic for improving sexual vigour. It has been mentioned in ancient Indian literature that the persons who take five to 10 grams of root powder of this vegetable with milk and 'misri' daily will never lose sexual vigour.

Dried dates, known as *chhuhara* in the vernacular, is a highly strengthening food. Pounded and mixed with almonds, pistachio nuts and quince seeds, it forms an effective remedy for increasing sexual power.

Black raisins are also useful for restoration of sexual vigour. They should be boiled with milk after washing them thoroughly in tepid water. This will make them swollen and sweet. Eating of such raisins should be followed by the use of milk. Starting with 30 grams of raisins with 200 ml. of milk, three times daily, the quantity of raisins should be gradually increased to 50 grams each time.

A vigorous massage all over the body is highly beneficial in the treatment of impotence as it will revive the muscular vigour which is essential for nervous energy. The nerves of the genital organs are controlled by the pelvic region. Hence a cold hip bath for 10 minutes in the morning or evening will be very effective.

Every effort should be made to build up the general health level to the highest degree and fresh air and outdoor exercise are essential to the success of the treatment. Yogasanas such as dhanurasana, sarvangasana and halasana are also highly beneficial.

The scheme of treatment outlined above will go a long way in restoring sexual vigour, but of course the results achieved will depend upon the age and condition of the sufferer. Longstanding cases will obviously not get such good results from the treatment as comparatively early cases; and younger men will naturally tend to do better than older men.

Where the trouble is of psychological origin, treatment should be just the same, but in these cases advice from a qualified psychotherapist would be desirable. The patient also requires gentle handling by a willing partner.

CHAPTER 124

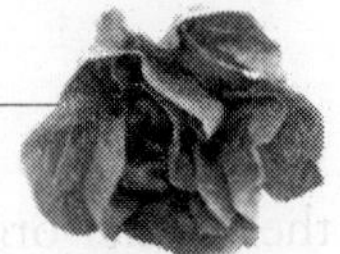

Sinusitis

Sinusitis refers to an inflammation of the mucous membrane lining the paranasal sinuses. It often follows the common cold, influenza and other general infections. Germs which are usually eliminated from the body sometimes find their way into these sinuses or chambers on either side of the nasal passage, leading to sinus trouble.

The sinuses consist of cavities or chambers contained in the bones situated in the head and face region. The frontal, maxillary, ethmoid and sphenoid sinuses are the paranasal sinuses which communicate with the nose. The frontal sinuses lie on the frontal bone directly above the eyes. The maxillary sinuses are located one on each side of the nose under the cheekbone. The ethmoid and sphenoid sinuses are situated behind the nose or either side of it. These air sinuses lighten the weight of the skull and give resonance to the voice.

Symptoms

The symptoms of sinusitis are excessive or constant sneezing, a running nose, blockage of one or both nostrils, headaches and pressure around the head, eyes and face. Sinus headaches are usually felt in the forehead and in the face just below the eyes. The patient may suffer from a low grade fever, lack of appetite, loss of sense of appetite, and toothache. He feels miserable because of difficulty in breathing. The voice is also affected because of the blocked nose.

Causes

Sinusitis results from the congestion of the sinus passages due to catarrh. It is caused by over-secretion of mucus in the membranes lining the nose, throat and head. This over-secretion is due to irritation caused by toxins in the blood.

A faulty diet is thus the real cause of sinus trouble. When a person consumes certain types of foods or drinks regularly, these, in due course, have a conditioning effect on the entire system. As a result, some persons become more sensitive to certain allergens, whose reaction ultimately turns into sinusitis.

The Cure

Correcting the faulty diet is of utmost importance in the treatment of sinusitis. Patients should take a balanced diet. Most persons with sinus trouble also suffer from acidity. Their diet should, therefore, veer to the alkaline side. The intake of salt should be reduced to the minimum as salt leads to accumulation of water in the tissues and expels calcium from the body.

In the acute stage of the disease, when fever is present, the patient should abstain from all solid foods and only drink fresh fruit and vegetable juices diluted with water on a 50 : 50 basis. After fever subsides, he may adopt a low-calorie raw fruit and vegetable diet with plenty of raw juices.

After the acute symptoms are over, the patient may gradually embark upon a well-balanced diet of three basic food groups, namely seeds, nuts and grains; vegetables and fruits. In persistent chronic conditions, repeated short juice fasts may be undertaken for a week or so at intervals of two months.

Those suffering from sinusitis should completely avoid fried and starchy foods, white sugar, white flour, rice, macaroni products, pies, cakes and candies. They should also avoid strong spices, meat and products. Butter and ghee should be used sparingly. Honey should be used for sweetening. All cooked foods should be freshly prepared for each meal. Vegetables should be taken in liberal quantities. All kinds of fruits can be taken with the exception of those belonging to citrus group such as lemon, lime, orange and grapefruit. Milk should be taken in liberal quantities as it contains calcium which has a marked effect in overcoming inflammation of the tissues.

A diet rich in vitamin A is the best insurance against cold and sinus trouble. Vitamin A is the 'membrane conditioner' as it helps build healthy mucus membranes in the head and throat. Some of the valuable sources of this vitamin are whole milk, curds, egg yolk, pumpkin, carrot, leafy vegetables, tomato, oranges, mango and papaya.

When the sinus trouble has already developed, relief can be obtained by taking vitamin A in large therapeutic doses of 25,000 I.U. per day. Vitamin C has also proved beneficial in the treatment of sinusitis and the patient should take one gram of this vitamin per day in two therapeutic doses of 500 mg. each.

One of the most effective remedies for sinus problems is to eat pungent herbs like garlic and onion which tend to break up mucous congestion all through the respiratory tract. One should begin with small mild doses and increase them gradually. Beneficial results can also be achieved by adding these herbs in moderate amounts to regular meals.

Carrot juice used separately or in combination with juices of beet and cucumber or with spinach juice is highly beneficial in the treatment of sinus trouble. 100 ml. each of beet and cucumber juice or 200 ml. of spinach juice should be mixed with 300 ml. of carrot juice in these combinations.

Water Treatment

Cold application over the sinus will give great relief; alternate hot and cold applications will also prove beneficial. Take pans of hot and cold water, bathe the whole face with hot water—as hot as you can bear—and then apply cold water for short duration. Nasal inhalation of steam for five minutes every hour will also give relief.

Yogasanas such as viparitakarani, bhujangasana, yogamudra and shavasana, yogic kriyas, such as jalaneti and sutraneti and pranayamas like anuloma-viloma and suryabhedan will be beneficial in the treatment of sinus trouble.

Plenty of sleep, adequate rest and fresh air are essential in the treatment of sinus trouble. Patients should avoid the use of perfumes and strongly scented hair oil.

CHAPTER 125

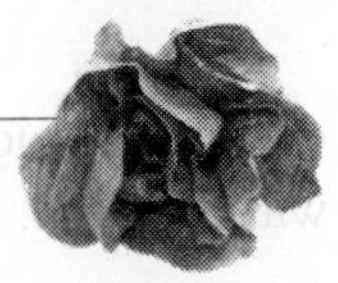

Sore Throat

Sore throat refers to the inflammation of the pharynx, or back of the throat. It occurs frequently when a person has a cold or an attack of influenza. This inflammation may also involve the tonsils and adenoids if these have not already been removed. An irritating condition of the throat may range from the harmless to the potentially serious.

Symptoms

In case of an acute sore throat, the patient complains of burning and dryness in the throat followed by chills, fever and some hoarseness or laryngitis. The lymph glands along the sides of the neck may become swollen and tender. The back of the throat may become very red and even covered with a greyish-white membrane. The patient may find difficulty in swallowing, especially during the acute stage. There may also be postnasal discharge if the irritation has spread to nasal passages. The patient with sore throat caused by 'Streptoccal' germs suffers from high fever and sharp pain with swelling.

Causes

Sore throat is mainly caused by bacteria or a viral infection. Many different kind of ailments can give rise to this condition. The most common of these ailments are common cold and influenza. Other diseases which can cause sore throat are tonsilitis, mumps, sinusitis, measles, and diphtheria. Even leukemia on rare occasions may lead to sore throat. Other causes of this disease are excessive smoking and talking, frequent use of voice as in certain professions like singing, acting and teaching.

Treatment

The patient suffering from sore throat should fast on orange juice and water for three to five days, depending on the severity of the condition. He should take orange juice diluted with warm water every two or three hours from 8 a.m. to 8 p.m. during this period. The bowels should be cleansed daily with warm water enema. This should be done twice daily in more serious cases.

A wet pack should be applied to the throat at two-hourly intervals during the day, and also one at night. The procedure is to wring out some linen material in cold water, wrap two or three times round the effected part, and cover with some flannel. The throat may be gargled several times with warm water mixed with a little salt. A hot Epsom-salt bath, taken daily during this period, will be highly beneficial.

When the more severe symptoms subside, the patient may further adopt an all-fruit diet for three or four days, taking three meals a day of juicy fruits such as orange, apple, pineapple and papaya at five-hourly intervals. Thereafter, he may gradually adopt a well-balanced diet, with emphasis on seeds, nuts and grains, raw vegetables and fresh fruits. The daily dry friction, deep breathing and other exercises should form part of the daily health regimen.

Home Remedies

Certain home remedies have been found to be beneficial in the treatment of sore throat. One such remedy is the use of mango (*aam*) bark which is very efficacious in sore throat and other throat disorders. Its fluid can be applied locally with beneficial results. It can also be used as a throat gargle. This gargle is prepared by mixing 10 ml. of the fluid extract with 125 ml. of water.

The herb *belleric myroblan* (*bahera*) is another valuable remedy for sore throat. A mixture of the pulp of the fruit, salt, long pepper (*pipli*) and honey should be administered in the treatment of this condition. The fried fruit, roasted after covering it with wheat flour, is also a popular remedy for sore throat.

Betel leaves (*pan-ka-patta*) have proved beneficial in the treatment of this disease. The leaves should be applied locally for obtaining relief. The fruit of the betel tree, mixed with honey, can also be taken beneficially to relieve irritating throat cough.

The bishop's weed (*ajowan*) is valuable in treating sore throat. An infusion of the seeds mixed with common salt can be used beneficially as a gargle in acute condition caused by colds. The spice cinnamon (*dalchini*) is also regarded as an effective remedy for sore throat resulting from cold. Coarsely powdered and boiled in a glass of water with a pinch of pepper powder and honey, it can be taken as a medicine in the treatment of this condition. The oil of cinnamon, mixed with honey, also gives immense relief. A gargle prepared from fenugreek (*methi*) seeds has been found to be a very effective remedy for treating sore throat. To prepare this gargle, two tablespoons' of fenugreek seeds should be put in a litre of cold water and allowed to simmer for half an hour over a low flame. It should be allowed to cool to a bearable temperature strained and used as a gargle.

The leaves of the holy basil (*tulsi*) have also been found beneficial in the treatment of this condition. The water boiled

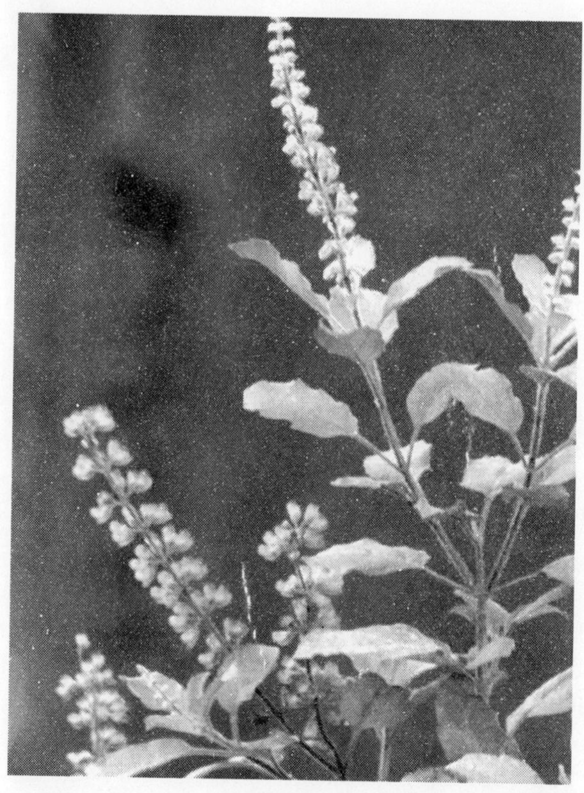

The leaves of holy basil are beneficial in the treatment of sore throat

with basil leaves should be taken as a drink and also used as a gargle in sore throat.

The patient should avoid rapid changes in temperature like hot sunshine to air-conditioned rooms. He should avoid cold and sour foods which may irritate his throat. To prevent the disease, a person should avoid touching tissues, handkerchief, towels or utensils used by the patients suffering from sore throat.

CHAPTER 126

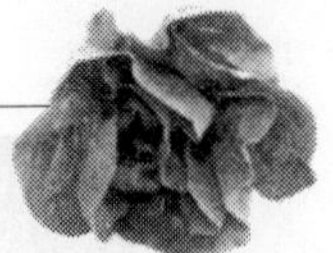

Stomatitis

Stomatitis refers to inflammation of the mucous membrane lining the mouth. It is a painful condition resulting from infection. Ulcers may form on the gums and the mouth, particularly between the teeth. These ulcers contain numerous germs. Simple ulcers in the mouth, however, come and go spontaneously. The disease is quite common both in adults and children.

Symptoms

A person suffering from stomatitis finds it very difficult to take his meals because of pain. At times, he has to go without food altogether. On other occasions, he has to be content with small quantity of liquid food which he gulps down with difficulty. He also feels pain and difficulty in talking. Other symptoms of stomatitis are excessive salivation, coated tongue, bright red mouth, irritability, vomiting after taking meals, reduced appetite and bad breath. The patient may also suffer from mild fever and constipation.

Causes

Stomatitis may arise from a variety of causes. The most important cause which leads to this condition are defective functioning of the stomach and indigestion. Poor oral hygiene and nutritional deficiencies are other main causes of stomatitis. The disease may also result from infection with Candida albicans (thrush) and infection with Vincent's Spirochaete (Vincent's angina). It may also be found in blood disease such as leukaemia.

Treatment

As stomatitis generally results from toxic condition of the system, the treatment for this disease has to be constitutional. It should aim at improving the digestive system. Temporary measures will only suppress the disease. To begin with, the patient should be placed on orange juice and water for three to five days. The procedure is to take the juice of an orange, diluted with water on 50 : 50 basis, every two hours during the day. If orange juice does not agree, carrot juice, diluted with water, may be taken. The bowels should be cleansed daily with a warm-water enema during this period. If this is not possible in case of children, a glycerine suppository may be applied.

After the juice diet, the patient should adopt an exclusive diet of fresh fruits for further three to five days. In this regimen, he should take three meals a day of fresh juicy fruits, such as apple, grapes, grapefruit, orange, pear, pineapple, peach and papaya. Thereafter, the patient may gradually embark upon a well balanced diet consisting of seeds, nuts, grains, vegetables and fruits. The emphasis should be on fresh fruits, whole grain cereals, raw or lightly-cooked vegetables and sprouted seeds, like alfalfa and mung beans. The patient should avoid meats, tea, coffee, white sugar, white flour and all products made from them. He should also avoid condiments, pickles, refined and processed foods, soft drink, candies and ice-cream.

Certain home remedies have been found beneficial in the treatment of stomatitis. The most important of these is the use of lemon (Bara nimbu). Taking a tablespoon of lemon juice daily before meals will correct the functioning of the stomach and help cure the condition. The patient should also gargle several times daily with lemon juice mixed in water. This gargle can be prepared by mixing 20 ml. of lemon juice in 100 ml. of hot water.

Another simple but effective home remedy for stomatitis is the frequent use of a mouth-wash containing a teaspoon each of salt and baking soda in a glass of warm water. This should be used every two to three hours to keep the mouth as clean as possible.

The use of alum (phitkari) is also valuable in stomatitis. The patient should gargle with alum diluted in hot water. Concentrated solution of alum may also be applied with the help of a swab on the ulcerated spots.

Other Measures

Proper oral hygiene is of utmost importance in the treatment of stomatitis. The patient should carefully brush his teeth and gums so as to remove any foul material. He should also take multi-vitamin tablets, especially those high in vitamin B complex. This will aid in recovery. Other helpful methods include fomentation every three hours over the mouth, cheeks and jaws and hot foot bath twice daily. In case of hot foot bath, the patient should keep his legs in a tub or bucket filled with hot water at a temperature of 40° to 45°C. Before taking this bath, a glass of cold water should be taken and the body should be covered with a blanket so as to ensure that no heat or vapour escapes from the foot bath. The duration of the bath is generally from 5 to 20 minutes. The patient should take a cold shower bath immediately after the bath.

CHAPTER 127

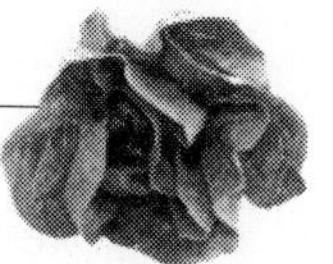

Stress

The term stress has been borrowed by biologists from engineering, where it implies an ability to withstand a defined amount of strain. Dr. Hans Selye, a great medical genius and noted world authority on stress, has described stress as "a state manifested by a specific syndrome which consists of all the non-specifically induced changes within a biological system."

The term implies any condition that harms the body or damages or causes the death of a few or many cells. The body immediately tries to repair the damaged cells but it can do so only if the diet is adequate, providing a generous supply of all the essential nutrients. If, however, rebuilding of cells is not able to keep pace with their destruction, the condition will result in disease. The most common diseases associated with stress are heart disease, diabetes, headache and peptic ulcer. Other diseases resulting from stress are ulcerative colitis, chronic dyspepsia, asthma, psoriasis and sexual disorders.

Reactions to stress are manifold. No one situation is stressful to all the people all the time. Some of the factors that can produce stress are children or the lack of them, the boss or the subordinate, the traffic, the telephone or the lack of it, over-work or not enough to do, too much money or too little of it, making decisions, a dull routine job, lack of authority and apprehensions about the future.

Symptoms

The body and the mind react to any stress factor. A large number of physical changes take place at the time of stress-induced arousal. The brain and nervous system become intensely active, the pupils of the eye dilate, digestion slows down, muscles become tense, the heart starts pumping blood harder and faster, blood pressure increases, breathing becomes faster, hormones such as adrenaline are released into the system along with glucose from the liver and sweating starts. All these changes take place in a split second under the direction of the nervous system. If the stress factors are immediately removed, no harm accrues and all the changes are reversed.

Stress in its earlier and reversible stage leads to poor sleep, bad temper, continual grumbling, longer hours of work with less achievement, domestic conflict with spouse and children, repeated minor sickness, absenteeism and prolonged absence for each spell of sickness, accident proneness, feeling of frustration and persecution by colleagues and complaints of lack of cooperation and increase in alcoholic intake.

It is essential that these symptoms are recognised early by the patients or their well-wishers and remedial measures taken to overcome them. If, however, stress is continuous or repeated frequently, a variety of symptoms appear such as dizziness, stiff muscles, headache, vision problems, breathing difficulties, asthma, allergies, palpitation, digestive disorders, blood sugar irregularities, backache, skin disorders, bowel disorders and sexual difficulties.

Causes

Stress may be caused by a variety of factors both outside the body and within. External factors include loud noises, blinding lights, extreme heat or cold. X-rays and other forms of radiation, drugs, chemicals, bacterial and various toxic substances, pain and inadequate nutrition. The factors from within the body include feelings of hate, envy, fear or jealousy.

Treatment

In dealing with stress, the patient should completely change his life style. He should adopt an optimum diet which should be able to meet the nutritional demands of stress. Such a diet should obviously be made of foods which, in combination, would supply all the essential nutrients. It has been found that a diet which contains liberal quantities of (i) seeds, nuts and grains, (ii) vegetables, and (iii) fruits would provide an adequate amount of all the essential nutrients. Each of these food groups should roughly form the bulk of one of the three meals. These three basic health-building foods should be supplemented with certain special foods such as milk; vegetable oils and honey.

There are many foods which are helpful in meeting the demands of stress and should be taken regularly by the patient. These are yogurt, blackstrap molasses, seeds, and sprouts. Yogurt is rich in vitamin A, B complex and D. It relieves insomnia, migraine and cramps associated with menstruation. Blackstrap molasses, a by-product of the sugar refining process, is rich in iron and B vitamins. It guards against anaemia and is good for heart diseases. Seeds such as alfalfa, sunflower and pumpkin and sprouts are rich in calcium and quite effective as deterrents of listlessness and anxiety. Steam cooked vegetables are best as boiling causes many vitamins and minerals to be dispelled into the water.

The leaves of holy basil, known as *tulsi* in the vernacular, are highly beneficial in the treatment of stress. They are regarded as adaptogen or antistress agents. Recent studies have shown that the leaves protect against stress significantly. It has been suggested that even healthy persons should chew 12 leaves of basil twice a day, morning and evening for preventing stress.

Certain nutrients are beneficial in relieving stress. These are vitamins A and B, minerals such as calcium, potassium and magnesium which reduce the feeling of irritability and anxiety. Vitamin A is found in green and yellow vegetables. Some of the valuable sources of vitamin B are cashews, green leafy vegetables, yeast, sprouts and bananas. An element of vitamin B complex, pantothenic acid is especially important in preventing stress. It has a deep effect on the adrenal glands and the immune system and adequate amount of this vitamin along with vitamin A can help prevent many of the changes caused by stress.

Potassium deficiencies are associated with breathlessness, fatigue, insomnia and low blood sugar. Potassium is essential for healthy heart muscles. Nuts and unrefined grains are good sources of potassium. Calcium is a natural sedative. Deficiencies can cause fatigue, nervousness and tension. Dairy products, eggs, almonds and soyabeans are rich sources of calcium. Magnesium is known as nature's tranquiliser and is associated with the prevention of heart attacks. Deficiencies may lead to excitability, irritability, apprehension and emotional disorders. Magnesium is also necessary for absorption of calcium and potassium and is found in many fruits, vegetables, seeds, dates and prunes.

There are certain foods which are associated with stress and anxiety and should be scrupulously avoided by patients. These foods are caffeine in coffee and many soft drinks, which causes nervousness, irritability and palpitation; salt which has been associated with heart diseases; cigarettes which cause tension, irritability and sleeplessness and which have been linked with cancer, and alcohol which depletes vitamins of B group considered essential for reducing stress.

Regular physical exercise plays an important role in the fight against stress. Exercise not only keeps the body physically and mentally fit, it also provides recreation and mental relaxation. It is nature's best tranquiliser. One can jog, run, walk or play games, depending upon one's liking. Walking is the simplest and safest exercise. One should take a brisk walk for 45 minutes or so daily. Yogic asanas, kriyas, and simple pranayamas, beneficial for maintenance of general health and mental relaxation, can serve as the best shock-absorbers against stress. These include asanas like pavanmuktasana, sarvangasana, halasana, ardhmatsyendrasana, bhujangasana, dhanurasana, yogamudra, padmasana, trikonasana, kriyas like kunjal and jalneti and pranayamas such as kapalbhati, anuloma-viloma, shitali, shitkari and bhramari.

Recreation and rest are equally important and patients should set a definite time for recreational activities. They should also take a holiday at regular intervals. And above all, they should simplify their life styles to eliminate unnecessary stress.

CHAPTER 128

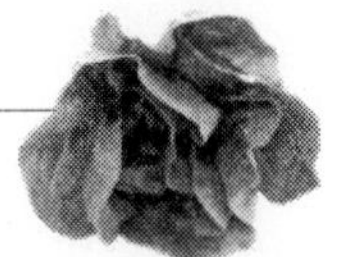

Stroke

A stroke, also known as apoplexy, is a sudden acute disturbance of brain function of vascular origin. It may result in loss of consciousness, paralysis or death. It is the most common form of brain disease, which can occur at any age, although, the risk increases greatly in the older years of life.

Symptoms

Usually, the first sign of stroke is dizziness, followed by nausea and vomiting, and later by weakness of the body. The patient may complain of a severe headache, and may even have a convulsion, or pass into a coma from which he cannot be aroused for some time. He may be completely paralysed on one side and may not be able to speak. He may be mentally alert, but for some time, he may not be able to recall the actual words he wants to use.

Many strokes occur suddenly and tend to clear after a few hours. In more serious cases, the patient may remain in a deep coma for several days. He may have a fever, a rapid pulse and difficulty in breathing. This condition may arise due to haemorrhage of the brain, if the coma lasts for more than six hours and the patient passes periods of convulsions with stiffness in the neck and his eyes are turned sharply toward the paralysed side. A severe haemorrhage may prove fatal in two or three days, especially if the patient has a high fever with a rapid pulse.

Most patients recover, if the stroke is due to thrombosis,

or if only a small vessel is involved. Many of them may not even lose consciousness, but the weakness or paralysis may continue for a long time. There may also be some permanent disability, even with the best of care.

Causes

The brain is a delicate organ requiring a constant supply of blood. A stroke occurs when one of the vessels leading to a portion of the brain becomes blocked by a blood clot. This may be due to inflammation, arteriosclerosis, or the presence of a clot or embolus from the heart. Occasionally one of the vessels leading to the brain may rupture because of a small aneurysm or enlargement in the wall of the vessel. This will cause a serious haemorrhage. A sudden rise in blood pressure caused by emotion like anger may rupture the aneurysm. Most strokes are due to thrombosis, or clotting of blood within the vessel. When this happens, that portion of the brain becomes necrotic and dies.

Treatment

Good nursing care is of utmost importance, especially during the acute stage. The patient should be made to rest in bed, and he should be turned frequently from side to side to prevent development of pressure sores. Cold compresses may be applied to the head to relieve pain. The patient should be protected from visitors and all forms of excitement. He should not return to work for several months.

The most important factor in treating this disease is fasting. The patient should fast for the first few days and he should be given only water to drink, if he can take it. Thereafter, he may be given orange juice and water. The fast should be continued till the severity of the stroke has passed off. He can then be allowed to take fresh fruits such as orange, apple, pineapple, pear, grapes, peach and papaya. The diet can be extended to include fresh and unboiled milk, and as convalescence progresses, the fruit and milk diet can be gradually followed by a well-balanced diet consisting of seeds, nuts and grains, with emphasis on fresh fruits and raw vegetables salad. The bowels should be cleansed twice daily with the warm-water enema for the first two or three days, and then daily until the bowels begin to function of their own accord.

The patient should be encouraged to use the paralysed limbs and move all the joints several times daily. The paralysed muscles should be gently massaged. As soon as possible, the patient should come out of bed and walk around the room.

The patient should avoid tea, coffee, white flour, sugar and all products made from them as well as all flesh foods. He should also avoid spices, condiments, pickles, tinned and frozen foods, fried foods and other foods which are difficult to digest. The consumption of alcoholic beverages and smoking, wherever habitual, should be stopped completely.

When the patient is able to move about, he should take breathing and other exercises daily, together with the daily friction and sponge. Prolonged neutral immersion bath will also be beneficial in the treatment of this disease. The procedure for this bath has been explained in the chapter on Therapeutic Baths.

Fresh air and outdoor exercises, as far as possible, correct diet along the lines outlined above, and clean wholesome living will prevent occurrence of further strokes. All undue nervous excitement, needless worry and excessive strain must be avoided.

CHAPTER 129

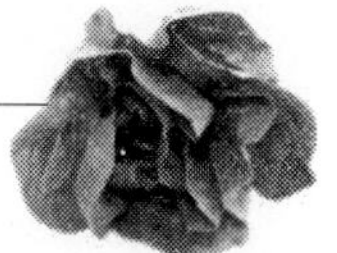

Styes

The term stye refers to a small painful boil, an inflammed hair follicle or an infection of a sebaceous gland in the edge of the eyelid. The infecting organism is usually a staphylococcus. This disease occurs due to debilitated condition of the system. Some persons seem more prone to these infections than others.

Symptoms

A stye gives rise to a throbbing pain which can be out of all proportions to its size. It can be felt for a day or two even before the stye is visible. It is accompanied by redness, swelling and oedema of the lid and conjunctiva. Sometimes, the infection disappears quickly without becoming a red swelling. But other styes worsen rapidly until the eyelid is very swollen. In the final stage, the stye will burst and discharge pus, causing the eyelids to stick together during a night's sleep in severe cases.

Causes

Stye results from an infection of the hair follicles. It may also result from blocking of the gland by dirt due to error of refraction. Recurrent styes occur because the infection is spread from one hair shaft to another often by the patient rubbing to relieve itching.

The real cause of styes is the toxic condition of the system brought about by wrong feeding habits, especially consumption of foods such as white bread, refined cereals, boiled potatoes, puddings, pies, pastries and confectionary. The disease makes its appearance when a person is in a run-down condition and below par. Eye strain is also a subsidiary factor in the onset of styes.

Treatment

The stye usually disappears on its own in two or three days. The progress of the condition can be curtailed by pulling the eye-lash at the site of the inflammation. Periodic application of moist warm compresses brings the pus out enabling its easy drainage. Sometimes it has to be evacuated by an incision with a knife. As stye can spread from an infected person to other members of the family, it is essential that the patient is given a separate face flannel and towel at least while his stye is at the discharging stage he should be discouraged from scratching.

To be effective, the treatment for stye should be constitutional. A thorough cleansing of the system and adoption of natural laws in diet and general living can help eliminate stye. To begin with, the patient should be placed on an exclusive diet of fresh fruits for two or three days. In this regimen, he should be given three meals a day of fresh juicy fruits such as orange, apple, pineapple, pear, peach and papaya. If possible, warm water enema should be given daily during this period to cleanse the bowels. Thereafter, he may be allowed to gradually embark upon a well-balanced diet. The emphasis should be on whole grain cereals, fresh fruits and raw or lightly-cooked vegetables.

The patient should avoid an excessive intake of starchy and sugary foods, meat and other protein and fatty foods, strong tea, coffee and too much salt, condiments and sauces.

Certain home remedies have been found beneficial in the treatment of styes. The most important of these is the use of clove (laung). This spice should be rubbed in water and applied over the eyes. This will give instant relief. The seed of a date rubbed with water can also be applied over styes with beneficial results.

The patient should be encouraged to adopt various methods of relaxing and strengthening the eyes. These include eye exercises like moving the eyes gently up and down, from side to side in a circle, clock-wise and anti-clockwise, rotating the neck in circles and semi-circles and briskly moving the shoulders clock-wise and anti-clockwise.

The patient should also resort to palming which is beneficial in removing strain and relaxing the eyes and its surrounding tissues. The procedure is as follows: sit comfortably in an arm chair or on a settee and relax with your eyes closed. Cover your eyes with your palms, right palm over the right eye and the left over the left eye. Do not, however press down on the eyes. With your eyes closed thus, try to imagine blackness, which grows blacker and blacker. Palming reduces strain and relaxes the eyes and its surrounding tissues.

Styes can be prevented by good hygiene, proper diet and by adopting various methods for relaxing and strengthening the eyes, as outlined above.

CHAPTER 130

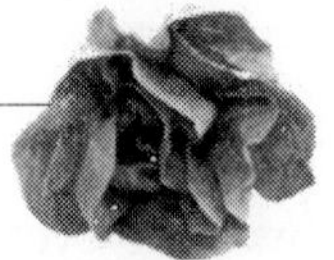

Thinness

Underweight, like overweight, is a relative term, being based on the ideal weight for a given height, built and sex. A person can be regarded as moderately underweight if he or she weighs 10 per cent below the ideal body weight and markedly so if 20 per cent below the ideal.

Appropriate body weight is among the most important physical attributes and has a deep influence upon the health and personality of an individual. For a healthy body, weight slightly above the average is favourable upto the age of 30 years, as it serves as a good defence measure against certain diseases, especially tuberculosis. Between 30 and 40 years of age, the endeavour should be to maintain the weight at the average level as during this period, many future diseases have their beginning. After the age of 40, it will be advisable to keep the weight slightly below the average, so as to lighten the burden on the heart, kidney and other vital organs.

There are two types of thin people. One type is wiry and energetic, who eat heartily but never put on weight. Presumably, they burn up energy due to constant activity. Such persons need not worry as chances are that they do not have any disease as such. The other type of thin persons lack energy and drive, are unable to take normal meals and find that rich food usually makes them sick. Their body lacks fat cells thus providing no storage place for added fat and the calories they consume are probably wasted.

Symptoms

Underweight due to an inadequate caloric intake is a serious condition, especially in the young. They often feel easily fatigued, have poor physical stamina and lowered resistance to infection. Diseases like tuberculosis, respiratory disorders, pneumonia, circulatory diseases like heart disorders, cerebral haemorrhage, nepthritis, typhoid fever and cancer are quite common among them. The occurrence of the complications of pregnancy in young women may result from malnutrition due to an inadequate energy intake.

Causes

Thinness may be due to inadequate nutrition or excessive bodily activity or both. Emotional factors or bad habits such as skipped meals, small meals, habitual fasting and inadequate exercise are some of the other causes of thinness. Other factors include inadequate digestion and absorption of food due to a wrong dietary pattern for a particular metabolism; metabolic disturbances such as an overactive thyroid and hereditary tendencies. Disorders such as chronic dyspepsia, chronic diarrhoea, presence of parasites like tapeworm in the alimentary canal, liver disorders, diabetes mellitus, insomnia, constipation and sexual disorders can also lead to thinness.

Treatment

Diet plays an important role in building up health for gaining weight. Nutrients which help keep the nerves relaxed are of utmost importance as nervousness causes all the muscles to become tense and the energy which goes into the tenseness wastefully uses up a great deal of food.

Although all vitamins and minerals are required for a sound health the most important ones are vitamin D and B_6, calcium and magnesium. The richest sources of vitamin D are milk, codliver oil and the rays of the sun. Calcium is also supplied by milk and yogurt. Magnesium can be obtained from green leafy vegetables such as spinach, parsley, turnip, radish and beet tops. These vegetables should preferably be taken in salad form or should be lightly cooked.

Lack of appetite can result from an inadequate supply of vitamin B, which leads to low production of hydrochloric acid by the stomach. Hydrochloric acid is essential for the digestion of food and absorption of vitamins and minerals into the blood. It is, therefore, necessary that the daily diet should be rich in vitamin B for normal appetite, proper digestion and absorption of foods and regular elimination. Foods rich in vitamin B are all whole grain cereals, blackstrap molasses, nuts, soyabean, eggs and butter. Vegetable oil is of special value to those wishing to gain weight as it is rich in vitamin E and essential fatty acids.

Underweight persons should eat frequent small meals as they tend to feel full quickly. Meals may be divided into six small ones instead of three big ones. These may consist of three smaller meals and three substantial snacks between them. The weight-building quality of a food is measured by the number of calories it contains. To gain weight, the diet should include more calories than are used in daily activities so as to allow the excess to be stored as body fat. The allowance of 500 calories in excess of the daily average needs is estimated to provide for a weight gain of one pound weekly.

All refined foods such as products containing white flour and sugar should be avoided, as they destroy health. Excessive intake of refined carbohydrates and fats may help the individual to put on weight but this will be detrimental to general health. The diet should be tilted towards alkaline-forming foods such as fruits and vegetables. Alkaline foods should comprise 80 per cent of the diet. The other 20 per cent should consist of acid-forming foods such as cereals and lentils. Beverages containing caffeine like soft drinks, coffee and tea should be curtailed. Smoking should be given up. Water should not be taken with meals but half an hour before or one hour after meals.

Milk Cure

An exclusive milk diet for rapid gain of weight has been advocated by some nature cure practitioners. In the beginning of this treatment, the patient should fast for three days on warm water and lime juice so as to cleanse the system. Thereafter, he should have a glass of milk every two hours from 8 a.m. to 8 p.m. the first day, a glass every hour and a half the next day, and a glass every hour the third day. Then the quantity of milk should be gradually increased so as to take a glass every half an hour from 8 a.m. to 8 p.m., if such a quantity can be tolerated fairly comfortably. The milk should be fresh and unboiled, but may be slightly warmed, if desired. It should be sipped very slowly through a straw. The milk should be unpasteurised, if possible.

Figs are an excellent food remedy for increasing weight in case of thinness. The high percentage of the rapidly assimilable sugar make them a strengthening and fattening food.

Regular exercises like walking and dancing, yoga, meditation and massage are also important as they serve as relaxants, reduce stress and induce good sleep. Yogasanas which will be especially helpful are sarvangasana, halasana and matsyasana.

A balanced diet together with adequate exercise, rest, emotional balance and the absence of acute diseases will enable an underweight person to build a healthy body and put on weight.

CHAPTER 131

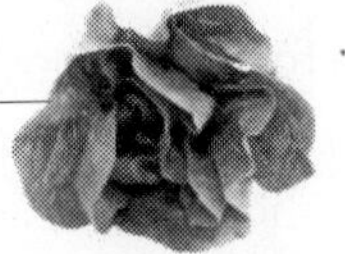

Typhoid Fever

Typhoid fever is an acute systemic disease caused by salmonella typhi bacteria. It is a condition in which there is a typical course of temperature, with marked abdominal symptoms consisting of ulceration of the bowels. The fever is of uncertain duration and liable to frequent relapses.

Typhoid fever is an infectious disease and persons contract it, through human carriers. The condition is common in tropical countries with poor sanitation and the menace of flies.

Symptoms

It takes from 10 days to two weeks for this disease to develop. The patient feels chilly, tired and weak. He suffers from headache and loss of appetite, followed by backache and diarrhoea or constipation.

Many patients also have bronchitis, so that in the early stages of typhoid, the disease may appear as pneumonia. The temperature rises and remains high for abut 10 days to two weeks. It has a tendency to rise in the evening and fall in the morning. Skin eruptions tend to appear in the second week and if proper care is not taken, inflammation of the bones and ulceration of the bowels may occur. The loss of appetite is more apparent. The tongue becomes dry and is coated with white patches in the central region of its surface. The fever gradually comes down to normal by the end of the fourth week.

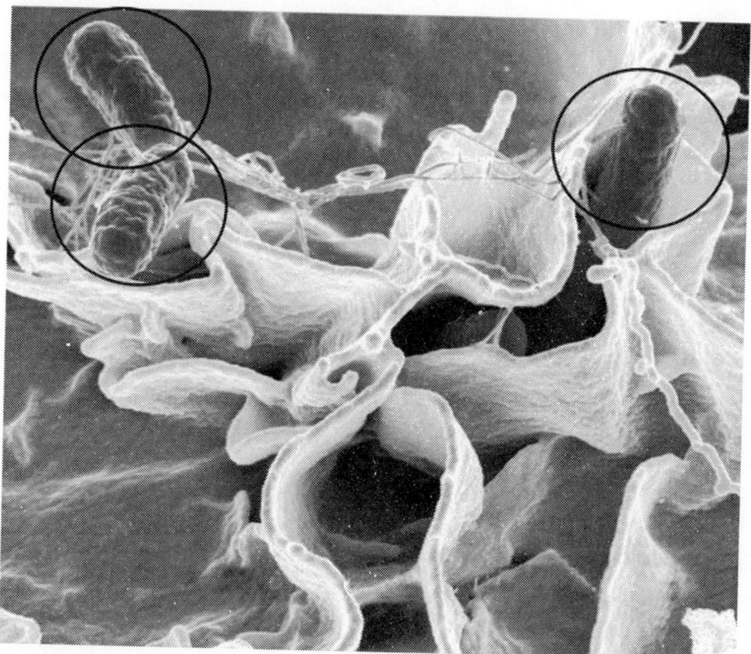

Electron micrograph showing Salmonella typhimurium (circled) invading cultured human cells.

Causes

Poor sanitation is most often responsible for this disease. Contaminated water is the usual source of infection. The next common cause is infected milk. Other foods may also be responsible for the disease. Sometimes, certain people, known as carriers, may spread the disease. After a patient has had the disease, the bacteria may survive in the gall-bladder for years, so that the patient becomes a carrier. If such a carrier is employed in preparing or serving food, the infection can spread. In a few cases, flies may bring the germs into the house and contaminate the food. Germs enter the body through the mouth, causing irritation and ulceration of the lower small bowel.

Typhoid fever usually develops in a person who has a great accumulation of toxic waste and other putrefactive material in his intestine, resulting from wrong dietary and faulty style of living. The germ of typhoid fever flourishes upon this morbid condition in the intestine. The disease is more common in persons who eat much meat or other flesh foods, as it is the nature of such foods to decompose and putrefy readily within the intestines.

Treatment

A complete bed rest and careful nursing is essential for the patient. He should be given liquid diet like milk, barley and fruit juices. Orange juice will be especially beneficial. In fact, the exclusive diet of orange juice diluted with water can be taken for first few days of the treatment with highly beneficial results. In typhoid fever, the digestive power of the body is seriously hampered and the patient suffers from blood poisoning called toxaemia. The lack of saliva coats his tongue and often destroys his thirst for water as well as his desire for food. The agreeable flavour of orange juice helps greatly in overcoming these drawbacks. It also gives energy, increases urinary output and promotes body resistance against infections, thereby hastening recovery. If possible, warm-water enema should be given daily during this period to cleanse the bowels.

Cold compresses may be applied to the head in case the temperature rises above 103°F. If this method does not succeed, to wring out a sheet or large square piece of linen material in cold water, wrap it twice around the body and legs of the patient and then cover completely with a small blanket or similar warm material. This pack should be applied every three hours during the day while temperature is high and kept on for one hour or so each time. Hot water compress may be applied to the feet and also against the sides of the body.

After the temperature has come down to normal and the tongue has cleared, the patient may be given fresh fruits and other easily digestible foods for two or three days. For drinks, unsweetened lemon water or plain water, either hot or cold, may be given. Thereafter, the patient may be allowed to gradually embark upon a well-balanced diet. The emphasis should be on fresh fruits and raw or lightly-cooked vegetables.

Prevention

The diseases can be prevented by ensuring a clean water supply, proper disposal of sewage and implementation of anti-fly measures. All drinking water should be either boiled or thoroughly purified. Milk should be pasteurized or boiled. People who handle food should be carefully screened to be sure that they are not carrying the germs of typhoid.

CHAPTER 132

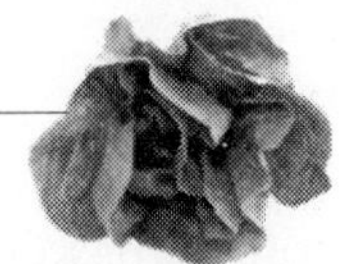

Thyroid Disease

Thyroid disease assumes various forms, the most frequent being hypothyroidism, also known as myxedema, and hyperthyroidism, also known as thyrotoxicosis or exophthalmic goitre. Hypothyroidism results from the withering or atrophy of the thyroid gland. Hyperthyroidism is a serious condition of the body, which results from overactivity of the thyroid gland.

Women are more prone to thyroid disease. They are especially likely to develop a sluggish thyroid after middle age. The disease is more common in women who are over worked and who do not get sufficient rest and relaxation. The period in older women's life, when she is more likely to be affected by this disease is at the menopause and thereafter, or when there is any extra physical strain on the body.

Symptoms

In hypothyroidism, the basal metabolism decreases below normal, with the result the patient tends to be slow in his movements. He is susceptible to cold, suffers from constipation and puts on weight. Other symptoms include dry, scaly and thickened hair, puffiness in the face. The pulse is slow and the patient often complains of vague pains in the back and stiffness in the joints.

The patient with hyperthyroidism is usually nervous, weak, sensitive to heat, sweats frequently, is over active and often underweight. There might be slight tremor in the fingers and

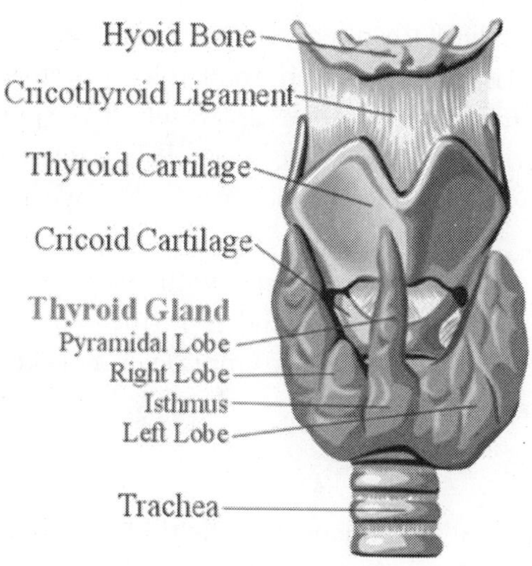

Thyroid Gland

palpitation of the heart. In many cases, there may be bulging of the eyes and passing excessive quantity of urine. The heart is over-active and usually enlarged. The pulse rate is rapid and may be irregular.

Causes

The main cause of hypothyroidism is insufficient production of thyroid hormone. Other causes of this disease are some pituitary deficiency and inborn error of the thyroid gland. The change usually comes gradually. The main cause of hyperthyroidism is the excess amounts of thyroid hormone produced by the overactive gland. This raises the metabolic rate of the body. Another important cause of this disease is physical or emotional stress. Heredity also plays a role and the disease seems to run in families.

The real cause of thyroid disease, however, is wrong feeding habits over a long period of faulty style of living, together with suppressive medical treatment of other diseases in the past. The thyroid gland plays an important role in destroying toxic matter generated in the intestines as a result of the putrefaction of animal protein material, like meat, fish, eggs, cheese and milk. The thyroid glands will be overworked when excessive quantities of these foods are consumed, resulting in the clogging of the intestinal tract with toxic matter. The overworking of the thyroid gland is further complicated by wrong living habits and excessive emotionalism, both of which weaken the system.

Treatment

The only real treatment for thyroid disease, whether hypothyroidism, hyperthyroidism or any other condition of thyroid gland, is cleansing of the system and adoption of a rational dietary thereafter, combined with adequate rest and relaxation. To begin with, the patient should take juices of fresh fruits such as orange, apple, pineapple and grapes every two hours from 8 a.m. to 8 p.m. for five days. The bowels should be cleansed daily with warm-water enema.

After the juice fast, the patient may spend further three days on fruits and milk, taking three meals a day of juicy fruits with a glass of milk, at five-hourly intervals. Thereafter, he may adopt a well-balanced diet consisting of seeds, nuts and grains, vegetables and fruits.

The patient should take plenty of rest and spend a day in bed every week for the first two months of the treatment. He should take physical exercise after the symptoms subside.

The appetite of the thyroid patient is usually very large and the weight reduction cannot be prevented for some time in case of hyperthyroidism. This is because until the heart beat slows down and the tremors stop, there will be incomplete assimilation of food. But as soon as the balance is restored, weight will slowly increase. To help the absorption of food, a narrow waist compress and, later, a neck compress should be worn for five nights a week. As weight increases, the almost constant hunger will gradually disappear.

Certain foods and fruits are extremely injurious for thyroid patients and should be avoided by them. These include white flour products, white sugar, flesh foods, fried and greasy foods, preserves, condiments, tea, coffee and alcohol.

Great care must be taken never to allow the body to become exhausted and any irritation likely to cause emotional upset should be avoided. The cure of thyroid disease is not a speedy one and there is often a recurrence of symptoms but these should gradually become less pronounced. Strict adherence to diet is essential for one year for complete cure. Half the daily intake of food should consist of fresh fruits and vegetables and the starch element should be confined to whole wheat products and potatoes. The protein foods should be confined to cheese, peas, beans, lentils and nuts. There might be slight recurrence of this extremely nervous complaint for some time, but the attacks will become less severe and of short duration as the treatment progresses.

CHAPTER 133

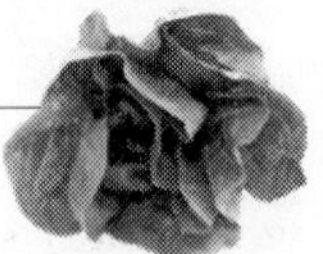

Tonsillitis

Tonsillitis refers to acute inflammation of the tonsils. It is also known as acute sore throat. Chronic tonsillitis is a term applied to cases in which there is enlargement of the tonsils accompanied by repeated attacks of infection.

The tonsils are two small lymphoid organs that lie one on each side of the throat. They can be seen just behind the back of the tongue between two folds of membrane running up to the soft palate. Normally, they are about the size of a lima bean but they can become very much larger if severely infected. They are valuable organs of selective elimination and perform a two-fold function. Firstly, they protect the throat against disease germs. Secondly, they serve as barometers for indicating infection elsewhere in the body, when they become sore and swollen.

Symptoms

The main symptoms of tonsillitis are sore throat, fever, headache, pain in various parts of the body, difficulty in swallowing and general weakness. The tonsils are seen to be inflamed and red when the mouth is opened wide. In many cases, spots of pus exude from them. Externally, the tonsillar lymph glands which lie just behind the angle of the jaw are tender and enlarged. In several cases there may be pain in the ear.

Causes

The chief cause of tonsillitis is a toxic condition of the

system generally and is brought to a head by a sudden lowering of vitality resulting from exposure and sudden chill. Tonsils enlarge and get inflamed when the toxins cannot be got rid of through the normal channels of elimination such as the bowels, kidneys and skin. Throat affliction of this kind is also associated with the result of chronic constipation, when toxins, which should have been ejected from the system in the normal way, are reabsorbed into the blood-stream.

Treatment

The treatment of tonsillitis on the lines of modern medical system by means of painting and spraying is both harmful and suppressive. It does not help to rid the system of the toxins, which are the root of the trouble. In fact it forces these toxins back into the system, which may cause more serious trouble later on. The correct way to treat the disease is to cleanse the system of toxic waste through proper dietary and other natural methods.

To begin with, the patient should fast for three to five days by which time serious symptoms would subside. Nothing but water and orange juice should be taken during this time. The bowels should be cleansed daily with a warm-water enema during the period of fasting. A cold pack should be applied to the throat at two-hourly intervals during the day. The procedure is to wring out some linen material in cold water, wrap it two or three times around the throat and cover it with some flannelling.

The throat may be gargled several times daily with neat lemon juice. Gargle made from the fenugreek seeds is very effective in severe cases. To make such a gargle, two tablespoonful of fenugreek seeds should be allowed to simmer for half an hour in a litre of water and then set aside to cool. The entire quantity should be used as a soothing gargle in a day with beneficial results. A hot Epsom-salt bath taken every day or every other day will also be beneficial.

After the acute symptoms of tonsillitis are over, the patient should adopt an all-fruit diet for further three or four days. In this regimen, three meals of fresh, juicy fruits such as apples, grapes, grapefruit, oranges, pears, pineapple, peaches and melon may be taken. The juice of fresh pineapple is most valuable in all throat afflictions of this kind. After the all-fruit diet the patient may gradually embark upon a well-balanced diet on the following lines.

Breakfast: Fresh fruits or grated raw carrot or any other raw salad, and milk. Prunes or other dried fruit may be added, if desired.

Lunch: Steamed vegetables, as obtainable, and whole wheat chappatis. Vegetables like bitter gourd and fenugreek are specially beneficial.

Dinner: A good-sized raw salad of vegetables as obtainable, sprouts seeds as mung beans and alfalfa seeds, wholemeal bread and butter or cottage cheese.

Raw vegetable juices are also valuable in the treatment of tonsillitis. Juice of carrot, beet and cucumber taken individually or in combination are especially beneficial. Formula proportion found to be helpful when used in combination are carrot 300 ml., beet 100 ml. and cucumber 100 ml.

The daily dry friction and hip bath as well as breathing and other exercises should all form part of the daily health regimen. A hot Epsom-salts bath once or twice a week can also be taken regularly with beneficial results.

Tonsillitis can be successfully treated by the natural methods outlined above. Surgery for the removal of the tonsils is necessary only in very rare cases, when tonsils are seriously diseased, rugged and contain hopelessly incurable pus pockets.

CHAPTER 134

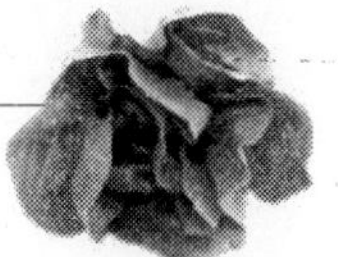

Tuberculosis

Tuberculosis is one of the most dreaded diseases. It is a major health problem in India and often rated the number one killer. Over five lakh people die of this disease every year.

Tuberculosis is caused by a tiny germ called *tubercle bacillus* which is so small that it can be detected only by a microscope. The germ enters into the body through the nose, mouth and windpipe and settles down in the lungs. It multiplies by millions and produces small raised spots called tubercles.

Tuberculosis is not hereditary but an infectious or communicable disease. Those suffering from the disease for a considerable time eject living germs while coughing or spitting and when these enter the nose or mouth of healthy persons, they contract the disease. Mouth-breathing and kissing as well as contaminated food and water are also responsible for spreading tuberculosis.

Symptoms

Tuberculosis is of four types, namely of lungs, intestines, bones and glands. Pulmonary tuberculosis or tuberculosis of the lungs is by far the most common type of tuberculosis. It tends to consume the body and the patient loses strength, colour and weight. Other symptoms are a raise in temperature especially in the evening, a persistent cough and hoarseness, difficulty in breathing, pain in the shoulders, indigestion, chest pain, and blood in the sputum.

Causes

Lowered resistance or devitalisation of the system is the chief cause of this disease. This condition is brought about mainly by mineral starvation of the tissues of the body due to an inadequate diet; and the chief mineral concerned is calcium. In many ways, therefore, tuberculosis is the disease of calcium deficiency. There can be no breakdown of the tissue and no tubercular growth where there is adequate supply of organic calcium in the said tissue. Thus an adequate supply of organic calcium in the system together with organic mineral matter is a sure preventive of the development of tuberculosis.

Lowered resistance also results from a variety of other factors such as suppression of the disease by drugs and medication, use of stale, devitaminised and acid forming foods, eating wrong combination of foods, such as taking fruits with starchy foods at one meal, causing fermentation in the stomach; wasting of energy through excessive loss of semen and living in ill-ventilated houses. Other causes include exposure to cold, loss of sleep, impure air, a sedentary life, overwork, contaminated milk, use of tobacco in any form, liquor of all kinds, tea, coffee and all harmful drinks. The factors prepare the ground for the growth of germs of various kinds, including tubercle bacillus. These germs may be present in the body but are quite harmless for those who are full of vitality and natural resistance.

Treatment

Tuberculosis is no longer considered incurable if it is tackled in the early stages. An all round scheme of dietetic and vitality building programme along natural lines is the only method to overcome the disease. As a first step, the patient should be put on an exclusive fresh fruit diet for three or four days. He should have three meals a day of fresh, juicy fruits, such as apples, grapes, pears, peaches, oranges, pineapple, melon or any other juicy fruit in season. Bananas, dried or tinned should not be taken. For drinks, unsweetened lemon water or plain water either hot or cold may be taken. If losing much weight on the all-fruit diet, those already under weight may add a glass of milk to each fruit meal.

After the all-fruit diet, the patient should adopt a fruit and milk diet. For this diet, the meals are exactly the same as the all-fruit diet, but with milk added to each fruit meal. The patient may begin with a litre of milk the first day and increase by quarter litre daily upto two to two and a half litres according to how the milk agrees. The milk should be fresh and unboiled, but may be slightly warmed if desired. It should be sipped very slowly. The fruit and milk diet should be continued for four to six weeks. Thereafter, the following dietary may be adopted:

Breakfast: Fresh fruits , as obtainable, and milk. Prunes or other dried fruits may also be taken, if desired.

Lunch: Steamed vegetables as available, one or two whole wheat chappatis and a glass of buttermilk.

Dinner: A bowl of raw salad of suitable vegetables with wholewheat bread and butter. Stewed fruit or cooked apple may be taken for dessert.

At bed-time: A glass of milk.

The chief therapeutic agent needed for the treatment of tuberculosis is calcium. Milk, being the richest food source for the supply of organic calcium to the body, should be taken liberally. In the dietary outlined above at least one litre of milk should be taken daily. Further periods on the exclusive fruit diet followed by fruit and milk diet should be adopted at intervals of two or three months depending on the progress.

During the first few days of the treatment, the bowels should be cleansed daily with the warm-water enema and afterwards as necessary.

The patient should avoid all devitalised foods such as white bread, white sugar, refined cereals, puddings and pies, tinned, canned and preserved foods. He should also avoid strong tea, coffee, condiments, pickles, sauces, etc.

The custard apple is regarded as an effective food remedy for tuberculosis. It is said to contain the qualities of rejuvenating drugs. The Ayurvedic practitioner prepares a fermented liquor called *sitaphalasava* from the custard apple in its season for use as medicine in the treatment of tuberculosis. It is prepared by boiling custard apple pulp and seedless raisins in water on slow fire. It is filtered when about one third of water is left. It is then mixed with powdered sugar candy and also the powder of cardamom, cinnamon and certain other condiments.

Indian gooseberry has proved to be an effective remedy for tuberculosis. A tablespoonful each of fresh amla juice and honey mixed together should be taken every morning in this condition. Its regular use will promote vigour and vitality in the body within a few days. Regular use of radish is also beneficial.

The patient should take complete rest of both mind and body. Any type of stress will prevent healing. Fresh air is always important in curing the disease and the patient should spend most of the time in the open air and should sleep in a well-ventilated room. Sunshine is also essential as tuber bacilli are rapidly killed by exposure to sun rays. Other beneficial steps towards curing the disease are avoidance of strain, slow massage, deep breathing and light occupation to ensure mental diversion.

Water Treatment

Certain water treatments are helpful in cases of tuberculosis. The patient's vital resistance can be built up by a carefully planned graduated cold bath routine twice a day. The intensity of the cold applications should be gradually increased to achieve satisfactory results. However, care must be taken to keep the patient from catching a chill. A short hot fomentation with alternate short cold application to the chest and back, and in the stomach region or a neutral immersion bath (water temperature 98° to 100°F) for an hour just before retiring at night is also beneficial.

Certain yogic practices are beneficial in the treatment of tuberculosis in its early stages. These include asanas like viparitakarani, sarvangasana and shavasana and jalneti kriya and anuloma-viloma pranayama.

CHAPTER 135

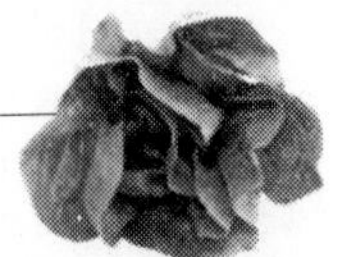

Urticaria

Urticaria is a common inflammatory affection, characterised by formation of wheals on the skin. The disease is also known as nettle-rash as the rash of Urticaria resembles the sting of a nettle. The disease may be acute, chronic or recurrent. It is considered to be an allergic reaction like hay fever and asthma.

Symptoms

Raised red and white patches appear on the skin. They are accompanied by burning, intense itching and stinging. Rubbing and scratching usually aggravates the hives. Itching is relieved by scratching, which results in new wheals. The outbreak of urticaria is sudden and the disease may affect either part or whole of the body. The eruptions may be as small as pin heads or as large as a rupee. They are usually much elevated, rounded, irregular and often surrounded by a reddened zone. The eruption may fade in a few minutes or an hour in one place, but may appear in another.

Other symptoms which accompany hives are fever, digestive disturbances and prostration. The disorder lasts from a day or two to a week. Recovery is rapid and complete, though recurring attacks take place at varying intervals. If the rash also attacks the throat, there is danger of blockage of the larynx.

Causes

There are several causes of urticaria. It may result from digestive disorders like mechanical irritation in the digestive tract or toxaemia. It may be caused by drugs like aspirin,

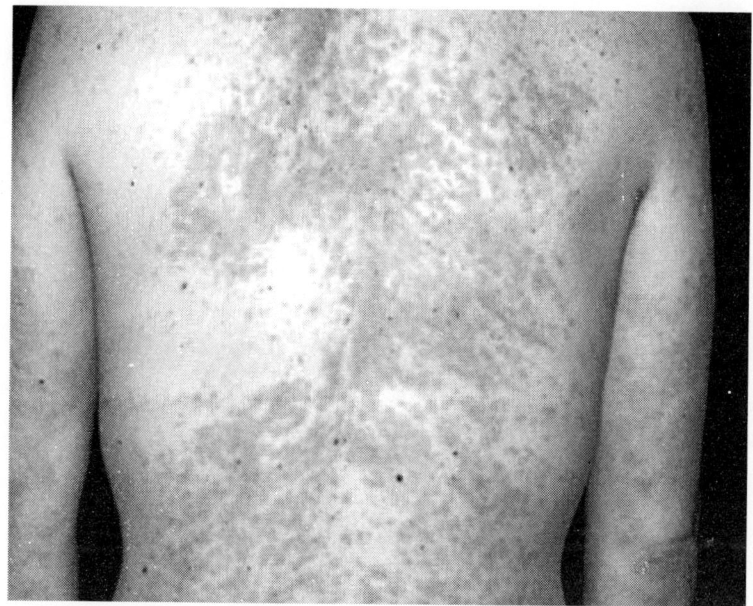

Urticaria

penicillin, serum, quinine, ipecac, turpentine and morphine. Certain foods often cause urticaria in susceptible individuals. These include strawberries, tomatoes, cucumbers, mushrooms, oatmeal, wheat, nuts, fish, eggs, chocolate, cheese, butter and sausage. The bites of bed-bugs, wasps, bees, mosquitoes, fleas and certain kinds of caterpillars may produce the disease. Irritations of the uterus or associate structures can also cause the disease. It may also result from emotional excitement.

Treatment

As urticaria has its origin in the gastro-intestinal tract, the best way to commence the treatment is to adopt an all-fruit diet for about five days. In this regimen, the patient should take three meals a day of fresh juicy fruits such as orange, apple, pineapple, grapes, pear, peach and papaya. A warm-water enema should be used daily during this period to cleanse the bowels, and later, if necessary. The patient should also drink a liberal amount of hot water.

After the all-fruit diet, the patient may embark upon a well-balanced diet consisting of seeds, nuts, grains, vegetables and fruits. The emphasis should be on fresh fruits and raw vegetable salad. The patient should avoid tea, coffee, alcohol, all flesh foods, refined foods and all foods which are difficult to digest. He should drink at least eight glasses of water daily between meals. A glass of water containing the juice of half a lemon may be taken one hour before each meals and also between meals.

The patient should spend two or three days on an all-fruit diet at regular intervals. This will further cleanse the system matters and help recovery.

Certain home remedies have been found beneficial in the treatment of Urticaria. The use of salt is valuable in urticaria accompanied by digestive disorders. In such a condition, about 12 grams of salt should be dissolved in water and taken by the patient. The throat should be tickled to induce vomiting. This will give relief and help in curing eruptions.

Equal quantity of alum (*phitkari*) and red ochere (*geru*) are found beneficial in the treatment of urticaria. These two substances should be ground together and the powder rubbed on the wheals.

The use of rosewater (*gulab jal*) in vinegar (*sirca*) is considered useful in case of severe itching on the eruption. About 35 ml. of rose water and 25 ml. of vinegar should be mixed and the mixture applied locally to the affected part. This will give immediate relief.

Mint (*pudina*) has also been found useful in relieving itching in urticaria. About seven grams of this leafy vegetable and 25 grams of brown sugar should be boiled together in water and drunk. This will relieve the itching.

Turmeric (*haldi*) is valuable in urticaria. The patient should take two teaspoons of turmeric powder mixed with water at regular intervals in treating this disease.

The patient should avoid exposure to cold and cold water. Fresh air and sunlight are also essential to the treatment and the patient should frequently expose his body to the sun and spend as much time outdoors as possible.

CHAPTER 136

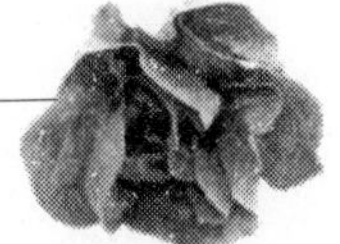

Varicose Veins

Veins are thin-walled vessels through which the impure blood is carried back to the heart. They usually have valves which regulate the flow of blood towards the heart. Varicose veins are a condition in which veins become enlarged, dilated or thickened.

Varicose veins can occur in any part of the body but generally appear on the legs. The veins of the legs are the largest in the body and they carry the blood from the lower extremities upwards towards the heart. The direction of circulation in these vessels is largely determined by gravity. Though there are no mechanical obstacles to blood-flow, it is usually the incompetence of the valve which leads to an increase in intervenous pressure.

Varicose veins have an unsightly appearance and can be dangerous. A blood clot within a large, greatly dilated vein may break away and move toward the heart and lungs, causing serious complications. Varicose veins are about thrice as common an occurrence in women as in men. This disease is rare in rural undeveloped societies.

Symptoms

The first sign of varicose veins is a swelling along the course of the veins. This may be followed by muscular cramps and a feeling of tiredness in the legs behind the knees. In some cases, the normal flow of blood towards the heart may be reversed when the patient is in an upright position. This results

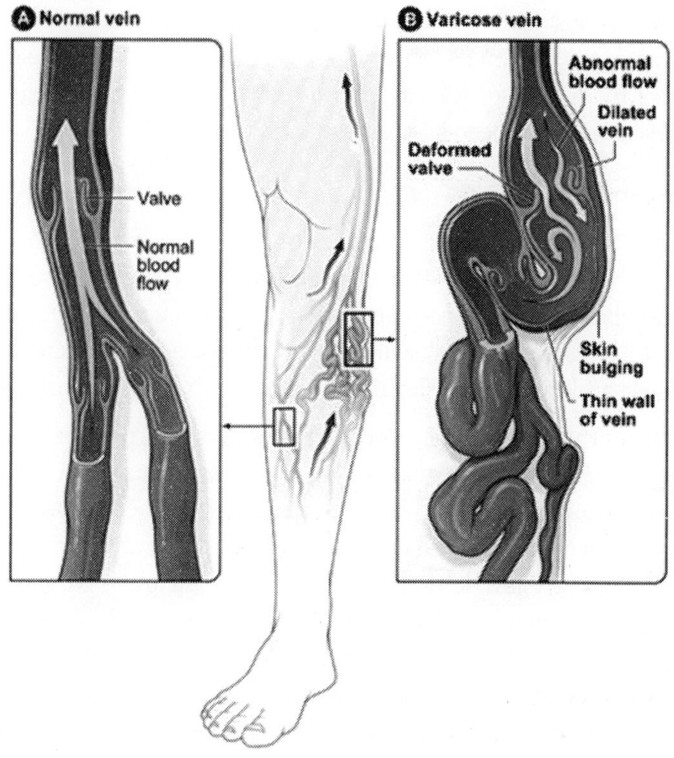

Varicose Veins

in venous blood collecting in the lower part of the legs and the skin becomes purplish and pigmented, leading to what is known as varicose eczema or varicose ulcers. Both conditions cause severe pain.

Causes

A varicose condition of the veins results from sluggish circulation due to various factors such as constipation, dietetic errors, lack of exercise and smoking. Standing for long periods and wearing tight clothing can also lead to sluggish circulation. Pregnancy may cause varicose veins due to increased pressure in the pelvis and abdomen, which slows down the flow of blood from the lower extremities to the heart. Women usually suffer from this condition in the early years of child-bearing. Obesity can also cause varicose veins.

Treatment

For a proper treatment of varicose veins, the patient should, in the beginning, be put on a juice fast for four or five days or on all-fruit diet for seven to 10 days. A warm water enema should be administered daily during this period to cleanse the bowels and measures should be taken to avoid constipation.

After the juice fast or the all-fruits diet, the patient should adopt a restricted diet plan. In this regimen, oranges or orange and lemon juice may be taken for breakfast. The midday meal may consist of a raw salad of any of the vegetables in season with olive oil and lemon juice dressing. Steamed vegetables such as spinach, cabbage, carrots, turnips, cauliflower and raisins, figs or dates may be taken in the evening. No bread or potatoes or other starchy food should be included in this diet, or otherwise the whole effect of the diet will be lost.

After the restricted diet, the patient may gradually embark upon a well balanced diet with emphasis on grains, seeds, nuts, vegetables and fruits. About 75 per cent of the diet should consist of raw vegetables and fruits. All condiments, alcoholic drinks, coffee, strong tea, white flour products, white sugar and white sugar products should be strictly avoided. A short fast or the all-fruit diet for two or three days may be undertaken every month, depending on the progress.

Raw vegetable juices, especially carrot juice in combination with spinach juice, have proved highly beneficial in the treatment of varicose veins. The formula proportion considered helpful in this combination are carrot 300 ml. and spinach 200 ml. to prepare 500 ml. of juice.

Certain nutrients, especially vitamins E and C have also been found effective in the treatment of this disease. The patient should take vitamin C in a therapeutic dose upto 3,000 mg. and Vitamin E in therapeutic doses from 600 to 1,200 I.U. daily. This will relieve him of pain and leg cramps associated with varicose veins.

The alternate hot and cold hip bath is very valuable and should be taken daily. The affected parts should be sprayed with cold water or cold packs should be applied to them. A mud pack may be applied at night and allowed to remain until morning. A hot Epsom-salts bath is also very valuable and should be taken twice a week.

Precautionary Measures

The following precautionary measures will help prevent varicose veins and ease symptoms if the disease has already developed:

1. When on a long plane or train trip, get up and walk around every half an hour. If on a long trip by car, stop once in a while and get out to stretch your legs.
2. When you are reading or watching television, elevate your feet and rest your legs on a chair or stool.
3. Mobility helps general circulation. Walking is beneficial as the movements of leg muscles help push the blood upward. Swimming or walking in deep water does much the same thing. The great pressures of the water against legs helps move the blood up the veins and protects against stagnation.
4. Sleeping with feet raised slightly above the level of the heart helps the blood flow away from ankles. In case of serious trouble with varicose veins, the bed should

be raised by placing blocks of six inches height under the posts at the foot. This is, however, not advisable for persons with heart trouble.

5. If confined to bed, movement of feet and legs should be encouraged to help keep circulation moving youthfully.
6. Round garters should never be worn. They cut off the venous circulation, thus raising pressure in the veins and increasing the risk of varicosities.
7. Elastic girdles should not be worn continuously, especially when seated for a long time, such as at a desk, or during a plane, train or auto trip. The girdles bunch up and hamper the return flow of blood.
8. Pregnant women should wear elastic stockings and lie down occasionally during the day. Getting up soon after delivery is also helpful in blood circulation.

These easy-to-follow flex-exercises are beneficial as they ease the cause of varicose veins and thereby relieve the resultant symptoms. Sun bathing and deep breathing exercises are also helpful.

Certain inverted yoga postures such as viparitakarani, sarvangasana and sirshasana are beneficial in the treatment of varicose veins as they drain the blood from the legs and reduce pressure on the veins. They help to relax the muscles and allow the blood to flow freely in and out of the lower extremities. Padmasana, gomukhasana, vajrasana and shalabhasana are also beneficial.

CHAPTER 137

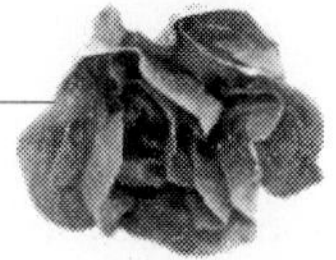

Venereal Diseases

There has been an alarming increase in venereal or sexually transmitted diseases (V.D. or S.T.D.) due to promiscuity and free sex. These diseases are caused by bacteria and germs and can become very serious if not treated properly and early. The most common diseases in this category are syphilis and gonorrhoea.

Syphilis is probably one of the oldest diseases of the human race. Sexual contact is the commonest way in which this disease is spread through a community. But many of those who contract the disease are innocent. Little children are sometimes born with this disease. It may also be transmitted from one person to another by kissing or handling infected clothing or other articles.

Symptoms and Causes

Syphilis usually begins as a small ulcering type of lesion which may occur anywhere in the body, the most common sites being the penis, the vulva or in the vagina. Violent or rough sex behaviour often results in abrasions and thus the virus comes in direct contact with the blood.

Gonorrhoea is usually transmitted by sexual contact. An acute inflammation of the male urethra or the vagina of the female due to infection through pus by the gonorrhoea germs is known as gonorrhoea. A person having a high degree of toxaemia and a low vitality may develop this condition with the slightest secretion. A clean blood stream and a high vitality on the other hand may protect one from this disease.

The wise plan, however, is to avoid all chances of infection.

The common chance is the sexual act in which one of the partners has this disease. Sometimes it may be contracted through other sources or it may be hereditary.

Gonorrhoea is a more difficult disease to identify than syphilis. About two-thirds of women with this disease have no symptoms at all or at most very trivial ones which may be passed off as an apparently harmless vaginal discharge. The usual symptom in the male is a discharge from the tip of the penis.

If the disease is neglected or improperly treated, it may spoil the entire blood stream which may produce gonorrheal rheumatism and cause infection of the eyes. Proper treatment is therefore, highly important soon after the occurrence of the infection.

Treatment

Syphilis and gonorrhoea are quite amenable to successful treatment by proper dietary and other natural methods, leaving no ill-effects to mar the future life and happiness of their victims. Suppressive drugs employed by the modern medical system in the treatment simply halts the active manifestations of the diseases in the victim's system for the time being. The disease-poisons and the metallic drugs used are still left in the patient's system and these have a most destructive effect upon the tissues and structures of the body, especially upon the nervous tissues.

The only safe way of treating venereal diseases is fasting. All cases of syphilis and gonorrhoea can be cured through the agency of the fast. This will not only prevent dreaded after-effects, but will also greatly enhance the whole general health level of the patient by a thorough cleansing of his system. The juice of an orange, in a glass of warm water, may be taken during this period. If orange juice disagrees, vegetable juices may be taken. Each day while fasting, it should be ensured that the bowels are cleansed of the poisonous matter thrown off by the self-cleansing process now set up by the body. This can be achieved through a warm water enema. The fast may be continued from seven to 14 days.

After the fast, the patient, may adopt an exclusive fruit diet for further five days. He should thereafter gradually embark upon a balanced diet for three basic food groups as outlined in the treatment for impotence (chapter 123), avoiding all the foods mentioned therein.

Major R. Austin, a doctor in the Royal Army Medical Corps in Great Britain in his book, *Direct Paths to Health* mentions a case of a syphilis patient aged 27 years who was cured only by dietetic treatment. Dr. Austin narrates the case as under:

"Mr. A., aged twenty-seven, came to me suffering from tertiary syphilis. The classic drugs had been used, but it had not stopped the ravages of the disease. His face and body were covered with rupial eruptions—ulcers covered with a scab—and the odour from his body was most unpleasant.

"I prescribed a fourteen-day fast with a saline purge daily, plenty of water and as much strained orange juice diluted with water as he liked to drink during the day. At the end of the fourteen days he was allowed two meals a day, one of them consisting of nothing but purely cooked vegetables and some butter, and the other of milk and fresh fruit.

"In six weeks from the date of commencing the treatment, all the eruptions had disappeared, as well as the foul odour of the body, and he was feeling remarkably well and has remained so ever since."

Vegetable juices are highly beneficial in the treatment of venereal diseases. Juices which are particularly helpful include those of carrot, cucumber, beet and spinach. The patient may make liberal use of carrot juice either in combination with spinach juice or cucumber and beet.

Amaranth (*chaulai ka saag*) is considered highly beneficial in the treatment of gonorrhoea. About 25 gms of the leaves of this vegetable should be given twice or thrice a day to the patient in this condition.

Fresh juice of the flowers of the drumstick is very useful in the treatment of gonorrhoea. For better results, this juice should be given twice daily with tender coconut water. It acts as a diuretic tonic in this disease.

A decoction of fresh lady's fingers has also been found useful in treating gonorrhoea. A cupful of mucilage of lady's fingers is mixed with a ripe banana and a glassful of buttermilk. This mixture is a very effective remedy for gonorrhoea. Four capsules of lady's finger are cut into 2.5 cm. pieces and are boiled in quarter litre of water for about 15 minutes. After cooling the pieces are squeezed and the mucilage is extracted and strained through a muslin cloth.

In case of syphilis, a 'T' pack should be employed for an hour for the local treatment of the initial sore and it should be repeated twice daily. All clothes, sheets and towels, used by the patient should be handled carefully to avoid new sores and to prevent infection to others. It is better to boil all such articles. In case of eruption on the different parts of the body, a wet sheet pack for an hour is beneficial. It will help bring out all the poisonous substances of the skin by producing more eruptions which will gradually dry up.

Application of pelvic packs occasionally for an hour is one of the most effective methods of treatment in case of gonorrhoea. As irritation in the prostate gland and urethra is present in this disease, a hot hip bath for eight minutes has a beneficial effect as it tends to relieve irritation.

An occasional steam bath for eight minutes is of outstanding value in both syphilis and gonorrhoea. It will help remove the poisonous substances from the body and enable the kidney to perform its work effectively. An overall massage has also beneficial effects upon the entire body.

CHAPTER 138

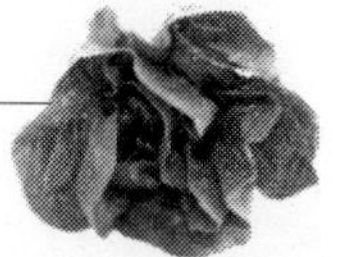

Warts

Warts refer to hard, dry growths in the skin. They are capable of spreading, but are usually harmless. They often disappear spontaneously. These small benign tumours of the skin are most common in childhood, but after infancy.

Warts come in various shapes and sizes. Common warts are raised cauliflower-like lesions which occur most frequently on the hands. They may be scattered or grouped. These warts usually resolve spontaneously eventually. Some warts are thread like and others flat.

Symptoms

Warts usually appear as rough elevation in the skin. These elevations occur more frequently on the fingers, elbows, knees, face and scalp. They usually appear as small raised painless lesion with a rough dry surface. Where there is pressure as on the soles of the feet, they may be hardly raised, but tend to be painful. They flourish in the moist areas of the body.

When warts occur on the feet, they are known as verrucae. They are particularly catching. They are most easily spread in swimming baths and bathrooms because the moist, warm atmosphere at these places is just right for this infection to be passed from person to person. Some swimming baths hold foot inspections and will not allow in any patient with a verrucae. Others insist that special 'verrucae-socks' are worn if a verrucae is present.

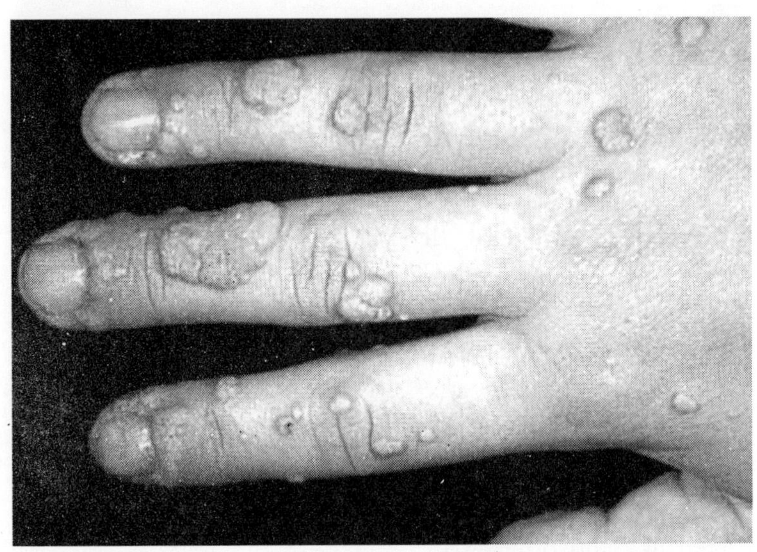

Common Warts—They occur as rough elevation in the skin.

Causes

Warts are mainly caused by virus infection. Viruses usually penetrate the skin via small abrasions. Warts are unpredictably contagious and the patient may infect himself in different places. Thus for instance, he may get wart on the lips, if he sucks a wart on the finger. Infection can also spread from one member of the family with a wart to other members. Constitutional factors also appear to be at the root of the troubles. These factors lead to some defects in the proper development of the skin surface in certain areas.

Treatment

It is important to treat a simple wart as soon as it appears, otherwise it may spread. Dietary measures can be helpful in treating this condition. To begin with, the patient should be kept on an all-fruit diet for about two or three days. During this period, he should take three meals a day of fresh juicy fruits such as grapes, orange, apple, pineapple, mango, pear and papaya. The warm-water enema should be taken to cleanse the bowels during this period and afterwards, if necessary.

After the all-fruit diet, the patient may gradually embark upon a well-balanced diet of natural foods consisting of seeds, nuts, grains, fruits and vegetables. The emphasis should be on fresh fruits and raw vegetable salad. Further short periods on all-fruit diet at monthly intervals may be necessary until the skin condition improves.

The patient should avoid tea, coffee, flesh foods, white flour, sugar and all products made from them. He should also avoid all refined foods, tinned and frozen foods, as well as spices, condiments and pickles.

Certain home remedies have been found beneficial in the treatment of warts. The most important of these is the use of castor oil (*arandi*). This oil should be applied generously over the affected parts every night. The treatment should be continued for several months.

Milky juice of the figs (*anjeer*) is another valuable remedy. This juice should be extracted from the fresh, barely ripe fruits and applied on warts several times a day. The treatment should be continued for two weeks.

Raw potatoes (*alu*) have been found beneficial in the treatment of warts. A potato should be cut and rubbed on the affected area several times daily. This should be continued for atleast two weeks. It will bring good results

Onions (*piyaz*) are also valuable in warts. They are irritating to the skin and they stimulate the circulation of the blood. Warts sometimes disappear when rubbed with cut onions.

The herb Indian squill (*jungli piyaz*) is useful in removing warts. A powder of the bulb of this herb should be applied locally over the affected area, with beneficial results.

The herb dandelion (*kukraundha*) is another valuable remedy for warts. The milk from the cut end of dandelion should be applied over the affected area two or three times daily.

The herb marigold (*saldbarh*) has been found beneficial in the treatment of warts. The juice of the leaves of this plant can be applied beneficially over warts. The sap from the stem has also been found beneficial in the removal of warts.

The oil extracted from the shell of the cashewnut (*kaju*) being acrid, vesicant and rubefacient, has proved useful in warts. It should be applied externally over the affected area in treating this condition.

Certain other applications have also proved beneficial in treating this condition. These include juices of papaya and pineapple fruits and chalk powder mixed with water.

CHAPTER 139

Whooping Cough

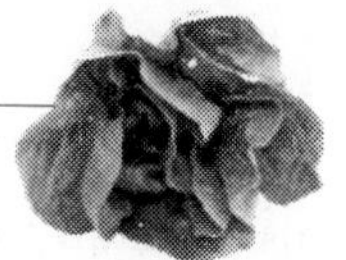

Whooping cough or pertussis, as it is called in medical parlance, is a contagious disease, Unlike some other diseases, a new born baby has no immunity to this disease, and can get it any time after birth. It commonly affects infants during the first year of their life, when it is very severe and most of the deaths due to it occur during this period. Many cases occur in children upto 5 years of age. In some cases children upto 12 years may also be affected. The disease may cause serious trouble in the lungs.

This highly infectious disease is caused by bacteria. It spreads rapidly from one child to another by droplet-infection. This is especially so during the early catarrhal stage, but once the typical spasmodic bout starts, the infectivity becomes negligible. This disease has a prolonged course of 8 to 10 weeks.

Symptoms

The disease has a catarrhal and a spasmodic stage. For the first week, the cough is like an ordinary upper respiratory catarrh. At the end of a week, it becomes spasmodic and comes in bouts, initially more often during the night, but later during the day as well. The child goes on coughing. His face becomes red and suffused, the tongue protrudes and the eyes begin to water. At the end of the bout, the child takes a deep breath, and there is a prolonged croaking sound which is called a whoop. This sound is produced by the air entering through a partially closed glottis (entrance to the larynx). This gives the disease its name. The child brings out a sticky secretion from his nose and mouth and very often vomits. At the end of the bout, the child lies back exhausted. Gradually, over the next three or four weeks, the bouts of cough and their duration become less and disappear in about 8 to 10 weeks from the beginning of the disease, in immunized children, the disease is mild.

Due to the severity of bouts of cough, bleeding can occur into the eyes, from the nose, the lung and, in rare cases, into the brain, resulting in convulsions. In many young children, lung complications such as collapse of a part of the lung are common because of the thick sticky nature of the secretions blocking the passage of air to a part of the lung. Secondary infection may result in pneumonia. There may be convulsions and, in rare cases, inflammation of the brain.

Causes

Whooping cough is caused by the micro-organisms *Bordetella pertussis and Bordetella parapertussis.* Of these, the first one gives rise to more severe infections. Whooping cough is also associated with various adinoviruses, para-influenza and respiratory viruses. The actual cause of the disease, however, is wrong feeding of children with refined and demineralised foods and the absence of a sufficient quantity of fresh fruits and salad vegetables in their diet. This results in accumulation of excessive quantities of catarrh and mucus in the child system. The disease is an attempt on the part of nature to throw out this catarrh and mucus. The use of drugs to treat other diseases can also lead to whooping cough.

Treatment

In the beginning of the treatment, the child should be placed on a fast, of orange juice and water for few days. He should be given the juice of an orange diluted with warm water on 50 : 50 basis. He should not be given milk or anything else. He should be given warm-water enema daily during this period to cleanse the bowels. In case of constipation, a mild laxative, preferably castor oil, should be administered. This will also relieve the pain in the abdominal muscles which are usually strained during the paroxysms of coughing. Cold packs should be applied to the throat and upper chest as required. Epsom-salt baths will be beneficial during this period.

After the more severe symptoms have cleared, the patient should be placed on an exclusive diet of fresh fruits for a few days. In this regimen, he should take fresh juicy, fruits such as apple, orange, pineapple and papaya. After further recovery, he can adopt a regular well-balanced diet, according to his age. The emphasis should be on fresh fruits, fruit and vegetable juices and milk. When the convalescent stage has been reached, the child should be encouraged to spend as much time as possible out doors.

Home Remedies

Certain home remedies have been found beneficial in the treatment of whooping cough. The most effective of these remedies is the use of garlic. The syrup of garlic should be given in doses of five drops to a teaspoon two or three times a day for treating this condition. It should be given more often if the coughing spells are frequent and violent.

Ginger (*adrak*) is another effective remedy for whooping cough. A teaspoon of fresh ginger juice, mixed with a cup of fenugreek (*methi*) decoction and honey to taste, is an excellent diaphoretic. It acts as an expectorant in this disease. A syrup prepared by mixing a teaspoon of fresh radish (*muli*) with equal quantity of honey and a little rock salt, is beneficial in the treatment of this disease. It should be given thrice daily.

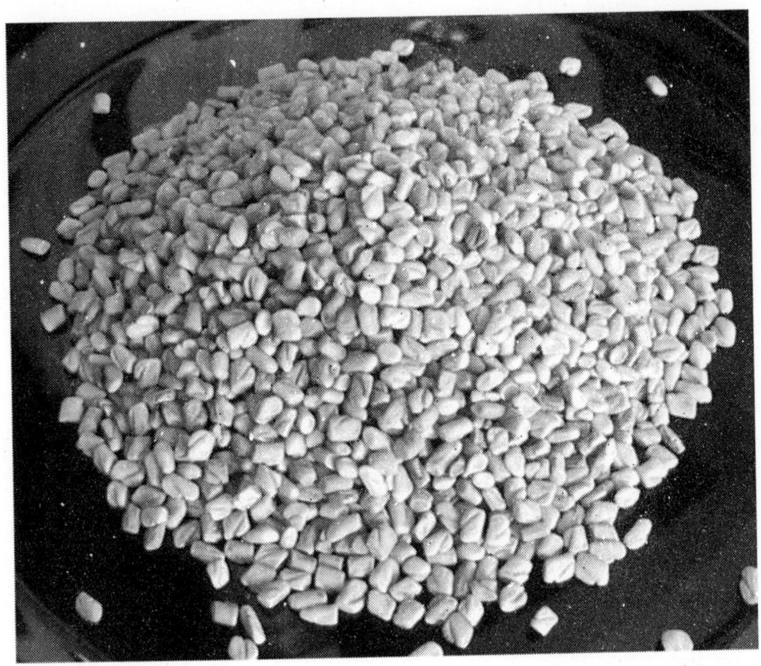

A decoction of fenugreek seeds is beneficial in whooping cough.

Almond (*badam*) oil is valuable in whooping cough. It should be given mixed with 10 drops each of fresh white onion juice and ginger juice, daily thrice for a fortnight. It will give relief.

Part IV

Women's Problems

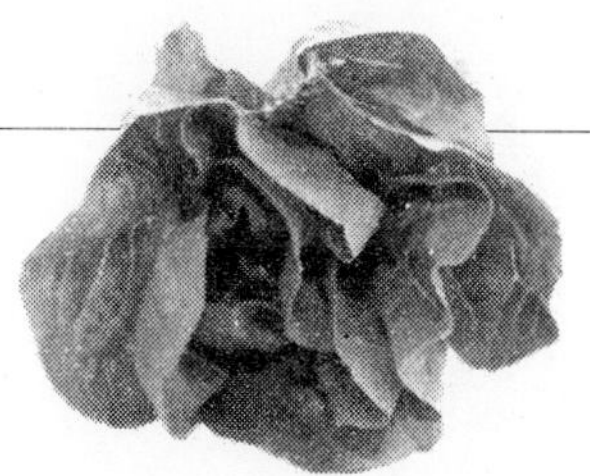

CHAPTER 140

Menstrual Disorders

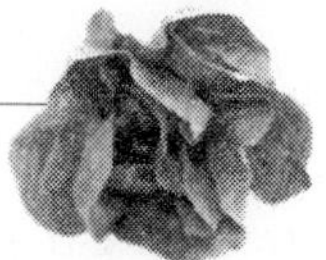

The maternal instincts of a woman arise almost entirely from the female hormones within her body. These hormones are produced in a pair of almond-shaped organs, known as the ovaries. They are situated deep within the pelvis, one on each side of the uterus or womb.

The two major female hormones are estrogen and progesterone. These hormones give the woman strength and stamina and are largely responsible for the peculiarly feminine shape of her body. The ovaries start producing large quantities of estrogen, the dominant female hormone when a girl reaches about 12 years of age. This enables her to grow rapidly and develop into a normal young woman. The commencement of menstruation at this time heralds the reproductive phase of her life, when she can have children. This phase may last for about 35 years.

The menstrual flow is connected with the female function of ovulation or the passing of the egg cell or ovum from the ovary to the womb ready for fertilisation. It is a provision of nature to cleanse the inner surface of the womb and enable reproduction to take place normally. The flow normally lasts for about four days and has a rhythm of 28 days.

The main problem relating to menstrual flow are painful menstruation, stoppage of menstruation and excessive menstruation, besides pre-menstrual tension which is discussed in the next chapter. These disorders are quite common, but they are not normal. Healthy women, living according to natural laws and eating diets of natural foods do not suffer from the monthly ordeal. Most menstrual disorders are caused by nutritional deficiencies which lead to deficiency and improper metabolism of the female sex hormones. These disorders are now discussed briefly.

Dysmenorrhoea: Painful menstruation or dysmenorrhoea, as it is called in medical parlance, is a very common occurrence these days. This disorder is traceable to a debilitated and toxic condition of the system in general and of the sex organs in particular due to a wrong diet, wrong style of living and nervous exhaustion. The pain may be felt either two or three days before or immediately before or during the flow.

Pain starting two or three days before the flow usually shows that the ovaries are not functioning properly. This is a glandular misfunction and a carefully planned natural diet will usually put matters right. For local treatment, hot hip baths on alternate nights for a week before the period is due will be highly beneficial. Between periods, cold hip baths will increase the tone of the ovaries.

Pain immediately before the flow commences is indicative of uterine flexion, which means that the position of the womb is abnormal. A professional examination should be arranged to ascertain the position of the womb and corrective exercises undertaken under professional advice. Uterine flexion often occurs in women who are so thin that they have lost internal fat and the ligament, on which the womb is suspended. General treatment along dietetic lines is essential along with corrective exercises.

When the pain occurs during menstruation, it usually means that the womb itself is inflamed. This condition can be relieved by proper attention to diet and hot hip baths just before the period is due and cold hip baths between the periods. The hot hip bath is generally taken for eight to ten minutes at a water temperature of 100°F which can be gradually increased to 120°F. The cold hip bath should be taken for 10 to 15 minutes at a water temperature of 50° to 65°F.

Amenorrhoea or stoppage of menstrual flow: Stoppage of menstruation is natural during pregnancy and at the menopause, but abnormal at any other time. It is true that some women have very infrequent periods but this seems to be peculiar to their particular type and cannot be termed as stoppage. If, however, the periods have been quite regular for a number of years and then suddenly stop or the cycle becomes frequently interrupted, it denotes a debilitated and devitalised condition of the system, especially of the sex organ. Causes contributing towards this condition are anaemia, worry, grief, fright or other serious emotional disturbances, malformation of the womb, tuberculosis, displacement of womb and debility, especially after a serious illness.

The treatment for amenorrhoea should be directed towards the rectification of the disease-condition responsible for causing the trouble in the first place. Along with this, a course of general health-building treatment should also be carried out. If serious emotional disturbance has caused the trouble, an initial period of quietness and rest is essential to the treatment. All excitement, excessive mental strain and study should be avoided for a considerable period.

Menorrhoea or excessive menstruation: Profuse menstrual flow is common in certain women and usually denotes a blood deficiency, especially blood calcium. A variety of causes may be responsible for this trouble, but toxic condition of the system is at the root of the matter. It is essential to keep the patient absolutely quiet and confined to bed. The bottom of the bed should be raised 10 cm to 13 cm. In case of excessive bleeding, a gauze may be inserted in the vagina as a temporary measure.

For the first few days the diet should consist only of milk and raw vegetables. No stimulants should be taken as they tend to increase the flow. When the bleeding has stopped, great care should be taken to avoid over exertion or straining the body in any manner. A full nature cure diet should then be adopted using fresh vegetables raw salads twice daily. As a long term measure, what is needed is a scheme of treatment which will thoroughly cleanse the system of toxic material.

Treatment

The various disorders relating to menstrual flow are indicative of the low level of a woman's health and a toxic condition of her sex organism, which has been brought about by wrong habits of living, especially wrong dietary habits. These disorders are made more deep-seated and chronic by modern medical efforts to deal with them through the suppressive agency of surgery and drugs. The disorders being systemic in origin, can be tackled only by treating the system as a whole so as to remove the toxicity from the body and build up the general health-level of the sufferer.

To undertake such a scheme of all round health-building treatment, the sufferer from menstrual disorders should begin with an all-fruit diet for about five days. In this regimen, the patient should have three meals a day of fresh, juicy fruits, such as apples, pears, grapes, papaya, oranges, pineapple, peaches and melon. No other foodstuff should be taken; otherwise the value of the whole treatment will be lost. However, if there is much weight loss on the all-fruit diet, those already underweight may add a glass of milk to each fruit meal. During this period the bowels should be cleansed daily with a warm water enema.

After the all-fruit diet, the sufferer should adopt a well-balanced diet on the following lines:

Upon rising: A glass of lukewarm water mixed with the freshly squeezed juice of half a lime and a spoon of honey.

Breakfast: Fresh fruits such as apple, orange, grapes, papaya, banana and milk.

Lunch: A bowl of freshly prepared steamed vegetable such as carrot, cabbage, cauliflower, squash, and beans, two or three whole wheat chappatis.

Mid-afternoon: A glass of carrot juice or sugar cane juice.

Dinner: A large bowl of fresh green vegetable salad using all available vegetable such as carrot, cabbage, cucumber, tomatoes, radish, red beets and onion and mung bean sprouts.

Bed-time snack: A glass of fresh milk or an apple.

The diet factor is of the utmost importance. Fruits and salads, nature's body-cleansing and health-restoring foods, must form the bulk of the future diet along with whole grains, nuts and seeds, especially in sprouted form. Frequent small meals should be taken instead of few large ones to prevent low blood sugar, which is common during menstruation. The foods which should be avoided in future are white-flour products, sugar, confectionery, rich cakes, pastry, sweets, refined cereals, flesh foods, rich, heavy, or greasy foods, tinned or preserved foods, strong tea, coffee, pickles, condiments and sauces. Smoking, if habitual, should be given up completely as it aggravates menstrual disorders.

A further short period on all-fruit, say two or three consecutive days, can be undertaken at monthly intervals, according to the need of the case. The morning dry friction and cold hip baths should form a regular feature of the treatment. All cold baths should however, be suspended during the menstrual period.

Certain remedies have been found useful in menstrual disorders. Cooked banana flower eaten with curd is one of the more important of such remedies. The banana flower appears to increase progesterone hormone and reduce the bleeding.

Beet juice has been found very effective for menstrual disorders. It should be used in small quantities of 60 to 90 grams, at a time two or three times a day in these conditions.

Coriander seeds are highly beneficial in the treatment of excessive menstruation. Six grams of these seeds should be boiled in half a litre of water. It should be taken off the fire when only half the water remains. Sugar candy should be added to it and the patient should drink it when it is still warm.

Ginger has been useful in menstrual disorders. A piece of fresh ginger should be pounded and boiled in a cupful of water for few minutes. The infusion sweetened with sugar should be used thrice daily after meals as a medicine for dysmenorrhoea, and amenorrhoea due to exposure to cold winds and taking cold bath.

Sesame seeds are also useful in menstrual disorders. Half a teaspoonful of powder of these seeds taken with hot water twice daily acts excellently in reducing spasmodic pain during menstruation in young unmarried anaemic girls. Its regular use, two days prior to the expected periods, cures scanty menstruation. Warm hip bath containing a handful of bruised sesame seeds should be simultaneously taken along with this recipe.

Safflower seeds have also been found to be beneficial in the treatment of painful menstruation. A decoction prepared by boiling two teaspoonfuls of powdered seeds in 120 ml. of water should be given as a remedy for this condition. Dried flowers mixed with confection of rose can also be given as a medicine for this purpose.

CHAPTER 141

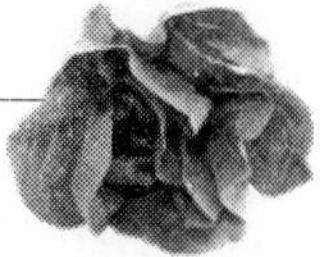

Premenstrual Syndrome

The premenstrual syndrome (PMS) refers to a variety of symptoms which recur in the same phase of the menstrual cycle. These generally make their appearance two to seven days before the onset of menstruation and are relieved once the menses start.

Approximately, 40 per cent of menstruating women suffer from premenstrual tension and it occurs mostly in women over 30 years of age. In some women, the onset of symptoms seems to coincide with ovulation and may then persist until menstruation commences. In some rare cases, relief from the premenstrual syndrome may be obtained only with the cessation of the menstrual flow.

Symptoms

The onset of this syndrome is abrupt, generally with a headache which is often accompanied by vomiting. A general feeling of depression and irritability permeate the entire experience. What is worse, these symptoms intensify progressively, making the last day of the PMS the worst.

Tension headaches are common during this period, but in some cases, migrainous attacks occur with severe pain and vomiting. The patient suffers from breast tenderness, which is sometimes so severe that it is almost unbearable. There may also be abdominal bloating, accompanied in some cases, by odema of the ankles and hands. Some women resort to dieting to get rid of the abdominal bloating but this only leads to fatigue and depression. Others may experience a craving for sweet foods.

Some of the less common symptoms are exacerbation of epilepsy dizziness, back ache, hoarse voice, greasy hair, acne and allergic reactions.

Patients suffering from premenstrual tension may show a weight gain of one kg or more in the latter part of the menstrual cycle due to salt and water retention. The retention of fluid is partly due to ovarian steroids, but there is also an increased output of antidiuretic hormone from the posterior pituitary gland.

Diagnosis

There is no specific laboratory diagnosis of the premenstrual syndrome. The problem can be diagnosed on the basis of past history showing a clear, recurrent relationship between a stage of the menstrual cycle and the onset of symptoms as well as the coincidence of relief with the start or cessation of menstruation. The patient may maintain a personal diary about her symptoms and feelings during those days. The record should be kept for at least three cycles.

Causes

The causes behind the premenstrual syndrome still remain unexplained. Some authorities believe that deficiency of the hormone progesterone may result in PMS but this has not yet been satisfactorily proved. Emotional stress can often contribute to the symptoms, and the social relationship of the patient needs to be reviewed.

A team of researchers at Sinai Hospital in Baltimore and John Hopkins University School of Medicine, London, through carefully controlled studies, concluded that dietary deficiencies, particularly that of vitamin E and vitamin B_6 or pyridoxine are the most common causes of PMS.

Treatment

Treatment depends on the severity of the symptoms. Where only mild symptoms are experienced, the problem can be alleviated by a change of routine. Extra work and stressful situations should be avoided. Fluids should be moderately restricted and care should be taken not to add extra salt to the food. The patient's partner and family members should be educated about all the facets of the PMS. The patient should not take any oral contraceptives as these may cause fluid retention and lowering of plasma levels. Hormonal imbalance and infections of the uterus can be helped by a natural diet regimen.

As most women feel tension arising from chronic constipation, it is essential to treat this condition first. In constipation, the putrefying faecal matter may be reabsorbed into the bloodstream, and the same blood, if supplied to the brain, will cause gradual enervation. Constipation can be relieved by a lukewarm water enema and liberal intake of seasonal fruits and vegetables and simple fibrous meals.

Other treatment for the PMS include regular cold hip baths for 10 to 15 minutes twice a day. This will relieve congestion and inflammation of the uterus and the connected organs. Tension will also be dissipated with this treatment. Hot foot baths followed by a cold compress to the lower abdomen and the inner surfaces of the thighs also help to relieve uterine congestion and tension.

If the cold hip bath is not practicable, a wet girdle pack applied twice a day on empty stomach is very beneficial for clearing up uterine congestion and improving bowel functions.

All these treatments should be suspended during the menstrual flow.

Diet plays a significant role in preventing premenstrual syndrome. The patient should avoid refined carbohydrates, sugars, coffee, tea, tobacco, other stimulants, oily, fried or spicy food and all meats.

A regular practice of yogasanas, especially those recommended for strengthening the genito-urinary system will be very useful in overcoming premenstrual syndrome. These asanas are bhujangasana, shalabasana, vajrasana, paschimotanasana, ardhamatsyendrasana and trikonasana. Other helpful measures are brisk walks and abdominal exercises which are good for strengthening the abdominal muscles and pelvic organs.

Great relief can also be obtained by manipulating the tender points gently, on the big as well as other toes of the feet. Manipulation on the middle portion of the left foot which relates to the uterus and vagina will help to correct the disorder of the uterus.

Mental poise is an important factor. Negative mental attitudes like fear, worry, anger, jealousy, tension and inferiority complex should be eliminated by positive thinking, meditation and good company.

CHAPTER 142

Menopausal Problems

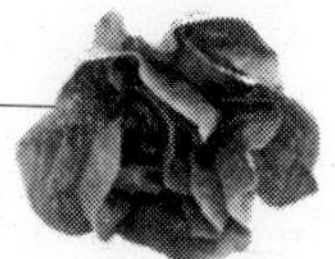

The menopause or a woman's change of life is a perfectly normal event which occurs in the mid or late forties. It signifies the end of the female reproductive period of life which commenced at adolescence in the early teens.

There are several misconceptions about menopause. Many women at this time feel that they are growing old and that they are well past their full physical vigour. Other women feel that the menopause brings a cessation of sexual pleasure. These apprehensions are far from true. Menopause may be considered an end to woman's fertility but certainly not to her virility. It does not decrease a woman's physical capacity or sexual vigour or enjoyment.

Symptoms

During the menopause, the entire chain of endocrine glands is disturbed, particularly the gonads, thyroid and pituitary. In a really healthy woman, the menopausal change takes place without any unpleasant symptoms. The only sign that the 'change' taking place is the cessation of menstrual flow. There are, however, many women who do not enjoy good health due to dietetic errors and a faulty style of living. In these cases, the menopausal change often leads to all kinds of distressing physical, emotional and nervous symptoms and manifestations.

Hot flashes, night sweats, nervous tension, menstrual disturbances, insomnia, diminished interest in sex, irritability and depression are the typical symptoms of menopause. Other symptoms are chilly feelings, fatigue, palpitation, dizziness, headaches and numbness. Not every woman will get these severe reactions. The severity of the symptoms depend on a variety of factors such as general health, previous surgery and radiation. Menopause and its problems are usually over when menstruation stops.

Causes

The annoying symptoms associated with menopause arise from the fact that the ovaries are no longer producing their normal amount of estrogen, the dominant female hormone. Anything which interferes with the normal functioning of the ovaries may also bring about these symptoms. The same strange feelings may occur if the ovaries are removed by surgery because of disease. This can also result from heavy X-ray therapy or the use of radiation.

A lack of normal hormone balance may also result in a severe backache. This is caused by thinning of the bones arising from the low level of estrogen in the bloodstream. Unless properly treated, this may eventually lead to a collapse of one or more of the vertebrae.

Treatment

Although menopause cannot be avoided, it can be postponed for as long as 10 to 15 years and it can be made a smooth affair when it comes, with a proper nutritional programme, special supplements and the right mental attitude.

When a woman is affected by the menopausal change to any marked extent, it is a sure sign that her body is in a toxic condition and in need of a thorough cleansing. For this purpose, she should undergo a course of natural health-building treatment.

Diet is of utmost importance in such a scheme of treatment. In fact the problems at menopause are often much more severe than that at puberty largely because the diet has been deficient for many years prior to its onset, in many nutrients such as protein, calcium, magnesium, vitamins D, E and pantothenic acid.

The diet should be made up from three basic food groups, namely (i) seeds, nuts and grains, (ii) vegetables and (iii) fruits. The emphasis should be on vitamin E-rich raw and sprouted seeds and nuts, unpasteurised high quality milk and home-made cottage cheese and an abundance of raw, organically grown fruits and vegetables. Plenty of freshly made juices of fruits and vegetables in season should also be included in the diet.

All processed, refined and denatured foods, such as white sugar, white flour and all articles made with them, should be completely eliminated. Take special supplements such as vitamins C, B_6 and pantothenic acid, which have a specific property of stimulating the body's own production of estrogen or enhancing the effect of the existing estrogen.

During menopause, the lack of ovarian hormones can result in a severe calcium deficiency. For this reason, a larger than usual intake of calcium may help greatly. Vitamins D and F are also essential for assimilation of calcium. Any woman having difficulty at this time should supplement her daily diet with 1,000 units of natural vitamin D, 500 milligrams of magnesium and two grams of calcium daily, which can be supplied by one quart of milk.

During the menopause, the need for vitamin E soars 10 to 50 times over that previously required. Hot flashes, night sweats and other symptoms of menopause often disappear when 50 to 100 units of vitamin E are taken daily. The symptoms recur quickly if the vitamin is discontinued.

Of late, it has become popular to take estrogen to prevent or postpone menopausal symptoms. Although hormone therapy is apparently successful and will, in many cases, help the patient to feel and act younger, it cannot be recommended in all cases because of its carcinogenic effect. If, however, estrogen therapy is undertaken, it should never be administered at the same time as vitamin E therapy. Ingestion of estrogen and vitamin E should be separated by several hours.

Beet juice has been found very useful in menopausal disorders. It should be taken in small quantities of 60 to 90 ml at a time thrice a day. It has proved much more permanently helpful than the degenerative effects of drugs or synthetic hormones.

Carrot seeds have also been found valuable in menopausal tension. A teaspoonful of the seeds should be boiled in a glassful of cow's milk for about 10 minutes and taken daily as a medicine in this condition.

Plenty of outdoor exercise, such as walking, jogging, swimming, horse-riding or cycling, is imperative to postpone menopause. Other helpful measures in this direction are avoiding mental and emotional stress and worries, especially worry about growing old, sufficient sleep and relaxation and following all general rules of maintaining a high level of health. The healthier a woman is, the fewer menopausal symptoms she will experience.

Menopause can be made a pleasant affair by building bodily health and a sane mental outlook. From puberty to menopause, a woman has been somewhat of a slave to her female glands. At specified intervals she was inconvenienced by her menstrual periods. She bore children, enduring the pain and discomfort of pregnancy. Menopause relieves her of this bondage to her femininity. She can now experience some of the happiest days of a woman's life. A whole new life is given to her, if she is wise enough to prepare for it and accept it as such.

CHAPTER 143

Childbirth the Natural Way

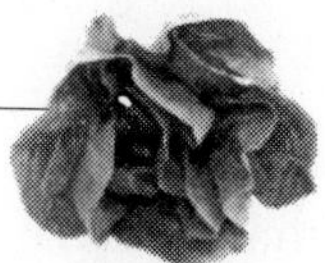

Childbirth, in the normal way, should be a purely natural function with very little pain or discomfort to the women concerned. It is so even today with primitive races. But many civilised women appear to find the bearing of children a task fraught with grave risk and suffering and attended by numerous minor or serious after-effects. This is solely due to wrong dietary habits and a faulty style of living. Really healthy mothers will always have an easy time when pregnant.

Pregnancy makes many demands on the prospective mother, the most important being her nutritional needs and those of the unborn child. Studies of nutrition of women during pregnancy shows a definite relationship between the diet of the mother and the condition of the baby at birth. These studies have also shown that some of the complications of pregnancy such as anaemia, toxemia and premature delivery may result from a diet inadequate in the nutritional needs of the mother and the baby.

The process of childbirth becomes painful mainly due to a large foetus in the womb. This results from an excessive intake of denatured foods such as white flour products, white sugar, refined cereals, meat and other flesh foods during pregnancy. Other factors contributing to the suffering of women include lack of exercise, unhygienic habits of living and restrictive garments.

It is quite wrong to assume that the larger the baby is at birth, the healthier it will be. The weight of the baby should be about three to three and a half kgs. at birth. If the weight is more than that, delivery will be painful for the mother. Such a child will also be covered with unnecessary fat and watery tissue, which is really waste matter and an impediment to health.

A proper diet during pregnancy is the most important factor for not only having a painless childbirth but also for giving birth to a healthy baby. The idea of 'eating for two', which is so prevalent today, is absurd and it leads to overeating, resulting in an unusually, heavy baby The diet during pregnancy should consist of natural, vital foods and minimum intake of today's denatured food products. The unborn child will require an adequate amount of organic minerals from its mother for building of bones and tissues and this can be supplied by natural foods such as fruits, raw vegetables, wholemeal bread and milk. Unnatural foods like white bread, sugar, meat, pudding and pies are very deficient in organic mineral matter and their intake during pregnancy leads to loss and decay of teeth, general debility and other ailments after childbirth.

Pregnancy is rendered more difficult in case of habitual constipation. In the advanced stage, this is aggravated by the pressure of the enlarged uterus on the bowels. This can be avoided by eating plenty of fresh fruits and vegetables of high fibre content. The expectant mother should drink eight to 10 glasses of water. She should not delay going to the lavatory when there is the urge. In severe constipation, a lukewarm water enema may be taken once every week.

The diet for expectant mothers should be planned along the following lines for securing a safe and easy childbirth and a healthy child:

Breakfast: Fresh fruit in season or grated raw carrot or any other raw salad and milk. Prunes or other dried fruit may also be taken, if desired.

Lunch: Steamed vegetables, as obtainable, whole wheat chappatis and a glass of buttermilk.

Dinner: A good-sized raw salad of any suitable vegetables, sprouted mung beans, whole wheat bread, butter or cottage cheese and prunes or other dried fruit as dessert.

Besides proper diet, the expectant mother should be given daily a dry friction and cold sponge during the first five or six months of pregnancy. A dry friction bath can be taken with a rough dry towel or with a moderately soft bristle brush, if a brush is used, the procedure should be as follows: take the brush in one hand and begin with the face, neck and chest. Then brush one arm, beginning at the wrist and brushing towards the shoulders. Now stoop down and brush one foot, then the ankle and leg. Then do the other foot and leg, and next the hips and certain portion of the body. Continue brushing each part until the skin is pink. Use the brush quickly backward and forward on every part of the body. If a towel is used, it should be fairly rough, and the same process should be followed.

The cold sponge is taken as follows: wring out a towel in cold water, and rub the whole body in the manner described for the friction bath, if, during the process of rubbing the towel becomes too dry, it should be wrung out again.

The expectant mother should also take breathing and other mild exercises. After the sixth month, tepid water may be used for the sponge. Exercises should either be modified or suspended altogether. A good walk should be taken daily right upto the end of the eighth month and all household duties should be performed in a normal way. This will keep the muscles of the womb and pelvis in good condition and will ensure safe and easy childbirth. The exercise should, however, always be well within the capacity of the prospective mother and all undue strain, worry or excitement should be avoided.

Recoupment

For the really healthy woman, recoupment after childbirth poses no problem. Women among primitive races are able to rise and go about their duties immediately after delivery. The women of civilised nations are however, seldom able to do so. In fact it is customary to keep them in bed for a considerable time after childbirth. It is usually due to the abnormal slowness with which the generative organs assume the former position.

As in the case of pregnancy, diet plays an important role in the recoupment after childbirth. The diet of the mother for the first two days after confinement should consist of only fresh juicy fruits with some warm milk. A salad with thin whole wheat bread and butter may be added to the diet the next day. The diet may thereafter be extended gradually until it approaches the pre-natal diet outlined above.

The diet should exclude white bread or white flour products, sugar, jam, pastries, puddings, pies, heavy, greasy and fried foods. Strong tea, coffee, alcohol, condiments, pickles and vinegar should be strictly avoided.

It is most essential that the baby nurses at the mother's breast to stimulate production of milk, especially during the critical period following birth. This is important for a number of reasons. The infant, nursing at the breast, causes the uterus to contract. The contraction of the uterus-will help expel any portion of the placenta which may still remain following delivery. It will also stop the mother from haemorrhaging. If those mothers who are afraid of losing their figures would try nursing their babies, they would discover their figures actually improve after childbirth.

Feeding of Children

During the first 48 hours immediately after birth, the

mother's breasts generally do not produce milk. This is in accordance with nature's plan that the infant should fast during this period. He will have no need for food and none should be given. All children after this period should be breast-fed when possible. Breast feeding is the natural and ideal way of feeding the infant. Mother's milk is pure, fresh and easily digestible. It helps the child to grow. The child should be given four feeds a day at four-hourly intervals but no feeds should be given during the night, if the child wakes up at night only water should be given. Babies should be breast-fed for at least eight months as this is nature's way of providing all the required nutrients during this period. Recent research has shown that the mother's body is able to react to infections in the child and the bacteria in the baby's mouth leads to the production of appropriate antibodies in the mother's milk. Breast-fed babies are, therefore, less prone to gastrointestinal and respiratory diseases. If for any reason, it is impossible to breast-feed the child, it should be fed on goat's milk or cow's milk, diluted with water, with milk sugar added. The child should not be given artificially prepared, patent or tinned milk foods. When a mother can partly feed the child, she should give it two feeds of her own and two bottle feeds or one of her own and three bottle feeds. Those mothers who suffer from diseases like high blood pressure, diabetes, heart trouble, should not breast-feed their babies.

Where children are entirely breast-fed, they need nothing more than the milk they receive from their mothers. Children on bottle feed, should be given some orange juice daily, in addition to the bottle feeds. No baby, whether breast-fed or bottle-fed, should be given anything except milk and orange juice for the first 10 to 12 months of existence. No starchy food or anything else should be given during this period. If they are given starchy foods such as bread, or oatmeal before weaning, it will lead to the early development of such child ailments as cough, colds, measles, whooping cough and so on as babies lack the proper enzymes needed for their digestion before that age.

At the age of one year, a baby should be given about a litre of milk with fruit juices daily. Never force a baby to take food if it does not want to, and never overfeed. If a baby shows no inclination for food on a certain day, it should be given as much as it wishes for and no more. The assumption that the baby should have a certain amount of food every day has no basis. On the other hand, if a baby does not appear to be satisfied with the quantity of its food and wants more at a feed, it should be given as much as it wants.

CHAPTER 144

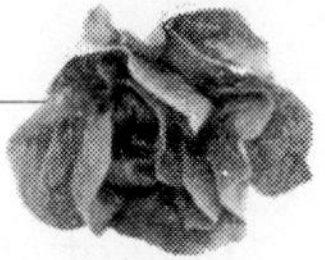

Habitual Abortion

The term abortion refers to the expulsion of the foetus from the uterus before the complete formation of the placenta. It is also commonly known as miscarriage. This may occur any time before 28 weeks of gestation but is most common during the first 12 weeks of pregnancy. One in five to ten pregnancies terminates in this way.

When miscarriage occurs repeatedly at a certain period of pregnancy, it is termed 'habitual abortion'. It is one of the most perplexing problems of gynaecology and a major cause of maternal mortality. A woman who has suffered two or more terminations of this sort consecutively is said to be a case of habitual abortion.

Symptoms

Pains of the same character as labour pains and bleeding are the two main symptoms of possible abortion. Bleeding may lead to the detachment of the ovum from the uterus. It now acts as a foreign body in the uterus which stimulates uterine contraction. This generates a lot of pain and the foetus is thrown out of the body. In later weeks when the foetus is well developed, if it dies in the uterus, it leads to maceration of the body. The abdomen is filled with blood and the skin colour appears red. Sometime after a few more days, the foetus gets dehydrated and the fluid surrounding the foetus gets dried away.

Causes

One of the most important causes of habitual abortion is a congenital malformation of the uterus. A hysterogram, before the woman becomes pregnant, will be useful in detecting any abnormality, so that she is made aware of her case. Deficient functioning of the thyroid is another important cause of habitual abortion.

Most cases of habitual abortion, however, result from an inadequate secretion of the female hormone progesterone. This hormone is responsible for the development of the placenta. In the early stage of pregnancy, the gonadotrophin secreted by the cytotrophoblast of the chorion, one of the foetal membranes, stimulates the corpus lotemum to produce more oestrogen and progesterone, both essential female hormones. At a later stage, by about the 12th week of pregnancy, the placenta takes over the production and secretion of the hormones. Any deficiency of these hormones at this stage is detrimental to the growth of the foetus. It is, therefore, during this critical period, when habitual abortions mostly occur. Lack of progesterone is especially instrumental in expelling the fertilised ovum and it results in an abortion.

Another important cause of habitual abortion may be chronic constipation which leads to putrefaction of morbid matter and wastes in the large intestines. This in turn causes auto-intoxication and inflammation of the reproductive organs, which can lead to a miscarriage.

Abortion may result from the excessive use of certain drugs. Drugs enter the foetus through the placenta. They may act quite differently on the foetus from the mother. Drugs which have adverse effects on the foetus are called 'tera-togenestic drugs' and may include painkillers, antibiotics, tranquilisers and hormones. A high dosage of such drugs may produce contraction in the uterus and induce abortion.

Other causes of habitual abortion are excessive physical exercise, mental excitement, sexual intercourse, syphilis infections, fibroid tumours, blood incompatibility of husband and wife, systemic disorders in the mother like hypertension, chronic nephritis, diabetes and even her mental condition.

Thorough examination of the pregnant woman's blood, urine, blood pressure and their related parameters help in detecting maternal disorders. Serological tests, for example, prove the presence or absence of syphilis infection. Pelvic examinations help to diagnose uterine displacements, fibroids or ovarian tumours. A hysterogram also helps to detect uterine malfunctions. The exact cause must be ascertained for prescribing correct treatment.

Treatment

Conditions such as hormonal imbalance, infections of the uterus and chronic constipation can be remedied by natural methods of treatment. For congenital uterine malformation, however, recourse may have to be taken to surgery.

On appearance of the first symptoms of possible abortion, the patient should be put to bed immediately and the bottom end of the bed raised. Cold compresses at 60°F temperature should be applied continuously to the inner portion of the thighs, the perinium, the vagina and the lumbar region. Compresses should be changed every 15 to 20 minutes. When the compress is removed for renewing, the surface should be rubbed with a warm dry flannel for half a minute or until reddened, before applying the compress again. Simultaneously, a hot application should be made to the feet.

A neutral or warm water enema is an effective remedy for a constipated colon which is a major cause for the toxaemic condition of the uterus. This will relieve the bowels and thus reduce any excessive pressure on the uterus and other pelvic organs. A regular cold hip bath for a duration of 10 minutes twice every day is very helpful in relieving congestion and inflammation of the uterus. Wet girdle packs, twice every day, on an empty stomach, also relieve congestions and infections in the uterus and other pelvic organs. It is advisable that women with a history of repeated abortions should adopt these techniques before conception and continue them during the first two months of pregnancy.

Hormonal imbalances can be set right by practising yogic exercise. Yogic asanas such as sarvangasana, vajrasana, bhujangasana, shalabhasana, dhanurasana, paschimottashana and trikonasna are especially useful in improving thyroid, pituitary, adrenal and gonaidal endocrine functions and should be practised regularly by women who suffer from imbalances of this sort, upto the first two months of pregnancy.

Dietary control is of utmost importance in the prevention of habitual abortion. Pregnant women should avoid refined carbohydrates, sugars, non-vegetarian food, coffee and tea. They should also avoid oily and fried foods as such foods lead to constipation, which is very detrimental to pregnancy. Smoking or chewing tobacco and drinking alcohol must be strictly avoided.

The pregnant woman's diet chart should be on the following lines:

Breakfast: Fresh fruits and a glass of milk mixed with a teaspoonful of honey.

Lunch: Steamed vegetables, boiled rice or whole wheat chappatis and soup or buttermilk.

Midafternoon: A glass of fruit juice or a whole fruit.

Dinner: Cooked diet similar to the afternoon meal may be taken till the seventh month. After that, fruits, nuts, germinated seeds and sprouts, milk, buttermilk and soups must form her diet because they reduce the workload on the digestive system and thus help avoid indigestion, constipation and related disorders.

Indian gooseberry, known as *amla* in the vernacular, is considered useful in preventing abortion. A teaspoonful of fresh amla juice and honey mixed together should be taken every morning during the period of pregnancy. It will also prevent infections and help in the absorption of iron. A brew made from safflower foliage is also said to prevent abortion.

Pregnant women with a history of repeated abortions should take all other precautions necessary to prevent miscarriage. They should avoid sexual intercourse, during early pregnancy. They should go to bed early and rise early and take regular exercise, but avoid fatigue. They should sleep on a hard mattress with their heads low, and remain calm and cool. All these measures will greatly help in correcting the phenomenon of habitual abortion.

CHAPTER 145

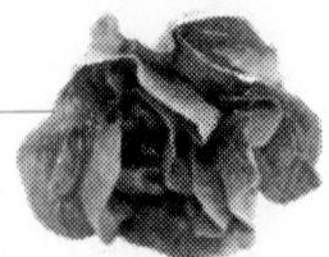

Female Sterility

Sterility in case of the female refers to the incapacity to conceive and give birth to a living baby. Sterility or failure to reproduce must be distinguished from frigidity which denotes failure to perform the sex act or performing it imperfectly.

It may be relevant to first examine the mechanism of conception. The sperms of the male are injected into the vagina during sexual intercourse. At the very same time an alkaline fluid is secreted from the vaginal walls. The sperms are able to move up the womb and through the fallopian tubes to fertilise the ova or the female egg only when this fluid is present.

Two factors are important in ensuring a normal secretion of this fluid. Firstly, there should be an adequate nerve supply to the vagina ducts. This is the reason why very nervous women fail to conceive. The nervous system in such cases must be strengthened by adequate rest, relaxation and a proper diet.

The second important factor is to ensure that the fluid flowing from the vaginal walls is alkaline. If this is not so, the sperms are destroyed by the acidic fluid, usually present in the vaginal canal and womb. To ensure the necessary alkalinity of the fluid, it is essential to take a predominantly alkaline diet, with a liberal intake of raw vegetables and fruits, and also to eliminate acid-forming foods.

Causes

Sterility in a female may be due to physical defects, physical debility and functional faults. Physical defects or structural abnormalities of the genitals and reproductive organs may be congenital or accidental and can result from malformation or sagging of the womb, collapse of the fallopian tubes and rigidity of the hymen.

Sterility due to physical debility can result from poor health as a consequence of certain acute or chronic diseases. These diseases may affect not only the physical body but also the genital organs. Complaints like gonorrhoea, syphilis and inflammation of the fallopian tubes also come under this category. Chronic anaemia, constipation and leucorrhoea aggravate these conditions.

Sterility may also be caused by loss of essential glands or organs of reproduction or a decrease in their functions, brought about by a variety of factors such as surgical injuries, tumour, excessive radiation and lack of normal menstrual cycle. Obesity or emaciation due either to dietetic errors or faulty metabolism are yet other factors which can contribute to female sterility.

Psychological factors like emotional stress, tension, mental depression, anxiety and fear may also result in psychosomatic sterility. This condition is generally temporary and can be corrected by psychotherapy.

Treatment

Structural defects can be ascertained by a thorough physical examination and radiology and can be set right by surgery. Physical debility and the functional faults of organic nature can be cured by simple and effective methods of natural treatment. These methods include hygienic living, optimum nutrition and following all the laws of nature.

Fasting is the best remedy for the treatment of disorders resulting from toxins in the system. A short fast of two or three days should be undertaken at regular intervals by women who are unable to bear children. The bowels should be cleansed by a warm water enema during the period of fasting and afterwards when necessary. This will have a beneficial effect not only on the digestive system but also on the surrounding organs of the urinary and genital system.

Diet is the most important factor in the treatment of sterility. It should consist of three basic health-building food groups, namely (i) seeds, nuts and grains, (ii) vegetables and (iii) fruits. These foods should be supplemented with milk, vegetable oils and honey. The best way to take milk is in its soured form, that is, curd and cottage cheese. Each food group should roughly form the bulk of one of three meals. About 70 to 80 per cent of the diet should consist of foods in their natural uncooked state, because cooking destroys much of the nutritional value of most foods. Sprouting is an excellent way of consuming seeds, beans and grains in their raw form as in the process of sprouting the nutritional value is multiplied, new vitamins are created and the protein quality is improved.

The daily menu of a health-building and vitalising diet may be on the following lines:

Upon rising: A glass of lukewarm water with the juice of half a lemon and a spoonful of honey.

Breakfast: Fresh fruits like apple, orange, banana, grapes and grapefruit and a glass of milk.

Lunch: A bowl of steamed vegetables seasoned with vegetable oil or butter and salt, two or three whole wheat chappattis and a glass of buttermilk.

Mid-afternoon: A glass of fresh fruit or vegetable juice.

Dinner: A large bowl of salad made up of fresh vegetables such as tomatoes, carrots, beetroots and onion, and sprouted moong or Bengal gram.

Bed-time: A glass of milk or an apple.

Excessive fat, spicy foods, strong tea, coffee, white sugar, white flour, refined cereals, flesh foods, greasy or fried foods should all be avoided. Smoking and drinking, where habitual, must be completely given up.

Certain nutrients, especially vitamins C and E and zinc, have been found helpful in some cases of sterility. The woman who is unable to conceive should take daily 1000 mg. of vitamin C, 100 I.U. of vitamin E and 30 mg. of zinc.

Certain remedies have also been found useful in the treatment of female sterility where there are no organic defects or congenital deformities. One such remedy is the tender roots of the banyan tree. These roots should be dried in the shade and finely powdered. This powder should be mixed five times their weight with milk and taken at night for three consecutive nights after the monthly periods are over. No other food should be taken with this. It should be repeated after the completion of the menstrual cycle every month till conception takes place.

An infusion of the fresh tender leaves of jambul fruit (*jamun*), taken with honey or buttermilk, is an excellent remedy for sterility and miscarriage due to ovarian or endometrium functional disorders. The leaves presumably stimulate the secretion of progesterone hormone and help the absorption of vitamin E.

The eggplant is also useful in overcoming functional sterility. Cooked tender eggplants, should be eaten with butter-milk everyday for a month or two for this purpose. It increases the capacity to absorb vitamin E and stimulates the secretion of progesterone.

Other helpful measures in overcoming female sterility are mud packs and cold water treatment like a hip bath and a wet girdle-pack. These treatments will greatly improve internal circulation in the genital organs and will relieve them of all kinds of inflammation and other abnormalities. Mud packs may be applied to the abdomen and sexual organs.

For a hip bath, a common tub may be used. The tub may be filled with sufficient water to cover the hips, when a person sits inside it. The cold hip bath should be taken for 10 minutes at a water temperature of 50° to 65°F. For wet girdle pack, a thin underwear wrung in cold water should be worn. Over this, a thick dry cotton or woolen underwear should be worn. All cold treatments should be suspended during menstruation.

Certain yogasanas which help tone up the gonads should also be practised regularly for overcoming female sterility. These asanas are saryangasana, matsyasana, ardhamatsyendrasana, paschimottanasana and shallabhasana.

All these practices together with clean habits, proper rest and relaxation will go a long way in overcoming female sterility.

CHAPTER 146

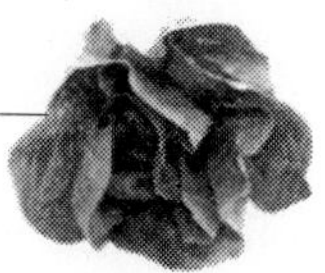

Leucorrhoea

Leucorrhoea, commonly known as whites, refers to a whitish discharge from the female genitals. It is an abnormal condition of the reproductive organs of women. If not treated properly in the initial stages, it may become chronic.

Investigations have shown that secretions from the uterus and upper part of the vagina flow down and are reabsorbed in the lower parts of the vagina. This is the normal constant flow within the female organs. The whitish discharge is caused by the presence of infection in any of these tissues and a variety of other factors. The condition may continue for weeks or months at a time.

Symptoms

In addition to the whitish discharge from the vagina, the patient feels weak and tired. She also suffers from pain in the lumbar region and the calves and a dragging sensation in the abdomen. Other symptoms are constipation, frequent headaches and intense itching. In the chronic form the patient feels irritable and develops black patches under the eyes.

Causes

Leucorrhoea does not develop suddenly in an acute form. It denotes a devitalised and toxic condition of the system generally. The condition also involves one or many parts of the reproductive organs. Whenever the body is loaded with toxins due to wrong dietary habits and the eliminative organs such as skin, bowels, lungs and kidneys are unable to eliminate the toxins, the body produces a profuse discharge or elimination through the mucous membrane of the uterus and vagina in the form of leucorrhoea. In the case of advanced, chronic inflammatory conditions of these organs, it leads to a discharge with pus, offensive in odour and colour varying from cream to yellow or light green.

In young girls, leucorrhoea may occur during the few years before and after the start of the menstrual flow. It may be due to an irritation of the genital organs caused by various factors such as dirt, soiled undergarments, intestinal worms and excessive mental stimulation of sex or masturbation. Some excess secretion is normal when the girl reaches puberty, due to overactivity in her sex glands and organs. This usually disappears within a short time.

In young women, leucorrhoea may occur during intermenstrual periods, due to thickening of the mucous membrane in the reproductive organs. Such a discharge is associated with painful menstruation and other menstrual disorders.

In mature women, a profuse yellowish discharge, associated with burning on urination, may be caused by gonorrhoea. This is a serious infection which should be treated promptly. During the child-bearing years, from adolescence to the mid-forties, the infection may sometimes follow the birth of a child due to damage of the cervix during delivery. This is increased by prolonged ill-health, anxiety, neurosis, sedentary occupation and standing for long periods. If not treated properly, this infection may continue for months or even years and may spread to other areas of the genital tract.

Leucorrhoea may also result from a chill. A chill causes inflammation of the womb and vaginal membranes. Other common causes are the displacement of the womb and unhygienic conditions which attract bacteria to the genital organs.

The Cure

A total health-building scheme is essential for the removal of the systemic toxicity which is primarily responsible for the disease. Such a scheme should consist of correct dietary habits, proper sleep, exercise, fresh air and sunshine.

To begin with the patient should fast for three or four days on lemon water or fruit juices for the elimination of the morbid matter from the body. During this period, the bowels should be cleansed daily with a warm water enema. In case of habitual constipation, steps should be taken for its eradication.

After a short fast, the patient may adopt an all-fruit diet for about a week. In this regimen, she should have three meals a day of fresh juicy fruits such as apples, pears, grapes, grapefruit, oranges, pineapple and peaches. If the patient is suffering from anaemia, or is very much underweight, the diet may consist of fruits and milk. The patient may then gradually embark upon a well-balanced diet consisting of three basic food groups namely (i) seeds, nuts and grains, (ii) fruits and (iii) vegetables.

Fresh fruits or fruit juices only should be taken between meals. All forms of white flour, white sugar, fried and greasy foods, condiments, preserves, tea and coffee should be avoided.

An effective home remedy for leucorrhoea is lady's fingers. A decoction of this vegetable is prepared by boiling 100 grams of the fresh capsules, cut transversely, in half a litre of water for 20 minutes and then strained sweetened. This decoction, given in doses of two to three ounces frequently, is highly beneficial in all irritable conditions of genito-urinary organs including leucorrhoea.

Fenugreek seeds are another excellent home remedy for leucorrhoea. They should be taken internally in the form of tea and also used as a douche. For a douche, the solution should be much stronger than tea. Two tablespoonful of fenugreek seeds should be put into a litre of cold water and allowed to simmer for half an hour over a low flame. It should then be strained and used as a douche.

Treatment through water is extremely beneficial in curing leucorrhoea. A cold hip bath twice a day for 10 minutes will help relieve congestion in the pelvic region and facilitate quick elimination of morbid matter. A warm vaginal douche at 30° to 40°C is beneficial for general cleansing and elimination of the purulent discharge. The procedure is to fill the douche can with 1½ litre of warm water and hang it at a level of three feet above the body. The patient should lie with the hips slightly raised above the body and a special nozzle applied for this purpose should be oiled and inserted slowly into the vagina. The flow can be regulated by the small valve at the nozzle. In severe cases of leucorrhoea, the douche should be done daily.

The passive inflammation of the affected organs can be cured by regular hot hip baths at 40°C for 10 minutes and regular use of wet girdle pack for 90 minutes every night. For a hot hip bath an ordinary bath tub may be used. It should be filled with water at 40°C . The patient should sit in the tub, keeping the legs outside, after taking a glass of cold water. The head should be covered with a wet cloth. A cold water bath should be taken after this treatment. For the wet girdle pack, a thin cotton underwear and another thick or woolen underwear are required. The thin underwear should be wrung in cold water and worn by the patient. The thick dry underwear should be worn above the wet underwear. If the patient feels chill, she should be covered with a blanket.

Yogasanas especially those which improve muscles of the abdomen and uterus are highly beneficial and should be practised regularly. These asanas are paschimottanasana, sarvangasana, halasana, padmasana, bhujangasana and shallabhasana.

The patient should completely relax and should avoid mental tension and worry. Abdominal exercises and walking are also helpful.

CHAPTER 147

Inflammation of the Uterus

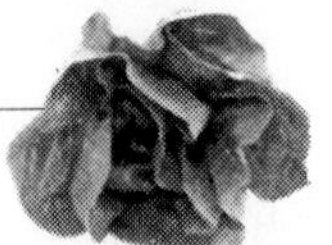

The uterus, often called the womb, is the most delicate organ of woman. It is liable to disorders of various kinds. Inflammation of this organ is a common occurrence in women. It may be acute or chronic.

The uterus is a hollow, pear-shaped muscular organ, situated in a bony frame called the pelvis. It is seven cm. long, five cm. in breadth and about 2.5 cm. thick. Its capacity is roughly three cubic centimetres. The lower narrow end of the uterus which opens into the vagina is called the cervix. The upper broad part is called the body of the uterus or the corpus.

The inflammation which may affect the lining membrane of the uterus is called endometritis. When it affects the muscular coat and substance of the uterus, it is termed metritis. Endometritis may be confined to the lining membrane of the cervix or neck of the uterus or it may attack the lining membrane of the entire organ. Commonly it is called catarrh of the uterus.

Symptoms

The symptoms of acute endometritis are slight fever, headache, general debility, loss of appetite, pain in the back and lower part of the abdomen and pelvis, and itching tendency in the vagina. In chronic endometritis, symptoms are the same, but not so severe as in the acute form. The only troublesome symptom is the discharge which may be either clear or opaque and yellow. This disease may produce sterility.

Chill, fever, rapid pulse and breathing, nausea, local pain and discharge are the symptoms of acute metritis. This is a very rare case, but it may occur after confinement on account of infection. Chronic metritis may occur for many reasons and is probably the most common disease among women. The symptoms are disorders of menstruation, more or less profuse leucorrhoea, constipation, lack of vitality, weakness in the back and the limbs, pain in the lower portion of the back and a tendency to abortion.

Causes

Inflammation of the uterus may be caused by sudden chill, or by exposure to cold during menstruation. The disease sometimes occurs because of the medicines applied for the purpose of stimulating the menstrual flow. Other causes are the use of irritants to produce abortion, the use of strong purgatives, the insertion of instruments and preventives, and excessive sexual indulgence. Sometimes bicycle riding, horse back riding and dancing may also cause inflammation of the uterus among weak and underweight women. The displacement of the uterus in any form may also lead to this condition.

Treatment

If the inflammation is caused by a chill or exposure to cold during menstruation, the patient should start the treatment with a hot leg bath. This may be replaced by a hot hip bath after two or three days. In case of pain, hot and cold hip baths will be beneficial. The water should be changed from hot to cold, every two minutes and this should be repeated thrice.

As this disease produces the tendency towards constipation, the patient should take an enema once daily with warm water as can be comfortably borne by the patient. It is also advisable to apply alternate compress on the abdomen just before employing enema.

In the chronic form the treatment should aim at increasing the general vitality. To begin with, the patient should resort to fasting on orange juice and water for two or three days. The procedure is to take every two hours from 8 a.m. to 8 p.m. the juice of an orange diluted with warm water on 50 : 50 basis. If the orange juice does not agree, juices of vegetables such as carrots and cucumbers may be taken. A warm water enema may be taken each day while fasting to cleanse the bowels.

After the short juice fast, the patient may adopt an all-fruit diet for about two days, taking three meals a day of fresh juicy fruits such as apples, pears, grapes, grapefruit, orange, pineapple, peaches and melon.

After the juice fast the patient should follow a well-balanced diet of seeds, nuts and grains, vegetables and fruits. This diet should be supplemented with milk, yogurt, butter-milk, vegetable oil and honey. A further short juice fast or periods on the all-fruit diet may be necessary at intervals of a month or two, according to the needs of the case. If constipation is habitual, all steps should be taken for its eradication.

The foods which should be avoided are: white flour products, sugar, confectionery, rich cakes, pastries, sweets, refined cereals, flesh foods, rich, heavy and greasy foods, tinned or preserved foods, pickles, condiments and sauces.

The patient should also undertake moderate exercise and walking in fresh air as it will help increase general health and vitality. Yogic asanas such as sarvangasana, bhujangasana, uttanasana and shavasana are also beneficial in the treatment of inflammation of the uterus.

No real cure is possible unless the system as a whole is treated. The blood has to be purified, the nerves strengthened and the waste deposits accumulated in the system eliminated before the trouble can be completely overcome.

CHAPTER 148

Prolapse of the Uterus

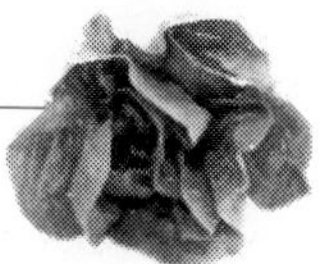

Prolapse of the uterus refers to the downward displacement of the vagina and uterus. The word prolapse is derived from the latin *procidere* which means with effect to fall. This disorder is more common in our country than in the western world.

The uterus is held in position by adequate ligaments. Besides, it has the support of the muscular structures of vagina and all other local tissues and muscles. Due to the laxity of support by muscles, tissues and ligaments, the uterus sags downwards.

Symptoms

A woman suffering from prolapse of the uterus feels that something is coming down through the vagina. She feels a sense of fullness in the region of the bladder and rectum. Other symptoms include dragging discomfort in the lower abdomen, low backache, heavy menses and mild vaginal discharge. There is also an increase in the frequency of urination and the patient feels difficulty in total emptying of the bladder. There may also be a burning sensation due to infection. The woman may experience difficulty in passing stools and complete evacuation of bowels. These symptoms become more pronounced before and during menstruation. The condition may also result in difficulty in normal sexual intercourse and sometimes sterility.

Causes

There are several factors which contribute to the

displacement of the uterus. These include continuous distension of the intestines with gas or excess food materials, leading to constant downward pressure on the womb, chronic constipation, leading to pressure from behind from an over-filled colon, tight clothing especially tight corsets, constant stooping, and a weakened condition of the internal muscles of the abdomen, through lack of exercise and bodily weakness.

Some of the other important factors responsible for prolapse of the uterus are prolonged labour, and interference in the delivery by inexpert people, lack of proper rest and diet in postnatal periods, repeated deliveries and manual work. An increased weight of the womb, tumours of the uterus, traction of the uterus and surgical injuries can also lead to this disorder. Menopausal atrophy may also precipitate it.

Prevention

It is easier to prevent prolapse of the uterus than cure it after its occurrence. The measures to prevent it should include good antenatal care in pregnancy, proper management and timely intervention during delivery, good postnatal care with proper rest, correct diet and appropriate exercise so as to strengthen the pelvic musculature.

Treatment

Treatment for a displaced womb must consist mainly of a suitable diet and exercise. The diet should be so planned as should aim at building up the internal musculature of the body. Of course, any tendency towards tight lacing, constant stooping, and heavy lifting must be carefully guarded against, once a natural regime is undertaken, as these will automatically tend to hold up the success of the treatment.

To begin with the patient should adopt an all-fruit diet for about five days. During this period she should take three meals consisting of juicy fruits such as orange, apple, pineapple, grapes at five hourly intervals. The bowel should be cleansed daily with a warm water enema,

After the all-fruit diet, the patient should gradually embark upon a well-balanced diet based on three basic food groups, namely (i) seed, nuts and grains, (ii) vegetables and (iii) fruits. The all-fruit diet should be repeated for three days at monthly intervals till the condition improves.

Carrots have proved useful in the treatment of prolapse of the uterus. For prolapse of the uterus, pulped carrot should be placed in a muslin bag and inserted in the vagina. This should be kept for some time, using fresh carrots every twelve hours. This will heal and strengthen the parts and help greatly in preventing any further disorders in the female reproductive system.

A hot Epsom-salts bath is also beneficial in the treatment of prolapse of the uterus and should be undertaken twice a week. This bath is prepared by dissolving one or one and a half kg. of Epsom-salts in an ordinary bath of hot water. The patient should remain immersed in the bath from ten to twenty minutes. This bath should be taken just before retiring to bed, and care should be exercised not to get chilled afterwards. No soaps should be used with the bath as it will interfere with its beneficial effects. The alternate hot and cold hip bath are also useful and should be undertaken at night on alternate days.

Exercise

Exercises to strengthen the pelvic musculature are extremely useful in the treatment of prolapse of the uterus. Lying on a couch with the legs raised higher than the rest of the body is very helpful in relieving pain and discomfort from a displaced womb. This should be done from half an hour to an hour two or three times daily. The feet should be raised about eighteen inches by placing cushions under them. When this is not possible, the patient can sit on a chair with the feet on another chair. The more this can be done during the day, the better will it be in every way. The patient should also perform other exercises aimed at strengthening the abdominal muscles. These exercises will help greatly in correcting the displacement of the uterus.

Women should always take precautions to space out their children so as to prevent repeated successive deliveries. This will allow the genital tissues to regain their strength and vitality and thereby prevent prolapse of the uterus.

CHAPTER 149

Vaginitis

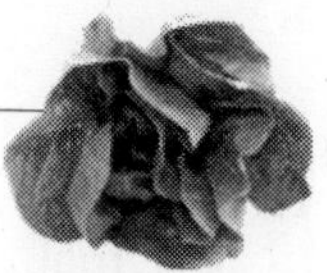

Vaginitis can be described as an inflammation of the vagina and vulva. It is a fairly common problem with women. This can be avoided by taking proper treatment in the initial stages itself. But women usually tend to hide this problem.

Changes in the activity of the vaginal epithelium and in the vaginal secretion at different ages have a profound influence on the defence against vaginal infection. In the adult, the normal vaginal moisture or secretion consists of mucous and discarded vaginal cells. This discharge generally causes no irritation, though the amount secreted and consistency vary. The variance is also due to the periodicity of the menstrual cycle and psychological conditions. Normal healthy women do not suffer from the sensations of itching, burning, pain or irritation.

In unhealthy women and in abnormal conditions the resident organisms (bacteria) multiply rapidly and produce excessive waste products. It causes tissue irritation in this region leading to itching, swelling and burning. There is increase in the frequency or discharge of urine which is accompanied with an unpleasant odour.

Symptoms

The symptoms of vaginitis are feeling of heat and fullness in the vagina, a dragging feeling in the groin, increased urinary frequency and vaginal discharge, that is, leucorrhoea. The clear or white secretion becomes purulent and yellow. The severity of leucorrhoea depends upon the degree of bacterial infection.

Causes

The main causes of vaginitis are irritation of the vagina by external factors, like cuts, abrasions in this region, constant wearing of tight-fitting clothes and wearing unclean clothes, using dirty or infected water and lack of hygiene.

Certain medications and treatments can increase susceptibility to infection. These include the use of antibiotics, hormones and excessive douching. Susceptibility is greater in cases of pregnancy, diabetes, and certain psychological conditions as well as during the latter half of the menstrual cycle. Irritation from contraceptive devices can also lead to this condition.

Unhygienic conditions combined with wrong dietary habits increase toxemia thereby lowering body resistance. According to the nature cure philosophy, whenever the body is loaded with toxins or morbid matter, it tries to eliminate it through the eliminative organs. In women, this elimination is established in the form of profuse discharge, that is leucorrhoea, initially. In later stages, the discharge can become offensive in cases of chronic inflammation.

Treatment

Maintenance of hygienic conditions is the most important factor in the treatment of vaginitis. It is only after this is achieved that morbidity and consequent inflammation and discharge can be prevented.

Another important factor is diet. The patient should be made to fast for three to five days. Depending upon the condition, the fasting period may be extended. During this period, she may take juices of lemon and other sub-acidic fruits. This will give the system an opportunity to divert its vital energies to check inflammation and infection.

After the juice fasting, the patient may adopt a restricted diet, consisting of raw vegetable salads, fruits and sprouts. This will ensure minimal mucous secretions. This restricted diet should be continued for 10 to 15 days, it will help reduce inflammatory conditions. Boiled vegetables which are easily digestible and wheat chappatis may be added gradually to this diet. Later, rice, dal, vegetable soup or buttermilk may be taken for lunch and an uncooked diet for dinner.

The patient should avoid coffee, tea, and other stimulants as well as sugar, fried and refined foods.

Hydrotherapy

Treatment through water plays an important role in overcoming vaginitis. The patient should be given an enema with lukewarm *neem* water to cleanse the bowels and prevent constipation which increases the toxemic conditions, inflammation and infection in the genital organs. For general cleansing and elimination of purulent vaginal discharge, *neem* water vaginal douche at 35°C—40°C followed by a cold douche will be highly beneficial.

In persistent cases, cold vaginal irritation provides relief. This treatment is best administered with a fountain syringe, containing water. The syringe should be placed two or three feet above the patient and water injected into the vagina. The patient should lie upon her back, with hips elevated and water should flow out of the vaginal canal.

A decoction of the herb chebulic myrobalan has proved very useful for vaginal irritation and inflammation. It should be used as an external douche to wash the vulvar parts. When there is a thick white discharge, washing the part with a decoction made with *neem* leaves and chebulic myrobalan fruits will greatly help.

A moderately prolonged cold hip bath accompanied with a hot foot bath is also helpful. The level of cold water must be 34 inches in height. The patient should sit in the tub in such a manner that legs remain out of the tub. This bath can be given for 20 to 30 minutes.

Another mode of treatment considered beneficial is the wet girdle pack for about an hour. For this treatment, a thin cotton underwear and another thick or woolen underwear are required. The thin underwear should be wrung in cold water and worn by the patient. The thick dry underwear should be worn above the wet underwear. If the patient feels chill, she should be covered with a blanket. This treatment helps reduce inflammation.

A cold douche on the perineal region for 10 to 15 minutes, twice a day helps reduce vaginitis. A mud pack on the abdomen for 10 minutes twice daily also helps reduce inflammation.

Chromotherapy can also be used to treat this complaint. Blue light treatment given to the afflicted region for an hour accompanied with vaginal irrigation using green coloured charged water helps reduce the infection.

After recovery, it is essential to adopt correct eating habits and hygienic living conditions. Proper rest and exercise are also important.

CHAPTER 150

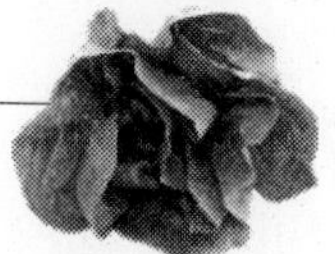

Pruritus Vulvae

Pruritus literally means a sensation of itching and vulva is the name given to the entrance to the vagina. It is a symptom, not a disease in itself. At least 10 per cent of women all over the world suffer from this complaint.

Pruritus vulvae is generally relieved through scratching in the initial stages. At a later stage, the patient develops a burning sensation in this region. This can intensify to such an extent that women suffering from this complaint prefer to remain indoors and refuse to go out. This problem occurs more during the night. The patient may scratch the area during sleep and wake to find that she has made herself bleed.

Causes

One of the main causes of pruritus vulvae is purulent and mucopurulent vaginal discharge. Due to this discharge, the vulva region chafes. The resulting tenderness causes pain. Over 80 per cent of the cases occur due to this cause. Pruritus without vaginal discharge occurs in 15 to 20 per cent of the cases.

In some cases pruritus vulvae may develop due to the presence of skin diseases not specific to the vulva such as psoriasis, seborrheic dermatitis and scabies. Other causes include animal and vegetable parasite infections which tend to cause pruritus pubic rather than pruritus vulvae, conditions of the urinary track like incontinence of urine and pyuria. Highly acidic urine sometime causes soreness which subsequently leads to pruritus. Glycosuria and diabetes also contribute to this condition.

Pruritus vulvae can result from skin sensitivity to various kinds of soaps, bath salts, deodorants and antiseptics which contain particular phenols and oresols and from certain drugs. These allergies may also be caused by nylons and tight-fitting clothes. In rare cases the disorders may develop as an offshoot of certain major problems like jaundice, uraemia, and other toxic conditions.

Many mental disturbances can affect the sexual bias and psychoneurosis results. The skin of the vulva region can also be a site of psychoneurosis, nervous fatigue and rough clotting. Sexual frustration and guilt feelings can also lead to pruritus vulvae.

Treatments

There is always some underlying cause for the onset of pruritus, but scratching soon damages the skin and causes secondary changes which may obscure the primary cause. In addition, the skin may become sensitized to some local application. In long standing cases, the diagnosis of both the initial cause and the reason for the maintenance of the irritation may become extremely difficult, particularly when more than one factor is involved. Successful treatment depends on two cardinal principles, namely, to remove any underlying cause and to stop further damage to the skin by scratching or by unsuitable application.

The most important factor in the treatment of pruritus vulvae caused by infections through fungus or parasites, is cleanliness. Bowels should be kept clean either through enemas or a natural diet. The patient must wear clean clothes to avoid this problem. After urination, the vagina should be thoroughly washed with plain cold water. In case of severe pruritus, it is advisable to wash the vulva with *neem* leaves decoction and apply green light charged coconut oil.

Treatments like *neem* water vaginal douches help kill bacteria and fungus. The affected region should be exposed to green coloured light or rays of the sun through green coloured glass for 25 to 30 minutes. This will help reduce infections.

Pruritus vulvae resulting from discharges from the uterus, cervix or vagina causes inflammations. This can be reduced by regular application of mud packs on the lower abdomen, twice or thrice a day. A cold hip bath may also be taken for 10 minutes. An alternate hot and cold hip bath is especially useful in reducing inflammation.

In cases of pruritus resulting from diabetes mellitus, glycosuria, uraemia, jaundice and other toxic states, specific diets and treatments for these complaints should be followed before pruritus could be cured.

Skin diseases like psoriasis, scabies, fungal infections should be treated through various nature cure methods. These include steam baths, mud baths, immersion baths, sun baths, spine baths and chromotherapy.

Diet plays an important role in the treatment of pruritus vulvae. Initially the patient should be put on a juice fast for a few days. She should drink fruit and vegetable juices, diluted with water on a 50 : 50 basis. A warm water enema should be used daily during the period of fasting to cleanse the bowels.

Fasting helps relieve the toxic conditions not in just the affected regions but also the entire body. Thus inflammation is reduced. The diet after the juice fast could include seasonal fruits, salads, sprouts, vegetables soups or buttermilk. Cooked food should be included in the diet only much later.

The patient should avoid all processed, refined and denatured foods such as white sugar, white flour and all products made from them as well as coffee, tea, eggs, meat, spicy and oily foods. Alcohol and smoking are to be completely eliminated.

A natural mode of life will go a long way in overcoming pruritus vulvae. It will also lead to improvement in health in general.

CHAPTER 151

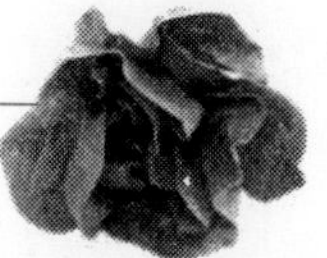

Hysteria

Hysteria is a mental and nervous disorder arising from intense anxiety. It is characterised by a lack of control over acts and emotions and by sudden convulsive seizures and emotional outbursts. It often results from repressed mental conflict.

This disorder appears in both sexes, but is far more common in young women of the age group between 14 and 25 years because of their natural sensitivity. In many cases it tends to occur around the period of adolescence and becomes less frequent after the age of 25. It is uncommon after the age of forty-five years.

Hysteria is an ancient disorder. The term is derived from the Greek word hystron, meaning uterus. The diagnosis dates back to ancient Greek medicine, according to which a variety of symptoms was attributed to a wandering of the womb through the body. The recorded history of the diagnosis begun in ancient Egypt with the Kahnus Papyrus dating from about 1900 BC, which enumerates a series of morbid states attributable to displacement of the uterus. In the Middle Ages hysteria was associated with ideas of demoniacal possession, witchcraft and religious fanaticism. Later it came to be solely related to the female sex.

Osler, an eminent psychiatrist defines hysteria as "a disorder chiefly of young women, in which emotional states control the body, leading to perversion of mental, sensory, motor and secretory functions."

Symptoms

A wide range of symptoms are regarded as hysterical. The onset of hysterical attacks may be sudden, provoked especially by strong feelings or may be heralded over a period of several hours by prodromal features. The main symptoms include inappropriate elation or sadness, crying without cause, almost convulsive laughter, deep sighing, cramps in the limbs, mild rumblings in the belly and sense of constriction in the throat.

The symptoms of hysteria are of two degrees. In the first degree, the patient may feel heaviness in the limbs, more severe cramps, strong feeling of ascending abdominal constriction, continual sighings, difficulty in breathing, constriction in the chest, palpitations, feeling of a foreign body lodged in the throat, swelling of the neck and of the jugular veins, suffocation, headache, clenched teeth, generalized and voluntary tensing of muscles of locomotion. The patient remains conscious during paroxysms. The convulsions are usually milder and occur more often during the bending and extending of limbs.

In the second degree, additional symptoms, besides the preceding ones, are noticeable and these may include wild and painful cries, incomplete loss of consciousness, enormously swollen neck, violent and tumultuous heart-beats, involuntary locomotor muscle contraction, frightening generalized convulsions, violent movement and frequent spitting. Sometimes the patient jumps about on his/her bed and at other times adopt almost tetanic postures. The attack may last several hours. There may be prompt return of consciousness immediately after the convulsions.

The psychical symptoms include a weakness of the will, a craving for love and sympathy and a tendency to emotional instability. Hysterical people tend to react too readily to suggestion and through this suggestibility they are swayed greatly by their surroundings. The morbid exaggerated moods lead to impulsive conduct which may often seem irrational. Such people are liable to be much misunderstood and misjudged. At times there may be much absent-mindedness, and loss of memory about events or for definite periods. If this mental dissociation is severe, one may develop hysterical wandering attacks, a state of double consciousness or dual personality.

Hysterical trances may last for days or weeks. Here the patient seems to be in a deep sleep, but the muscles are not usually relaxed. In the most severe instance of this, the heart's action and breathing may be scarcely apparent that death may be suspected and the person buried alive. Somnambulism or sleep-walking and catalepsy, where limbs remain in any position in which they are placed, are other hysterical states.

Causes

The most common causes of hysteria are sexual excess, or sexual repression, perverted habits of thought and idleness. Heredity plays an important part in its causation. A nervous family, taint and faulty emotional training, when young, are predisposing causes. The emotional shocks may have been caused by mental or physical factors such as mental strain, stress, fear, worry, depression, traumatism, masturbation and prolonged sickness.

Hysteria is an extremely complex mental phenomenon which may take varying forms. In certain types the disorder may result from some situation to which one is unable to adapt oneself such as marriage, engagement, position of responsibility, the death of relations or loss of love. Factors involving the sexual life in some way are frequently present.

A number of studies have indicated a possible connection between hysterical symptoms and organic brain disease. A patient with epilepsy has often been found to get hysterical attacks. Drug intoxication is another organic brain disease closely associated with hysteria.

Treatment

Hysteria is curable in nearly all cases. Since the causes of hysteria are both physical and mental, treatment should be directed toward both the body and the mind. Regard for one's physical welfare is of primary importance. A healthy, well-functioning body is best able to keep the reasoning mind in control of the total organism.

The measures on the physical side should include a well-ordered hygienic mode of living, a nutritious and bland diet, adequate mental and physical rest, daily exercise, agreeable, occupation, fresh air, regular hours of eating and sleeping, regulation of the bowels and wholesome companionship with others.

On the mental plane, the patient should be taught self-control and educated in positive thinking. Her mind must be, by some means, drawn away from herself. Proper sex education should be given immediately, especially as regards sublimation of sexual desire or normal sexual indulgence for the married patient.

In most cases of hysteria, it is desirable for the patient to start treatment by adopting an all-fruit diet for several days. She should have fresh juicy fruits such as orange, apple, grapes, grape-fruit, papaya and pineapple during this period. The all-fruit diet should be followed by an exclusive milk diet for about a month.

Most hysteria patients are considerably run down and the milk diet will help build better blood and nourish the nerves. If the full milk diet is not convenient, a diet of milk and fruits may be adopted. The patient may, therefore, gradually embark upon a well balanced diet of seeds, nuts and grains, vegetables and fruits. The patient should avoid alcohol, tea, coffee, tobacco, white sugar and white flour and products made from them.

Jambul fruit, known as *jamun* in the vernacular, is considered an effective home remedy for hysteria. Three kgs. of this fruit and a handful of salt should be put in a jug filled with water. The jug should be kept in the sun for a week. Women suffering from hysteria should take 300 grams of these fruits on an empty stomach and also drink a cup of water from the jug. The day she starts this treatment, 3 kgs. more of these fruits together with a handful of salt should be put in another jug filled with water, so that when the contents of the first jug are finished, contents of the other may be ready for use. This treatment should be continued for two weeks.

Honey is regarded as another effective remedy for hysteria. Two of the main causes of hysteria are irregularity of the menstrual cycle and insanity. Honey is invaluable for both these conditions. It causes good bleeding during the cycle, cleans the uterus, tones up the brain and the uterine musculature and keeps the body temperature at a normal level. It is advisable to use honey regularly and increase the quantity after the fits start. It will bring down body temperature thus preventing further fits.

Exercise and outdoor games are important in the prevention and cure of hysteria. They take the mind away from one's self and induce cheerfulness. Yogasanas which are useful in hysteria are bhujangasana, shallabhasana, matsyasana, sarvangasana, dhanurasana, halasana, paschimottanasana, yogamudra and shavasana. Weak patients, who are not able to take much active exercise, may be given massage three or four times a week.

Other measures useful in the treatment of hysteria are air and sun baths. They are calming and at the same time invigorating to the nerves. Daily cool baths are also an excellent tonic. Suitable physical activity must be balanced with adequate rest and sleep.

In case of a hysterical fit, the clothing of the patient should be loosened and her head lowered by laying her out flat at once. She should not be allowed to assume an erect position for sometime after the fit. She should be slapped gently in the face and mustard plasters applied to the soles of the feet and the wrists. In ordinary cases no further treatment is necessary and the symptoms will soon pass off or cease if the patient is left alone.

In a genuine hysterical attack, the most effective means of interrupting the paroxym is the application of cold water in some form to the head and spine. Either the cold water may be poured or cold pack or ice pack may be applied to the hand and the back of the neck. If this cannot be done, cold water may be splashed on the face. The patient should be provided with plenty of fresh air and some of her clothing should be removed to facilitate easy breathing and to expose the skin to fresh air.

In a violent seizure of hysteria, pressure on the ovaries often checks the attack. The patient should be made to lie on the back and the fist forcibly pressed into the iliac region. As soon as possible, a neutral immersion bath at 98° to 100°F. may be given and continued until the excited condition subsides. If this is not convenient, a hot foot-bath, with cold applications to the head, may be used instead. Following an attack, the patient should have rest, quietness, darkness and if possible, sleep until the lost energy has been gradually recovered.

Part V

Charts and Tables

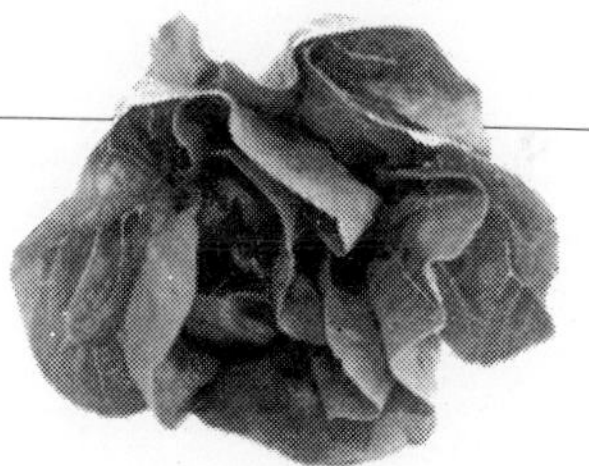

VITAMIN CHART

VITAMIN	FUNCTION IN THE BODY	VALUABLE SOURCES	RECOMMENDED DAILY ALLOWANCE		DEFICIENCY SYMPTOMS	SIDE EFFECTS OF OVER DOSAGES
			Adults	Children		
A	Essential for normal growth and vitality. Necessary for good sight and healthy skin. It protects the body against disease, especially of the respiratory tract.	Cod liver oil, whole milk, curds, butter, egg yolk, pumpkin, carrots, green leafy vegetables, tomatoes, mango, papaya orange, melon.	5,000 I.U.	2,000 to 4,000 I.U.	Eye infection, poor vision, night blindness, frequent colds, lack of appetite and skin disorder.	Loss of appetite, vomiting, headache, dryness of skin and hair loss.
B_1 or Thiamine	Essential for normal functioning of nervous system. Regulates carbohydrate metabolism, appetite and aids	Wheat germ, Brewer's yeast, outer layer of rice, wheat & other whole grain cereals, pulses, nuts,	1.2-3.0 mg.	0.4-1.2 mg.	Serious impairment of nervous and digestive systems, neuritis, beriberi, loss of weight diabetes, mental depression	Rapid heartbeat, low blood pressure, restlessness & trembling.

VITAMIN CHART

VITAMIN	FUNCTION IN THE BODY	VALUABLE SOURCES	RECOMMENDED DAILY ALLOWANCE		DEFICIENCY SYMPTOMS	SIDE EFFECTS OF OVER DOSAGES
			Adults	Children		
	in digestion.	peas, lime, legumes, kidney, dark green leafy vegetables, milk, egg, banana, apple.			and weakness of heart.	
B_2	Essential for growth and general health, healthy eyes, skin, nails and hair.	Green leafy vegetables, milk, cheese, wheat germ, egg, citrus fruits, banana, tomato. Brewer's yeast almonds and sunflower seeds	1.6-2.6 mg.	0.6-1.0 mg.	Burning sensation in the legs, lips and tongue, cracking at the angles of the mouth, premature wrinkles and eczema.	Itching and tingling in extremities.

VITAMIN CHART

VITAMIN	FUNCTION IN THE BODY	VALUABLE SOURCES	RECOMMENDED DAILY ALLOWANCE		DEFICIENCY SYMPTOMS	SIDE EFFECTS OF OVER DOSAGES
			Adults	Children		
B_3 or Niacin or Nicotinic Acid	Essential for proper circulation, healthy functioning of the nervous system and proper protein & carbohydrate metabolism	Yeast, liver, fish, whole wheat, green leafy vegetables, tomatoes, nuts, sunflower seeds and peanuts.	12-20 mg.	4.8-12.0 mg.	Pellarga, diarrhoea, insomnia, anaemia and mental disorders.	Nausea, vomiting, flashes and tingling sensations.
B_6 or Pyridoxine	Helps digestion and absorption of fats and proteins.	Liver, rice, milk, Brewer's yeast, cereals, legumes, meat, green leafy vegetables, carrots and peanuts.	1.3 mg	0.6 mg	Anaemia, skin disorders, migraine, kidney stones and mental disturbances.	Poor coordination, staggering, numbness, decreased sensation to touch, temperature, and vibration, and tiredness.

VITAMIN CHART

VITAMIN	FUNCTION IN THE BODY	VALUABLE SOURCES	RECOMMENDED DAILY ALLOWANCE		DEFICIENCY SYMPTOMS	SIDE EFFECTS OF OVER DOSAGES
			Adults	Children		
B_{12} or Cyanocobalamin	Essential for production of red blood cells and for several metabolic and enzymatic processes.	Milk, eggs, liver, bananas, peanuts, and sunflower seeds.	2.4 mg	1.8 mg	Certain types of anaemia, poor appetite and chronic fatigue.	Panic anxiety attacks, heart palpitations, hyperthyroid.
B_9 or Folic Acid	Essential for the growth and division of all body cells, healing processes and protein metabolism.	Whole grains, nuts and fresh green leafy vegetables such as asparagus, green beans and peas.	400 mcg	300 mcg	Certain types of anaemia, skin disorders and impaired circulation.	Loss of appetite, nausea, flatulence.
B_5 or Panthothenic Acid	Aids normal growth of hair and prevents dermatitis.	Wheat germ, whole grain bread, green vegetables,	5 mg	3 mg	Mental depression, irritability, muscular weakness,	Severe persistent diarrhea

VITAMIN CHART

VITAMIN	FUNCTION IN THE BODY	VALUABLE SOURCES	RECOMMENDED DAILY ALLOWANCE		DEFICIENCY SYMPTOMS	SIDE EFFECTS OF OVER DOSAGES
			Adults	Children		
		peanuts, liver and eggs.			insomnia and skin disorders	
C or Ascorbic Acid	Essential for normal growth and maintenance of body tissues especially those of the joints, bones, teeth and gums. Protects against infection and helps in quick healing of wounds.	Citrus fruits, green leafy vegetables, *amla*, sprouted Bengal and green grams.	50-75 mg.	30-50 mg.	Scurvy, anaemia, tooth decay, bleeding gums, painful and swo-llen parts, slow healing of wounds and premature ageing.	Formation of kidney stones, menstrual bleeding in pregnant women, activation of peptic ulcers.
D	Essential for proper bone & teeth formation	Rays of the sun, fish, milk, butter, eggs &	400-800 I.U.	400-800 I.U.	Rickets, tooth decay, pyorrhoea muscular	Irritability, nausea, vomiting, constipation, high

VITAMIN CHART

VITAMIN	FUNCTION IN THE BODY	VALUABLE SOURCES	RECOMMENDED DAILY ALLOWANCE		DEFICIENCY SYMPTOMS	SIDE EFFECTS OF OVER DOSAGES
			Adults	Children		
	& metabolism of calcium and phosphorus.	sprouted seeds	400 I.U.	400 I.U.	weakness and gross deficiencies of bones.	blood pressure and calcium deposits in arteries.
E	Essential for normal reproductory function, fertility & physical vigour. It dilates blood vessels and improves circulation.	Wheat or cereal germ, whole grain products, green leafy vegetables eggs, milk and all whole raw or sprouted seeds.	15 mg	7-11 mg	Degeneration of reproductive tissues, liver disorders & sluggish circulation.	High blood pressure
K	Necessary for proper clotting of blood & for prevention of bleeding.	Green leafy vegetables, spinach, cabbage & tomato.	65-80 mcg	300 mcg	Certain types of anaemia, skin disorders & impaired circulation.	Diarrhoea, nausea, vomiting, liver damage

MINERAL CHART

MINERAL	FUNCTION IN THE BODY	MAIN SOURCES	RECOMMENDED DAILY ALLOWANCE		DEFICIENCY SYMPTOMS	SIDE EFFECTS OF OVER DOSAGES
			Adults	Children		
1. Boron	Helps regulate the body's use of calcium, phosphorus and magnesium. Control cell growth. Thereby preventing abnormalities in growth.	Fruits & vegtables, especially apples, pears and carrots.	2 mg for adult & children —adequate in average diet.		Tumours, cysts & other abnormal growth.	Over 100 mg per day may produce toxic symptoms.
2. Calcium	Essential for proper development of bone & teeth, for normal action of heart and all muscle activity. Aids	Milk and milk products, green vegetables, mustard seeds, dried coconut, finger millet and almonds.	400 mg	600 mg.	Changes in the bones & muscles, listless, laziness, nervousness, mental derangement, fragile bones, tooth	Hypercalcemia

MINERAL CHART

MINERAL	FUNCTION IN THE BODY	MAIN SOURCES	RECOMMENDED DAILY ALLOWANCE		DEFICIENCY SYMPTOMS	SIDE EFFECTS OF OVER DOSAGES
			Adults	Children		
	clotting process of blood, stimulates enzymes in digestive process, ensures proper foetal growth & speeds healing processes.				decay, heart palpitations, muscle cramps, insomnia and irritability.	
3. Chlorine	Essential for proper distribution of carbon dioxide, manufacture of glandular hormone secretions, regulates the alkali-acid balance in the blood	Barley, wheat, and other grains & pulses, green leafy vegetables, and fruits.	300-900 mg	160-500 mg	Heat cramps, loss of hair & teeth, impaired digestion of foods and derangement of fluid levels in the body.	Chlorine fumes are poisonous.

MINERAL CHART

MINERAL	FUNCTION IN THE BODY	MAIN SOURCES	RECOMMENDED DAILY ALLOWANCE		DEFICIENCY SYMPTOMS	SIDE EFFECTS OF OVER DOSAGES
			Adults	Children		
	and prevents the building of excessive fat and auto intoxication.					
4. Chromium	Essential for metabolism of carbohydrates & fats. Increases effectiveness of insulin, takes protein where needed and aids in growth.	Betel leaves, arecanut and nuts.	50-200 mg	20-200 mg	Impairment of glucose tolerance, suspected factor in arterioclerosis & protein-energy malnutrition.	Occupational dermatitis (eczema) and lung cancer.
5. Copper	Helps conversion of iron into haemoglobin, stimulates the growth	Molluscs, shellfish, betal leaves, areca-nuts and other nuts.	2 mg	0.05-0.1 mg	Weakness of the body, digestive disturbances, and impaired respiration.	Poisonous

MINERAL CHART

MINERAL	FUNCTION IN THE BODY	MAIN SOURCES	RECOMMENDED DAILY ALLOWANCE		DEFICIENCY SYMPTOMS	SIDE EFFECTS OF OVER DOSAGES
			Adults	Children		
	of red blood cells. Essential for utilisation of vitamin C.					
6. Fluorine	Essential for healthy teeth	Bengal gram, cereals especially rice, leafy vegetables and dry tea leaves.	4 mg	2.5 mg	Dental caries	Dental fluorosis, fluorine intoxication
7. Iodine	Thyroxine secreted by thyroid gland, which is the chief stone house of iodine, controls the basic metabolism & oxygen consum-	Iodised salt, sea foods and spinach.	150 mcg	83 mcg	Cretinism in children characterised by dwarfness, mental retardness, and enlarged thyroid gland. Myxoedema in adults cha-	No effects from natural iodine.

MINERAL CHART

MINERAL	FUNCTION IN THE BODY	MAIN SOURCES	RECOMMENDED DAILY ALLOWANCE		DEFICIENCY SYMPTOMS	SIDE EFFECTS OF OVER DOSAGES
			Adults	Children		
	ption of tissues, utilisation of sugars, regulates rate of energy production & body weight and promotes growth.				racterised by slower rate of metabolism, thickening of skin. Dietary lack may lead to fatigue, lethargy and low blood pressure.	
8. Iron	Necessary for production of haemoglobin. Increases resistance to stress & disease, aids, growth and prevents fatigue.	Wholegrain cereals, pulses and legumes, fish, green leafy vegetables, fruits.	28 mg	26-40 mg	Anaemia, lowered resistance to disease, general run-down condition, pale complexion, shortness of breath on manual exertion, loss of interest in sex, mental depression and irritability.	Excess storage of iron in the body is harmful.

MINERAL CHART

MINERAL	FUNCTION IN THE BODY	MAIN SOURCES	RECOMMENDED DAILY ALLOWANCE		DEFICIENCY SYMPTOMS	SIDE EFFECTS OF OVER DOSAGES
			Adults	Children		
9. Magnesium	Helps keep nerves relaxed, necessary for all muscular activity, activator of enzymes involved in metabolism, fat and protein. It also helps utilisation of vitamin B and E.	Nuts, soyabeans, alfalfa, apples, figs, lemons, peaches, almonds, wholegrains, brown rice, sunflower seeds, sesame seeds, cereals & vegetables.	350 mg	150-200 mg	Kidney damage & kidney stones, muscle cramps, atherosclerosis, heart attack, epileptic seizures, nervous irritability, marked depression & confusion, impaired protein metabolism, and premature wrinkles.	Large amounts over an extended period of time can be toxic.
10. Manganese	Helps nourish nerves and brain and assists in coordinative action between	Nuts, whole grains & dried legumes.	3 mg	1.6 mg	Retarded growth, digestive disorders, abnormal bone development and deformities.	Blurred speech, tremors of hands, & spastic gait.

MINERAL CHART

MINERAL	FUNCTION IN THE BODY	MAIN SOURCES	RECOMMENDED DAILY ALLOWANCE		DEFICIENCY SYMPTOMS	SIDE EFFECTS OF OVER DOSAGES
			Adults	Children		
	brain, nerves & muscles; metabolism of carbohydrates, fats & proteins.					
11. Moybdenum	Essential for synthesis of haemoglobin & absorption of iron. Aids in carbohydrate & fat metabolism.	Whole grains, pulses & legumes, leafy vegetables and nuts.	500 mcg	266 mcg	Dental caries and sulphite sensitivities.	High intake through local plants can lead to gout.
12. Phosphorus	Essential for hair growth helps counteract fatigue, regular functioning of heart & for normal	Wholegrain cereals, milk, fish, carrots, leafy vegetables, black currants, raesp-	800 mg	440 mg	Loss of weight, retarded growth, reduced sexual powers & general weakness.	hyperphosphatemia or high blood phosphate levels

MINERAL CHART

MINERAL	FUNCTION IN THE BODY	MAIN SOURCES	RECOMMENDED DAILY ALLOWANCE		DEFICIENCY SYMPTOMS	SIDE EFFECTS OF OVER DOSAGES
			Adults	Children		
	functioning of kidney and regulates acid-alkaline balance in blood.	berries, raisins, apricots, soya beans, lentils & pulses and legymes.				
13. Potassium	Essential for muscle contraction, proper functioning of heart, maintains acid-alkaline balance in blood, prevents hyperacidity, promotes secretion of hormones, helps kidneys in detoxification of	Pulses such as green gram, cow peas, red gram black gram; & vegetables like lotus stems & sword beans, legumes, leafy vegetables and fruits.	1.7-5.5 g	0.9-3 g	Undue body tiredness, palpitations of heart, cloudiness of mind, nervous shaking, excessive perspiration of hands & feet, and great sensitivity of nerves to cold.	Muscular weakness, mental apathy, renal failure and adrenal insufficiency.

MINERAL CHART

MINERAL	FUNCTION IN THE BODY	MAIN SOURCES	RECOMMENDED DAILY ALLOWANCE		DEFICIENCY SYMPTOMS	SIDE EFFECTS OF OVER DOSAGES
			Adults	Children		
	blood, prevents female hormonal disorders, helps overcome fatigue & reduces blood pressure.					
14. Selenium	Aids in maintaining youthful elasticity in tissues, prevents or slows down ageing process and hardening of tissues.	Wholegrain cereals like wheat germ, barley and wholewheat bread.	40-70 mcg	20-30 mcg	Cancer, cardiovascular disease, inflammatory diseases, premature ageing & cataract formation.	Patchy baldness (alopecia), abnormal nails, emotional instability & lassitude.
15. Silicon	Essential for proper functioning of nerve cells & tissues, &	Apples, oranges, cherries, raisins, almonds, peanuts,	20-50 mg	—	Soft brittle nails, ageing symptoms of skin such as wrinkles,	Chronic fibrosis of lungs.

MINERAL CHART

MINERAL	FUNCTION IN THE BODY	MAIN SOURCES	RECOMMENDED DAILY ALLOWANCE		DEFICIENCY SYMPTOMS	SIDE EFFECTS OF OVER DOSAGES
			Adults	Children		
	synthesis of vitamin or thiamine in body, controls transmission of nerve impulses, enhances strength & integrity of bones, essential for growth of hair, nails, teeth; benefits in all healing processes.	B,raw cabbage, onions, endives, carrots, eggplants, pumpkin, red beets, celery, cucumber, fish, honey, corn & whole grains.			thinning or loss of hair, poor bone development, osteoporosis & sensitiveness to cold.	
16. Sodium	Maintains acid-base equilibrium, in transmitting nerve impulses, in relaxing	Vegetables like dry lotus stems, leafy vegetables, pulses & legumes, fruits,	10-15 g	5-10 g	Nausea, muscular weakness, heat exhaustion and mental apathy.	Water retention, high blood pressure and stomach ulcers.

MINERAL CHART

MINERAL	FUNCTION IN THE BODY	MAIN SOURCES	RECOMMENDED DAILY ALLOWANCE		DEFICIENCY SYMPTOMS	SIDE EFFECTS OF OVER DOSAGES
			Adults	Children		
	muscles, regulates osmotic pressure, maintains water balance.	fish and meat.				
17. Sulphur	Essential for synthesis of vitamin B_1, helps digestion of fats, controls metabolism of carbohydrates, essential for healthy skin, hair and nails, aids liver in bile secretion.	Red gram, green gram & leafy vegetables.	Adequate in diet	High-protein	Unhealthy growth of hair & nails.	Asthma joint degeneration.
18. Vanadium	Helps in metabolism of	Cereals, vegetables, nuts &	1-4 mcg	—	—	Toxic if taken in synthetic form.

MINERAL CHART

MINERAL	FUNCTION IN THE BODY	MAIN SOURCES	RECOMMENDED DAILY ALLOWANCE		DEFICIENCY SYMPTOMS	SIDE EFFECTS OF OVER DOSAGES
			Adults	Children		
	cholesterol and sugar thereby preventing occurrence of heart attacks.	oilseeds and fruits such as apples and plums.				
19. Zinc	Essential for healthy skin and hair, proper healing of wounds, successful pregnancies, male virility, guards against disease and infection, & transports vitamin A to retina.	Cereals, nuts, oilseeds, vegetables and fruits.	10-15 mg	10 mg	Anaemia, retardation in growth, and delayed genital malnutrition.	Loss of iron and copper in body, inhalation of zinc fumes can result in toxicity.

AMINO-ACID CHART

AMINO ACID	FUNCTION IN THE BODY	MAIN SOURCES	RECOMMENDED DAILY ALLOWANCE			DEFICIENCY SYMPTOMS	SIDE EFFECTS OF OVER DOSAGES
			Adults	Children	Infants		
1. Argin-ine	Essential for normal growth and proper fun-ctioning of im-mune system in the body and helps detoxify & eliminate urea.	Peanuts, cash-ew nuts, piyal seeds, water-melon seeds, walnuts, green and root vegetables.	—	—	—	Reduces sex imp-ulse and can ca-use impotence.	Reversible thicken-neing and coarsening of skin.
2. Histid-ine	Essential for growth and rep-air of human tissues, & conv-ersion of glucose into glycogen in liver.	Fruits such as bananas and grapes, meat and poultry, milk and milk products and root and green vegetables.	—	—	33 mg	Pain in bony jo-ints and rheuma-toid arthritis.	Taken orally, it can stimulate hydrochl-oric acid secretion in stomach.
3. Isoleu-cine	Essential for production and	Eggs, chicken, pork, mutton,	12 mg	28 mg	80 mg	—	—

AMINO-ACID CHART

AMINO ACID	FUNCTION IN THE BODY	MAIN SOURCES	RECOMMENDED DAILY ALLOWANCE			DEFICIENCY SYMPTOMS	SIDE EFFECTS OF OVER DOSAGES
			Adults	Children	Infants		
	maintenance of body proteins, regulates metabolism & functioning of thymus gland in neck, spleen & pituitary gland & useful in formation of haemoglobin.	pulses, soya beans, cottage checse, milk, piyal seeds, cashew nuts, and cereal grains.					
4. Leucine	Regulates protein metabolism in the body, and controls the net synthesis of protein.	Whole grains, milk and milk products, eggs, pork, beef, chicken, pulses soya beans	16 mg	42 mg	128 mg	—	Pellagra

AMINO-ACID CHART

AMINO ACID	FUNCTION IN THE BODY	MAIN SOURCES	RECOMMENDED DAILY ALLOWANCE			DEFICIENCY SYMPTOMS	SIDE EFFECTS OF OVER DOSAGES
			Adults	Children	Infants		
		and leafy vegetables.					
5. Lysine	Inhibits proliferation of viruses and eliminates virus infections.	Leafy vegetables, pulses & legumes, meat, poultry, milk and milk products, and ripe fruits.	12 mg	44 mg	97 mg	Poor appetite, reduction in body weight, anaemia, reduced ability to concentrate, headaches, nausea, dizziness, pneumonia, nephrosis, acidosis malnutrition and rickets.	—
6. Methionine	Protects liver from fatty degeneration, helps dissolve cholesterol and	Whole grains, meat, poultry, milk and milk products, leafy vegetables,	10 mg	22 mg	45 mg	Chronic rheumatic fever in children, hardening of lines (cirrhosis),	—

AMINO-ACID CHART

AMINO ACID	FUNCTION IN THE BODY	MAIN SOURCES	RECOMMENDED DAILY ALLOWANCE			DEFICIENCY SYMPTOMS	SIDE EFFECTS OF OVER DOSAGES
			Adults	Children	Infants		
	assimilates fat, essential for synthesis of haemoglobin, necessary for maintenance of normal body weight and proper nitrogen balance and prevents turnover formation.	peaches and grapes.				and nephritis of kidneys.	
7. Phenylalanine	Effective for weight control, controls appetite & efficient functioning of kidneys & bladder.	Curd, milk, cottage cheese, pulses and legumes, poultry, piyal seeds, groundnuts,	16 mg	22 mg	132 mg	Bloodshot eyes, cataract and several behavioural changes such as psychotic &	Harmful for hypertension, if taken over 100 mg.

AMINO-ACID CHART

AMINO ACID	FUNCTION IN THE BODY	MAIN SOURCES	RECOMMENDED DAILY ALLOWANCE			DEFICIENCY SYMPTOMS	SIDE EFFECTS OF OVER DOSAGES
			Adults	Children	Infants		
		pistachio nuts, almonds, leafy vegetables & whole grains.				schizophrenic. behaviour	
8. Threonine	Essential for development & proper functioning of brain and has powerful anti-convulsive effect.	Poultry, pork, leafy vegetables, whole grains, pulses, nuts, apples, peaches and figs.	8 mg	28 mg	63 mg	Irritability in children.	—
9. Thyptophan	Essential for blood clotting and formation of digestive juices, induces sleep, relaxes nervous	All seeds, nuts, vegetables.	3 mg	4 mg	19 mg	Increased sensitivity to light, pellagra.	Supplement may prove harmful during pregnancy.

AMINO-ACID CHART

AMINO ACID	FUNCTION IN THE BODY	MAIN SOURCES	RECOMMENDED DAILY ALLOWANCE			DEFICIENCY SYMPTOMS	SIDE EFFECTS OF OVER DOSAGES
			Adults	Children	Infants		
	system, wards off signs of premature ageing such as cataract of eyes, baldness, deterioration of sex gland functioning & malformation of tooth enamel.						
10. Valine	Essential for proper performance of the nervous system, prevents nervous & digestive disorders & is	Leafy vegetables, finger millet, rice and other cereals, kidney beans and other legumes & pulses,	14 mg	25 mg	89 mg	Sensitive to touch and sound.	Hallucinations and a sensation of insects crawling over the skin.

AMINO-ACID CHART							
AMINO ACID	FUNCTION IN THE BODY	MAIN SOURCES	RECOMMENDED DAILY ALLOWANCE			DEFICIENCY SYMPTOMS	SIDE EFFECTS OF OVER DOSAGES
			Adults	Children	Infants		
	important for body growth.	piyal seeds, pistachio, cashew nuts, peaches, poultry & milk.					

Calorie Chart – I

Requirement

(Based on Recommendation of Nutrition Experts Group of Indian Council of Medical Research (CMR) in 1989)

(A) Indian Man and Woman

(Kcal/day)

Particulars		KCAL
Man (60 kg):	Sedentary Work	2425
	Moderate Work	2875
	Heavy Work	3800
Woman (50 kg):	Sedentary Work	1875
	Moderate Work	2225
	Heavy Work	2925
	Latter half of pregnancy	+300
	Lactation	+700

(B) Children

(Kcal/day)

Age Group	Boys	Girls
1 – 3 years	1287	1193
4 – 6 years	1752	1630
7 – 9 years	2075	1833
10 – 12 years	2194	1965
13 – 15 years	2447	2056
16 – 18 years	2642	2064

(C) Infant

(Kcals/kg)

Age	Kcal/kg
0 – 3 months	116
3 – 6 months	99
6 – 9 months	95
9 – 12 months	101
Average during the first year = 103 Kcal/kg)	

Calorie Chart – II

Calorific Value of Common Foods

Per 100 grams of Edible Portion

S. No.	Food	Calories	S. No.	Food	Calories
1	ALMOND	655	34	FRENCH BEANS, DRY	346
2	AMARANTH	45	35	GARLIC	145
3	APPLE	59	36	GINGER	67
4	APRICOT (FRESH)	53	37	GRAPE-FRUIT	45
5	AVOCADO	215	38	GRAPES	71
6	BAEL FRUIT	137	39	GROUNDNUT	567
7	BANANA	116	40	GUAVA	51
8	BARLEY	336	41	HONEY	319
9	BEET ROOT.	43	42	INDIAN GOOSEBERRY	58
10	BENGAL GRAM (WHOLE)	360	43	JACK FRUIT	88
11	BENGAL GRAM (DAL)	372	44	JAMBUL FRUIT	62
12	BITTER GOURD	25	45	LADY'S FINGERS	35
13	BLACK GRAM	347	46	LEMON	57
14	BOTTLE GOURD	12	47	LENTIL	343
15	CABBAGE	27	48	LETTUCE	21
16	CARROT	48	49	LITCHI	61
17	CASHEWNUT	596	50	LIME	59
18	CELERY	37	51	LINSEED	530
19	COCONUT	444	52	LOQUAT	43
20	COLOCASIA	97	53	MAIZE	342
21	CORIANDER	288	54	MANGO	74
22	CUCUMBER	13	55	MILK	67
23	CURD	60	56	MUSK MELON	17
24	CUSTARD LEAVES	108	57	MUSTARD SEEDS	541
25	CUSTARD APPLE	104	58	OAT MEAL	374
26	DATE (DRIED)	317	59	ONION	50
27	DRUMSTICK	26	60	ORANGE	48
28	EGGPLANT	24	61	PAPAYA	32
29	FENUGREEK LEAVES	49	62	PARSLEY	87
30	FENUGREEK SEEDS	333	63	PEACH	50
31	FIG	37	64	PEAR	52
32	FINGER MILLET	328	65	PIGEON PEAS	335
33	FRENCH BEANS	26	66	PINEAPPLE	46

S. No.	Food	Calories	S. No.	Food	Calories
67	PISTACHIO NUT	626	81	SNAKE GOURD	18
68	POMEGRANATE	65	82	STRAWBERRY	44
69	POTATO	97	83	SUGAR CANE	39
70	PUMPKIN	25	84	SUNFLOWER SEEDS	620
71	RADISH	17	85	SWEET POTATO	120
72	RAISINS	308	86	TOMATO	20
73	RICE, RAW, HANDPOUND	346	87	TURNIP	29
74	RICE, RAW, MILLED	345	88	WALNUT	687
75	RIDGE GOURD	17	89	WATER CRESS	33
76	SAFFLOWER SEEDS	356	90	WATER MELON	16
77	SESAME SEEDS	563	91	WHEAT, WHOLE	346
78	SORGHUM	349	92	WHEAT, FLOUR, WHOLE	341
79	SOYA BEAN	432	93	WHEAT, FLOUR, REFINED	348
80	SPINACH	26	94	ZIZYPHUS	74

Height/Weight Chart

(A) Male

Height (in cm)	Age Group 25-29	30-34	35-39	40-44	45-49	50-54	55-59	60-64	65
150.0	56.5	58	59	60	60.5	60.5	60.5	59	58.5
152.5	57	58.5	59	60.5	61.5	61.5	61.5	60.5	59.5
155.0	58	59	60	61	62.5	62.5	62.5	62	61
157.5	59	60.5	61.5	63	63.5	63.5	63.5	63	63
160.0	61	62.5	63	64.5	65	65.5	65.5	65	64.5
162.5	62.5	63.5	64.5	66	66.5	67.5	67.5	67	66.5
165.0	64	65.5	66.5	67.5	68	69	69	69	68
167.5	66.5	67.5	68.5	69.5	70	71	71	71	70
170.0	68	69	70.5	72	72.5	73.5	73.5	73.5	73
172.5	69.5	71.5	73	74.5	75	75.5	76	76	76
175.0	71.5	74	75.5	76	76	77.5	78	78.5	78.5
177.5	74	76	78	79	79.5	79.5	80	81	81
180.0	76.5	81.5	80.5	81	82.5	82	82.5	82	82

(B) Female

Height (in cm)	Age Group 20-24	25-29	30-34	35-39	40-44	45-49	50-54	55-59	60-64
147.5	51	51.5	52.5	53.5	55	53.5	58	58	57
150.0	51	52.5	53.5	55	56.5	58	58.5	59	58.5
152.5	52	53	54.5	56	58	59	60	60.5	59.5
155.0	53	54	55.5	57.5	59.5	60.5	62	62	61.5
157.5	55	56	57.5	59	61	62.5	63.5	63.5	63
160.0	56.5	57.5	58.5	60.5	62.5	64	65.5	65.5	65
162.5	58	59	61	63	64.5	66.5	67.5	67.5	67
165.0	59.5	61	63	64.5	66	68	69	69	68.5
167.5	61	63	64.5	66.5	67.5	69	70.5	70	70
170.0	63	64.5	66.5	68	69.5	71	72.5	73.5	72
172.5	71.65	66.5	68	69.5	71.5	73.5	75	75	74

(C) Children

MALE			FEMALE		
AGE (Yrs)	HEIGHT (cms)	WEIGHT (kgs)	AGE (yrs)	HEIGHT (cms)	WEIGHT (kgs)
1½	81.8	11.4	1½	80.9	11.1
2	87.5	12.6	2	86.6	12.3
3	96.2	14.6	3	95.7	14.4
4	103.4	16.5	4	103.2	16.4
5	108.7	18.4	5	109.1	18.4
6	118.9	22.1	6	117.3	21.4
7	123.3	24.5	7	122.7	24.8
8	127.9	26.4	8	126.8	26.1
9	133.6	30.0	9	132.3	26.7
10	138.5	32.4	10	138.5	33.5
11	143.4	35.3	11	144.1	36.5
12	148.9	38.8	12	150.3	42.6

Statement Showing Names of Common Foods in Indian Languages

Sr. No.	English	Hindi	Bengali	Gujarati	Kannada	Malayalam	Marathi	Tamil	Telugu
1	Almond	Badam	Badam	Badam	Badam	Badam	Badam	Badam	Badam
2	Amaranth	Chaulai-ka-saag	Kanta-not ya	Kantalo Dabho	Mulla dantu	Vullancheru-cheera	Kante-math	Vullu Keerai	Vulla thota-hoord
3	Apple	Seb	Seu	Safarjan	Sebu	Apple	Safarchand	—	Amruta phalamau
4	Apricot	Khumani or Zordalu	—	—	Jinde-hannu	Apricot	—	—	Kurbani pandlu
5	Avocado	Kulu Naspati	Kulunashpati	—	—	—	—	—	—
6	Bael Fruit	Bel or Siriphal	Bel	Bil	—	Koovalam-kaya	Bel	Bilwa pazham	Maredu pandu
7	Banana	Kela	Kela	Kash	Bale hannu	Vazha pazham	Kela	Vazha pazham	Arati pandu
8	Barley	Jau	Job	Jau	Jave godhi	Yavam	Jau	Barli	Barli biyyam
9	Beet root	Chukandar	Beet	Beet	Beet	Beet	Beet	Beet	Beet
10	Bengal Gram	Channa	Chola	Chana	Kadale	Kadala	Harbara	Kothuka-dalai	Sanagalu
11	Bitter Gourd	Karela	Karela	Karela	Hagal kai	Kaippakka	Karle	Pavakkai	Kakara kayi

Sr. No.	English	Hindi	Bengali	Gujarati	Kannada	Malayalam	Marathi	Tamil	Telugu
12	Black Gram	Urad	Mashkalair dal	Aalad	Uddina bele	Uzhunnu parippu	Uddachi dal	Ulutham paruppu	Minapa pappu
13	Bottle Gourd	Lauki	Lau	Dudhi	Sore kai	Charanga	Dudhi	Surai kai	Anapakaya
14	Cabbage	Bandgobhi	Bandha	Kobi	Kosu	Mutta gose	Kobi	Muttai kose	Gos koora
15	Carrot	Gajar	Gajar	Gajar	Gajri	Carrot	Gajar	Carrot	Gajjara
16	Cashewnut	Kaju	Hijli badam	Kaju	Geru beeja	Kasu andi	Kaju	Mundiri paruppu	Jeedi pappu
17	Celery	Ajwain-ka-patta	Randhumi sag	Ajmana pan	—	Sellery	—	—	—
18	Coconut	Narial	Narkel	Nariyal	Thengini kai	Thenga	Naral	Thenga	Kobbari
19	Coriander	Dhania	Dhane	Kothmer	Kothambari	Kothamalli	Kothimbir	Kothamalli	Kothimiri
20	Cucumber	Khira	Sasha	Kakdi	Southe kayi	Vellarika	Kakadi	Kakkari-kkai	Dosa kayi
21	Curd	Dahi	Doyi	Dahi	Mosaru	Thayir	Dahi	Thayir	Perugu
22	Custard Apple	Sitaphal	Ata	Sitaphal	Seetha-phalam	Seetha-phalam	Sitaphal	Seetha-phalam	Seetha-phalam
23	Date (dried)	Khajur	Khejur	Khajur	Kharjoora	Eethapazham	Khajur	Pericham pazham	Kharjoora pandu
24	Drumstick	Sanjana	Sajna danta	Saragava	Nugge kayi	Muringakkai	Shevaga sheng	Muringa-kkai	Mulaga kada
25	Eggplant	Baingan	Begun	Ringna	Badane	Vazhuthininga	Vangi	Kathirikai	Vankaya

Sr. No.	English	Hindi	Bengali	Gujarati	Kannada	Malayalam	Marathi	Tamil	Telugu
26	Fenugreek	Methi	Methi	Methi	Menthe	Uluva	Methi	Venthayam	Menthulu
27	Fig	Anjeer	Dumoor	Anjeer	Anjura	Atti pazham	Anjeer	Atti pazham	Athi pallu
28	Finger Millet	Ragi	Madua	Bhav	Ragi	Moothari	Nachni	Kezhva-ragu	Ragulu
29	French Beans	Farash Beans	—	Fansi	Haruli kayi	—	Pharashee	—	—
30	Garlic	Lahasoon	Rashun	Lasan	Bellulli	Vellulli	Lasson	Ullipoondu	Vellulli
31	Ginger	Adrak	Ada	Adu	Shunti	Inji	Ale	Inji	Allam
32	Grape-fruit	Chakotra	Bilati batabi	Chakotra	—	Mundri pazham	Bedaana	—	—
33	Grapes	Angoor	Angoor	Draksha	Draksha	Mundiranga	Draksha	Draksha	Draksha
34	Groundnut	Mungphali	China Badam	Bhoising	Kadale kayi	Nilakkadalai	Bhui mug	Nilakka-dalai	Verusa-naga
35	Guava	Amrud	Payra	Jamphal	Seeba	Perakka	Peru	Koya pazham	Jami pandu
36	Honey	Shahad	Mou	—	Ten thuppa	Then	Madh	Then	Thene
37	Indian Gooseberry	Amla	Amlaki	Amla	Nelli kai	Nelli kai	Anvla	Nelli kai	Usirikayi
38	Jambul Fruit	Jamun	Kalojam	Jambu	Neralai	Naga pazham	Jambhool	Naga phazam	Neredu pandu

Sr. No.	English	Hindi	Bengali	Gujarati	Kannada	Malayalam	Marathi	Tamil	Telugu
39	Lady's Finger	Bhindi	Dherash	Bhinda	Bende	Vendakkai	Bhendi	Vendakkai	Benda kayi
40	Lemon	Bara Nimbu	Pati lebu	Moly limbu	—	Poo naranga	Limbu	Elimich cham	Nimma kaaya
41	Lentil	Masur	Masoor	Masur dal	Masur bele	Masur parippu	Mysur dal	Mysore paruppu	Misur pappu
42	Lettuce	Salad Patta	Salad pata	Salat	Hakkarike-soppu	Uvar cheera	—	—	—
43	Lime	Nimboo	Lebu	Kadgi limbu	Nimbe	Cherunaranga	Musumbe	Elumichai	Nimma pandu
44	Linseed	Alsi	Tishi	Alsi	—	Cheruchana-vithu	Jawas	Ali vidai	Avise gindalu
45	Maize	Makka	Bhutta	Makai	Musikino	Cholam	Maka	Makka cholam	Mokka jonnalu
46	Mango	Aam	Aam	Keri	Mavinahannu	Mam pazham	Amba	Mam pazham	Mamidi pandu
47	Milk	Doodh	Doodh	Doodh	Halu	Pal	Doodh	Pal	Palu
48	Musk Melon	Kharbuza	Kharmuj	Kharbooja	Kharbuz-hannu	—	Kharbooja	Mulam pazham	Kharbooja
49	Mustard Seeds	Raye	Sorse	Rai	Sasuve	Kadugu	Mohori	Kadugu	Valasulu Avalu
50	Oats Meal	Jai	Jai	Jav	—	—	Jav	—	Yavalu

Sr. No.	English	Hindi	Bengali	Gujarati	Kannada	Malayalam	Marathi	Tamil	Telugu
51	Onion	Piyaz	Pyaza	Kando	Eerulli	Ulli	Kanda	Vengayam	Neerulli
52	Orange	Sangtra	Kamala lebu	Santra	Kithilal	Madhura naranga	Santre	Kichili pazham	Kamala pandu
53	Papaya	Papita	Pepe	Papaya	Pharangi	Omakai	Popai	Pappali	Boppayi pandu
54	Parsley	Prajmoda	—	—	Achu mooha	Kuthambelari	—	—	—
55	Peach	Arhu	Peach	Peech	Marasebu	Pochad poxam	Peech	Aru	—
56	Pear	Naspati	Nashpati	Nashati	Beri kai	Sabarjil	Nashpati	Berikai	Berikai
57	Pigeon Pea	Arhar	Arhar dal	Tuver	Thugare bele	Tuvara parippu	Tur dal	Tuvaram paruppa	Kandi pappu
58	Pineapple	Ananas	Anarash	Ananas	Ananas	Kayitha chakka	Ananas	Anasi pazham	Anasa pandu
59	Pistachio nut	Pista	Pesta	Pista	Pista	Pista	Pista	Pista	Pista
60	Pomegra-nate	Anar	Dalim	Dalamb	Dalimbari	Mathalam pazham	Dalimb	Mathalam pazham	Danimma pandu
61	Potato	Aloo	Gol alu	Batata	Alu gadda	Urula kizhangu	Batata	Urula kizhangu	Alu gaddalu
62	Pumpkin	Kumra	Kumra	Kohlu	Kumbala	Mathan	Lal bhopla	Parangi-kkai	Gummadi kayi
63	Radish	Muli	Mula	Mula	Mullangi	Mullangi	Mula	Mullangi	Mullangi

Sr. No.	English	Hindi	Bengali	Gujarati	Kannada	Malayalam	Marathi	Tamil	Telugu
64	Raisins	Munaqqa	Kishmish	Kishmish	Drakshi	Mundiringa	Manuka	Drakshai	Kishmish
65	Rice, raw, hand-pounded	Chawal	Chowl	Chokha	Akki	Ari	Tandool	Arisi	Biyyam
66	Ribbed gourd	Torai	Jhinga	Turia	Heerai kai	Peechinga	Dodka	Pirkkankai	Beera kayi
67	Safflower Seeds	Kusum	Kajireh	Kusumbe	Kusme bija	Chandura kam	Kardi	Sendur kam	Kusuma ginzalu
68	Sesame Seeds	Til	Til	Tal	Ellu	Ellu	Til	Ellu	Nurvulu
69	Sorghum	Jowar	Juar	Juar	Jola	Cholam	Jwari	Cholam	Jonnalu
70	Soyabean	Bhat	Garikalai	—	—	—	—	—	—
71	Spinach	Palak	Palang sag	Palak	Basalay-soppu	Basala cheera	Palak	Pasalai keerai	Bachchali koora
72	Snake Gourd	Chachinda	Chichinga	Pandola	Padavala	Pandavalanga	Padval	Padava-langai	Pottakayi
73	Strawberry	Straberi	—	—	—	—	—	—	—
74	Sugarcane	Ganna	Ikkhu	Sherdine	Kabbina	—	—	—	—
75	Sunflower Seeds	Suryamukhi	Suraj mukhi	—	—	Suryakanthi	Surya mukhi	Surua-kanthi	Podduthi-ru gudu Pu-vuginzalu

Sr. No.	English	Hindi	Bengali	Gujarati	Kannada	Malayalam	Marathi	Tamil	Telugu
76	Tomato	Tamatar	Tamater	Tameton	Tomato-hannu	Thakkali	Belwangi	Semi-takkali	Seema vankaya
77	Walnut	Akhrot	Akhrot	Akhrot	—	—	Akhrod	—	—
78	Watercress	Jal-kumbhi	Chandra-sana	Asalia	Alvi	Thutta-kaya-kamikal	Ahliv	Alli Illai	Adityayalu
79	Water-melon	Tarbuz	Tarmuj	Tarbuj	Kallangadi	Thannir mathan	Kalingad	Darbusini	Puchakayi
80	Wheat	Gehun	Gom	Ghau	Godhi	Gothambu	Gahu	Godumai	Godhumaly
81	Zizyphus	Ber	Ber	—	Bore	Badoram	—	Illandai	Cangarenu

Glossary

Abdomen: The part of the body between the chest and the pelvis, containing the digestive organs.

Abortion: Expulsion of immature baby from the womb before the 28th week of pregnancy.

Abscess: Localised collection of pus in the body tissues.

Absorption: The process by which digested foods from the intestine enter into the blood or lymph.

Acidosis : A condition in which there is increase in circulating acid substances or a reduction in alkali reserve in the body.

Acne: A pimple or small boil.

Acute: Any process which has sudden onset and runs a relatively severe and short course.

Addiction: Habituation to certain drugs, foods or drinks.

Adenoid: Swelling formed by the overgrowth of lymphatic glandular tissue at the back of the nose and throat.

Adrenal glands: two endocrine glands located on the top of the kidneys. They are divided into two sections, the cortex and the medulla.

Adrenalin: A hormone secreted by the adrenal medulla in response to nervous stimulation or lowered blood sugar.

Adolescence: The period of growth from 13 to 18 years of age.

Ageing: The process or the effects of growing mature or old.

Albumin: Main protein found in the blood.

Allergy: Sensitiveness of the body to a substance which does not normally affect other persons.

Allergen: Any substance capable of producing allergic reactions.

Alleviate: Relief from symptoms.

Alveoli: Air containing vesicles.

Alopecia: Patchy baldness.

Amenorrhoea: Absence of menstruation.

Amino acids: Chemical compounds out of which proteins are formed.

Amoeba: A microscopic animal consisting of one single cell.

Anaemia: Deficiency of oxygen carrying red blood cells.

Androgen: Male sex hormone.

Angina pectoris: A pain in the chest caused by diminished supply of blood to the heart.

Antibiotic: A chemical substance having the power to retard the growth of certain germs.

Antibody: Substances capable of counteracting the bacteria or bacterial products.

Anorexia: Loss of appetite.

Antidote: A substance used to counteract effect of poison or diseases.

Antigen: A protein which induces a reaction in the body and produces antibodies.

Antioxidant: A substance that has the ability to prevent or delay deterioration caused by the oxygen.

Antiseptic: A substance which inhibits the growth of or destroys micro organisms.

Antispasmodic: Drugs relaxing the contracted muscles.

Anus: Outlet of alimentary canal.

Appendicitis: Inflammation of the vermiform appendix.

Apoplexy: Brain hemorrhage or stroke.

Arteriosclerosis: Hardening and narrowing of arteries with impediment to circulation of blood.

Arthritis: Painful swelling of joints.

Aura: A sensation occurring prior to the onset of an epileptic fit.

Autonomic system: The part of the nervous system which controls the, vital organs, and which is involuntary.

Bacillus: A rod-shaped bacteria.

Bacteria: Microbe, micro organism.

Barium: An opaque chemical compound for visualising the gastrointestinal tract under X-ray.

Benign Tumor: Tumor or condition which is not malignant or cancerous.

Beta cells: Cells that make insulin. These cells are found in the islets of Langerhans in the pancreas.

Beri-Beri: A vitamin deficiency disease.

Bile: A greenish-brown fluid secreted by the liver.

Biopsy: Removal of a piece of tissue from the patient for the purpose of gross and microscopic examination to diagnose a disease.

Boil: A painful abscess at the hair root.

Bowl: Intestine, often applied to large intestine.

Bronchiectasis: Abnormal permanent dilation of the bronchi or breathing-tubes.

Bronchiole: Tiny branches of the bronchus.

Caecum: A blind sac at the junction of the small and large intestines.

Calcification: A process by which organic tissue becomes hardened by disposition of calcium salts within its substance.

Calculus: A stone or stony mass of minerals formed within the body.

Calorie: A unit of heat used for measuring the energy value of food.

Capillary: A tiny blood-vessel, connecting a vein and artery.

Cancer: Uncontrolled devastating growth of cells.

Carbohydrates: One of three basic sources of energy in the food and is found in grains, vegetables and fruits.

Carbuncle: Infection of skin and deep tissues that results in suppuration and discharge of pus from many openings.

Carcinogen: Any substance capable of causing cancer.

Carcinoma: Malignant or cancerous tumour of the skin or internal organs.

Cardiac: Pertaining to the heart.

Caries: Tooth decay.

Cell: The basic unit of which body is made.

Cerebral: Related to the brain.

Cervical spine: The top portion of the spine (neck), composed of seven vertebrae.

Cholesterol: A yellowish fatty substance synthesized in the liver and supplied in the diet.

Chronic: Long and continuous course of disease.

Cirrhosis: Fibrous scar replacing the cells.

Coma: An unconscious state from which the patient cannot be aroused.

Complication: A condition developing during a disease process.

Constipation: Difficult or infrequent bowel movements.

Convalescence: Gradual recovery from illness.

Convulsions: A violent and involuntary contraction or series of contraction of the voluntary muscles.

Cornea: The transparent circular portion of the front of the eye ball.

Coronary: Of or relating to heart.

Coronary thrombosis: A blockage of the blood flow caused by a blood clot in a coronary artery.

Cortisone: A steroid hormone secreted by the outer part of the adrenal glands.

Cramp: Sharp muscular pain.

Congestion: Accumulation of blood in the vessels of an organ or tissue.

Cystitis: Inflammation of the urinary bladder.

Decoction: A process of boiling down so as to extract some essence.

Dehydration: Abnormal loss of body fluids.

Delirium: State of mental confusion and excitement.

Deodorant: A substance which counteracts offensive odours.

Dermis: True skin lying beneath surface skin.

Diabetes: A disease resulting from the body's inability to produce or use insulin, characterised by high blood glucose levels.

Diagnosis: Identification of disease by patients symptoms and other methods.

Diaphragm: Muscle separating chest from abdomen.

Diastolic: Lower level of the blood pressure within the arteries when the heart is at rest.

Dimention: Loss of intellectual function.

Disease, functional: The abnormal functioning of the body organ when there is no defects in its structure.

Disinfection: Process of destroying pathogenic or harmful micro organisms.

Diseases organic: A structural defect in a body tissue leading to illness.

Diverticulosis: Abnormal pockets or pouches within a mucus membrane of the colon.

Douche: Washing with a stream of water.

Dropsy: Accumulation of water in tissue.

Ductless Glands: Glands which pour their secretion directly into the blood stream without benefit of a connecting tube.

Duodenum: First part of the small intestine adjacent to stomach.

Dysmenorrhoea: Painful or difficult menstruation.

Electrocardiograph: Diagnostic instrument used to record the electrical currents generated in the heart.

Embryo: Organism developing from conception to the end of the second month.

Enamel: Outer covering of the visible part of tooth.

Endemic: Disease prevalent in a particular area.

Endocrine: Glands secreting hormones.

Endocrine glands: A group of organs which secretes hormones directly into the blood.

Enema: Injection of water or other liquid into the colon via the anus.

Enzyme: Secretion of the special cells of the body for digestion of foods.

Epilepsy: A chronic disease usually functional, characterised by brief convulsive seizure and loss of consciousness.

Estrogen: One or two hormones secreted by the ovaries.

Excretion: Process of elimination of waste matter from the body.

Expectoration: The act of coughing up and spitting out materials from the lungs and trachea.

Expiration: Process of breathing out.

Fallopian tube: Tube carrying eggs from the ovaries to the womb.

Fats: The most concentrated source of calories in the diet found in daily products, flesh foods, nuts, oils and some vegetables.

Fatty acids: One of the end products of fat digestion.

Fibre: Indigestible material in grains, vegetables and fruits.

Fissure: A crack in the membrane lining the rectum.

Flatulence: Distension of the stomach or intestines with air or gases.

Follicle: A pocket in the dermis containing a hair root.

Fomentation: A hot, moist pack or application to the body.

Frigidity: Females sexual unresponsiveness.

Gangrene: Localised death of tissues due to loss of blood supply.

Gastric: Pertaining to the stomach.

Gene: Hereditary factor present in all cell.

Genetic: Inherited.

Gingiva: Gum.

Glucose tolerance: Method to measure the ability of patient to metabolize glucose.

Glutamic acid: A naturally occurring amino acid, a constituent of many proteins.

Glycaemia: Amount of glucose in the blood.

Goitre: Enlargement of thyroid.

Gonads: Testicles and ovaries.

Haemoglobin: Oxygen-carrying pigments found in red blood cells.

Hallucination: A mental impression having no foundation in fact.

Hay fever: Seasonal allergic reaction to pollen.

Heart burn: Burning sensation in upper abdomen and chest.

Hepatitis: Inflammation of the liver.

Heredity : The transmission of traits from parents to offspring.

Hernia: Rupture or protusion of organ or part of an organ through the wall of a body cavity.

Hormone: A glandular secretion that regulates body functions.

Hyperacidity: Digestive malfunction characterised by excessive secretions of acid by the digestive glands in the stomach and intestines.

Hypertension: Increase level of Blood pressure.

Hypoglycemia: A condition in which blood glucose level is too low, generally below 60 mg.

Ileum: Terminal portion of the small intestine.

Immunity: Capacity of the body to resist infection.

Impotence: Inability to have a erection.

Infarction: Death of tissue due to interruption of its blood supply.

Infection: Invasion of the body by micro-organisms.

Infestation: The invasion of the body by parasites.

Infusion: A process in which boiled water is poured over dried herbal leaves or flowers and allowed to steep from half an hour to two hours.

Inflammation: A reaction of the body tissues to injury, infection or irritation.

Ingestion: The act of taking food, medicines, etc. by mouth.

Inhalation: The drawing in of air or other vapour into the lungs.

Insomnia: The inability to sleep.

Insulin: The hormone of the pancreas which controls the blood sugar level.

Intercellular: In between the cells.

Islets of Langerhans: Clusters of cells in the pancreas that include the beta cells, which make insulin.

Jaundice: A yellow coloration of the skin due to excessive of bilirubin pigments in the blood.

Jejunum: Middle part of the small intestine concerned with digestion and absorption of food.

Kidneys: Two organs located behind the stomach that secrete urine by removing wastes from the blood.

Lactation: The period during which milk is produced.

Lactose: Milk sugar.

Larva: A stage in animal development after the egg.

Larynx: Voice Box.

Laxative: A mild purgative.

Lesion: A localised tissue damage caused by injury or diseases.

Leukaemia: A blood disease in which the white blood cells increase enormously in number.

Ligaments: A tough fibrous band connecting bones or other tissues of the body.

Lymph: The clear, liquid part of the blood which enters the space between body cells.

Malignant Tumour: Cancer with spreading power.

Marrow: The soft tissue in the hollow spaces of the bones.

Mastication: Chewing.

Masturbation: Sexual satisfaction derived by stimulation of ones own genitalia.

Maxilla: Upper jaw bones.

Meninges: The membranes of the brains and spinal cord.

Metabolism: The sum of the body processes involving the building up and breaking down of tissues.

Micturition: Process of passing urine.

Miscarriages: Interruption of pregnancy, spontaneous abortion.

Mucilage: A sticky substance extracted from certain plants.

Mucus: Lubricating fluid secreted by the mucus membrane of the body.

Mucous membrane: Smooth, soft lining of the passage and cavities of the body.

Myocardial: Pertaining to the heart muscle.

Myopia: Short Sight.

Nausea: Vomiting sensation.

Neuralgia: Pain in a nerve.

Neurone: Nerve Cell.

Neurosis: Emotional disorder caused by some inner conflict.

Node: A knot or swelling.

Nutrient: A food substance.

Nutrition: The process of assimilating food.

Oedema: An abnormal amount of fluid in the body tissues.

Oesophagus: Gullet, the tube leading from the mouth to stomach.

Ointment: A fatty medical preparation for external use.

Orgasm: Climax of sexual intercourse.

Osteoporosis: Thinning of the bones.

Ovulation: Release of a matured egg from an ovary.

Ovum: Egg.

Oxidation: A process of transforming one substance into another in which oxygen is used and energy is liberated.

Oxygen: A gaseous element which is essential for life and metabolism.

Palpitation: Conscious heating of the heart.

Pancreas: A large, glandular organ which secretes digestive enzymes into the intestine and insulin to the blood.

Parasite: An organism which lives in or on another organism.

Paralysis: Loss or impairment of motor function in a part.

Pathogenic: Causing disease.

Peristalsis: Wavelike muscular contractions of the walls of the stomach and intestine.

Peritoneum: The lining membrane of the abdominal cavity.

Peritonitis: Inflammation of the peritoneum.

Pharynx: Cavity behind and communicating with nose, mouth and larynx.

Pimple: A small elevation in the skin caused by localised bacterial infection.

Pituitary gland: A small endocrine gland located in the midbrain, which secretes hormones that regulates the functions of all the other endocrine glands.

Plasma: Liquid part of the blood.

Pneumonia: Inflammation of the lungs.

Progesterone: Pertaining to the lungs.

Purgative: Strong laxative which flushes the large intestine rapidly.

Pus: A yellow viscid matter produced by inflammation.

Polyuria: Excessive formation and excretion of urine.

Protein: One of three major sources of calories in the diet. It builds up bones, muscles and connective tissues.

Rash: A temporary eruption on the skin.

Rectum: Lower end of the large intestine.

Respiration: Process of breathing.

Retina: Light sensitive area at the back of the eye.

Rhinitis: Inflammation of the mucus membrane lining the nose.

Sclerosis: Hardening of the tissues.

Sebaceous gland: Glands secreting or conveying oily matter to lubricate the skin or hair.

Secretion: Any substance which is released into the body by a gland or organ.

Sedative: A drug or a substance which reduces excitement, irritation and pain.

Serum: The clear portion of blood separated from its clot.

Sinuses: Hollow cavities in the nasal bones.

Sphygmomanometer: An instrument that measures blood pressure.

Sprain: Injury to the ligament surrounding the joint.

Sprue: Chronic inflammation of the digestive tract, marked by indigestion and morning diarrhoea.

Sputum: Material coughed up from the lungs.

Stomatitis: Inflammation of the mouth.

Syndrome: A set of signs and symptoms occurring together as an expression of a disorder of function.

Systolic: Upper level of the blood pressure indicating the greatest force exerted by the heart.

Tendon: A tough strand which attaches a muscle to a bone.

Thrombosis: Clogging of a blood-vessel caused by the formation of a clot.

Thyroid glands: An important endocrine gland located in the throat, which secretes thyroxin.

Tissue: A collection of mass of cells of one kind.

Toxin: A poisonous substance produced by the action of micro organisms.

Tranquilizer: Drug used to quieten the nerves.

Tumor: Abnormal growth of a mass of cells in the body.

Ulcer: An open sore on the skin.

Urea: Chief nitrogenous constituent of the urine and final product of protein metabolism of the body.

Uric acid: A normal constituent of blood and urine metabolism.

Vaccine: Biological material injection into the body to protect against disease.

Vagina: A small sac containing liquid. A narrow elastic canal that extends from the cervix to the outside of the female body.

Wart: A small growth on the skin, usually caused by a virus.

Wheezing: Noisy and difficult breathing usually due to bronchial asthma.

Whitlow: Infection of the base of the fingernail.

Index

JAICO PUBLISHING HOUSE

Elevate Your Life. Transform Your World.

Established in 1946, Jaico Publishing House is the publisher of stellar authors such as Sri Sri Paramahansa Yogananda, Osho, Robin Sharma, Deepak Chopra, Stephen Hawking, Eknath Easwaran, Sarvapalli Radhakrishnan, Nirad Chaudhuri, Khushwant Singh, Mulk Raj Anand, John Maxwell, Ken Blanchard and Brian Tracy. Our list which has crossed a landmark 2000 titles, is amongst the most diverse in the country, with books in religion, spirituality, mind/body/spirit, self-help, business, cookery, humour, career, games, biographies, fiction, and science.

Jaico has expanded its horizons to become a leading publisher of educational and professional books in management and engineering. Our college-level textbooks and reference titles are used by students countrywide. The success of our academic and professional titles is largely due to the efforts of our Educational and Corporate Sales Divisions.

The late Mr. Jaman Shah established Jaico as a book distribution company. Sensing that independence was around the corner, he aptly named his company Jaico ("Jai" means victory in Hindi). In order to tap the significant demand for affordable books in a developing nation, Mr. Shah initiated Jaico's own publications. Jaico was India's first publisher of paperback books in the English language.

In addition to being a publisher and distributor of its own titles, Jaico is a major distributor of books of leading international publishers such as McGraw Hill, Pearson, Cengage Learning, John Wiley and Elsevier Science. With its headquarters in Mumbai, Jaico has other sales offices in Ahmedabad, Bangalore, Bhopal, Chennai, Delhi, Hyderabad and Kolkata. Our sales team of over 40 executives, direct mail order division, and website ensure that our books effectively reach all urban and rural parts of the country.

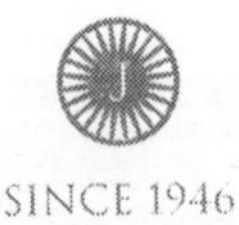

SINCE 1946